6 WEEK LOAN

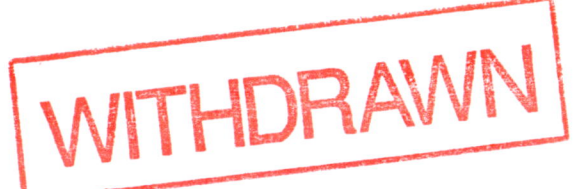

An Atlas of Investigation and Management
OSTEOPOROSIS

An Atlas of Investigation and Management

OSTEOPOROSIS

Anthony D Woolf

Professor, Department of Rheumatology
Royal Cornwall Hospital
Truro, Cornwall, UK

Kristina Åkesson

Professor, Department of Orthopaedics
Malmö University Hospital
Lund University
Malmö, Sweden

CLINICAL PUBLISHING

OXFORD

Clinical Publishing
an imprint of Atlas Medical Publishing Ltd
Oxford Centre for Innovation
Mill Street, Oxford OX2 0JX, UK

Tel: +44 1865 811116
Fax: +44 1865 251550
Email: info@clinicalpublishing.co.uk
Web: www.clinicalpublishing.co.uk

Distributed in USA and Canada by:
Clinical Publishing
30 Amberwood Parkway
Ashland OH 44805 USA

Tel: 800-247-6553 (toll free within U.S. and Canada)
Fax: 419-281-6883
Email: order@bookmasters.com

Distributed in UK and Rest of World by:
Marston Book Services Ltd
PO Box 269
Abingdon
Oxon OX14 4YN UK

Tel: +44 1235 465500
Fax: +44 1235 465555
Email: trade.orders@marston.co.uk

A catalogue record of this book is available from the British Library

ISBN-13   978 1 904392 26 2
ISBN e-book 978 1 84692 535 1

The publisher makes no representation, express or implied, that the dosages in this book are correct. Readers must therefore always check the product information and clinical procedures with the most up-to-date published product information and data sheets provided by the manufacturers and the most recent codes of conduct and safety regulations. The authors and the publisher do not accept any liability for any errors in the text or for the misuse or misapplication of material in this work.

Printed by T G Hostench SA, Barcelona, Spain

Contents

Preface

Osteoporosis is a growing public health problem world wide. A large proportion of the population from middle age onwards are at risk of suffering a fracture during their remaining lifetime. With a predicted dramatic increase of the older population in both developed and developing countries, the numbers of those with osteoporosis and suffering fractures is set to increase dramatically unless effective methods of prevention and treatment are implemented.

Knowledge of the causes of osteoporosis, who is most at risk of suffering fractures, how to case find, and of the means of prevention and treatment – including the recent development of very potent interventions that can stimulate bone formation or block bone resorption – have increased dramatically over the past two decades. There are evidence-based strategies for the prevention and treatment of osteoporosis, but still the majority people who are at high risk of the condition are either not treated or do not continue treatment for long enough to gain a real benefit.

There are various reasons for this, but one is lack of knowledge and understanding by clinicians about osteoporosis, which leads to a failure to appreciate that there are effective ways to prevent fractures.

The aim of this Atlas of Investigation and Management is to bridge the gap by giving an update on current knowledge and thinking in a format that makes information readily accessible. This Atlas also aims to address clinical issues in the care of fracture patients from different perspectives. Detailed information on fractures and their treatment is given in order to create a greater understanding of the specific questions that need to be considered when a patient presents with a fracture.

We hope this Atlas will therefore be a useful contribution towards the fight against preventable fractures.

Anthony Woolf
Kristina Åkesson

Abbreviations

ALP alkaline phosphatase

BALP bone specific alkaline phosphatase

BMD bone mineral density

BMI body mass index

BMP bone morphogenetic protein

BSP bone sialoprotein

BUA broadband ultrasound attenuation

CI confidence interval

CRP C-reactive protein

CTR calcitonin receptor

CTx C-terminal type I collagen telopeptide

Dpd deoxypyridinoline

DVT deep vein thrombosis

DXA dual energy X-ray absorptiometry

DXR digital X-ray radiogrammetry

ER oestrogen receptor

ERT oestrogen replacement therapy

ESR erythrocyte sedimentation rate

FSH follicle-stimulating hormone

GnRH gonadotrophin-releasing hormone

hPTH human parathyroid homone

HRT hormone replacement therapy

ICF International Classification of Functioning

ICTP type I collagen telopeptide

IGF insulin-like growth factor

IL interleukin

iv intravenous

LH luteinizing hormone

MORE Multiple Outcomes of Raloxifene Evaluation (trial)

MRI magnetic resonance imaging

NICE National Institute for Clinical Excellence

NTx N-terminal type I collagen telopeptide

OC osteocalcin

OPG osteoprotegerin

OPN osteopontin

PICP carboxy terminal propeptide type I procollagen

PINP amino terminal propeptide type I procollagen

PGE2 prostaglandin E2

PPAR peroxisome proliferator-activated receptor

PROOF Prevent Recurrence of Osteoporotic Fractures (trial)

PSA prostate specific antigen

PTH parathyroid homone

Pyr pyridinoline

(p)QCT (peripheral)quantitative computed tomography

QUS quantitative ultrasound

RA rheumatoid arthritis

RANKL receptor activator of nuclear factor kB ligand

RCT randomized controlled trial

rhPTH recombinant human parathyroid homone

RR risk ratio

SERMs selective oestrogen receptor modulators

SHBG sex hormone binding globulin

SOS speed of sound

SOTI Spinal Osteoporosis Therapeutic Intervention (trial)

STAR Study of Tamoxifen and Raloxifene (trial)

SXA single energy X-ray absorptiometry

TGF transforming growth factor

TNF tumour necrosis factor

TROPOS Treatment of Peripheral Osteoporosis Study (trial)

TRAP 5b tartrate resistant acid phosphatase

WHI Women's Health Initiative

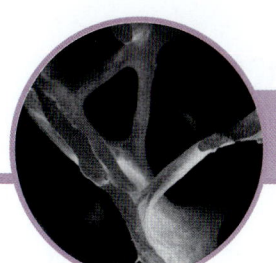

What is osteoporosis?

Introduction

Osteoporosis is a condition characterized by low bone mineral density and compromised microarchitectural integrity leading to structural failure of the skeleton even at low loads. The clinical consequence of osteoporosis is fracture.

Osteoporosis is common in the population and it has been estimated that 1 in 2 women and 1 in 5 men above the age of 50 years will suffer a fracture during their remaining lifetime. These fractures occur usually after the age of 65 years, the mean age of hip fracture in Sweden being 81 years. The number of people over 65 years and over 80 years is increasing dramatically. It is estimated that the population over 65 years of age will increase from the current 16% to between 20 and 25% by 2050 in Europe. There is also a predicted dramatic increase in the older population in less developed countries. Risk factors are also increasing such as reduced physical activity, less balanced diets, smoking, and alcohol consumption. These demographic changes are predicted to result in a dramatic increase in fractures with subsequent morbidity and mortality.

Definition of osteoporosis

Osteoporosis is a condition that is characterized by low bone mass and microarchitectural deterioration of bone tissue, leading to enhanced bone fragility and a consequent increase in fracture risk[1]. Bone quality and its strength is not only a reflection of density and microarchitecture but there are other factors that influence this and fracture risk[2] which need to be considered.

Bones grow in size during the first two decades of life,

with an acceleration during adolescence (**1.1**). This is followed by a period of consolidation. Peak adult bone mass is reached at about the age of 35 years for cortical bone and a little earlier for trabecular bone. Bone mass subsequently declines with ageing. This is a universal phenomenon, occurring in both sexes and in all races. At all ages, women have less bone mass than do men. With ageing this difference becomes more pronounced.

With ageing there are changes in the microarchitecture of bone (**1.2, 1.3**). There is thinning of the cortex and of trabeculae, and a loss of connectivity, in particular of the

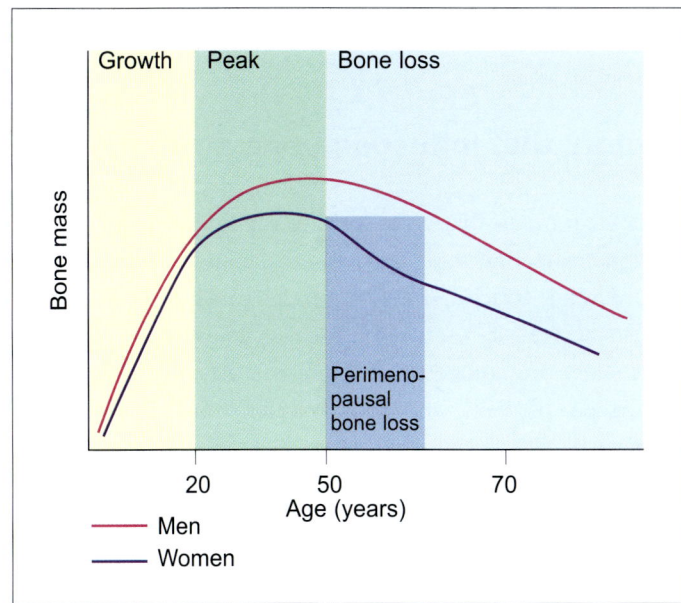

1.1 Changes in bone mass over life.

horizontal trabeculae. The operational definition of osteoporosis is in terms of bone mass[1] (*Table 1.1*), although this is not the only factor that determines bone strength or fracture risk. Bone mass or density is measured by dual energy X-ray absorptiometry in the hip or spine, but various techniques can be used at different sites which correlate with this.

Aetiology of fractures

The cause of fractures is multifactorial. The principal factors that interact are the strength of bone, the event of an injury (usually a fall), and the force on the skeleton from that injury (**1.4**). Various factors influence each of these.

Bone strength is dependent on the structural and dynamic characteristics of the bone – its density, quality and rate of turnover (**1.5**). The quality of bone tissue relates to its composition and microstructure, whereas its quality as an organ depends also on its macrostructure. Fractures usually follow an injury, in particular peripheral fractures. In young people this is usually related to sport or road traffic accidents, but in an older person typically is as a result of a fall. Falls become increasingly common with age and the causes are many (**1.6**). The causes can be considered as intrinsic, extrinsic, and environmental factors but usually there are several factors that contribute to a person falling. As people age, the impact of any fall increases for a variety of reasons (**1.7**), which increases the chance of a consequent fracture. These factors will be considered in more detail.

Factors that influence bone strength

Bone is an organ that gives form to the body, supporting its weight, protecting vital organs, and facilitating locomotion by providing attachments for muscles to act as levers (**1.8**). It also acts as a reserve for ions, especially calcium and phosphate, the homeostasis of which is essential to life. It is composed of cells and extracellular matrix, like other connective tissues, but the matrix has the unique ability to be calcified.

The strength of a bone and its ability to perform these physical functions depend on its structure and the intrinsic properties of the materials of which it is composed. The amount of bone (bone size, mass, and density), its spatial

Table 1.1 WHO definition of osteoporosis
Relates to peak bone mass (T-score)
• Osteopaenia: T-score -1 to -2.5 SD
• Osteoporosis: T-score ≥ -2.5 SD
• Established osteoporosis: osteoporosis + fracture

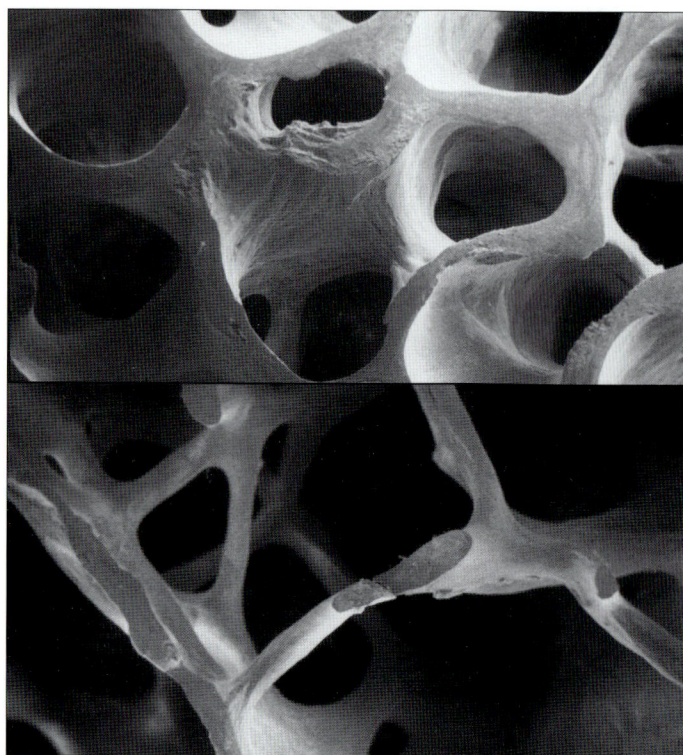

1.2, 1.3 Normal trabecular bone (top), and osteoporotic trabecular bone (bottom). (From Dempster DW, *et al.* (1986). A simple method for correlative light and scanning electron microscopy of human iliac crest bone biopsies: qualitative observations in normal and osteoporotic subjects. *J Bone Mineral Res* **1**:15–21).

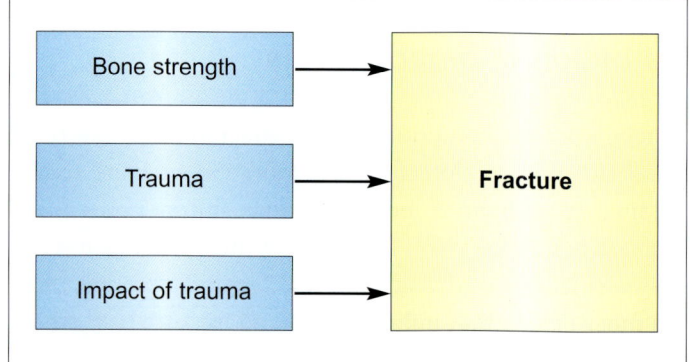

1.4 Principal factors causing fracture.

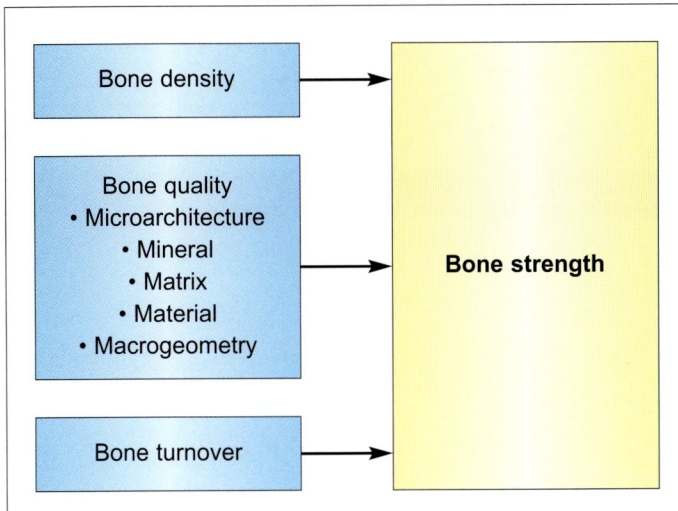

1.5 Factors that influence bone strength.

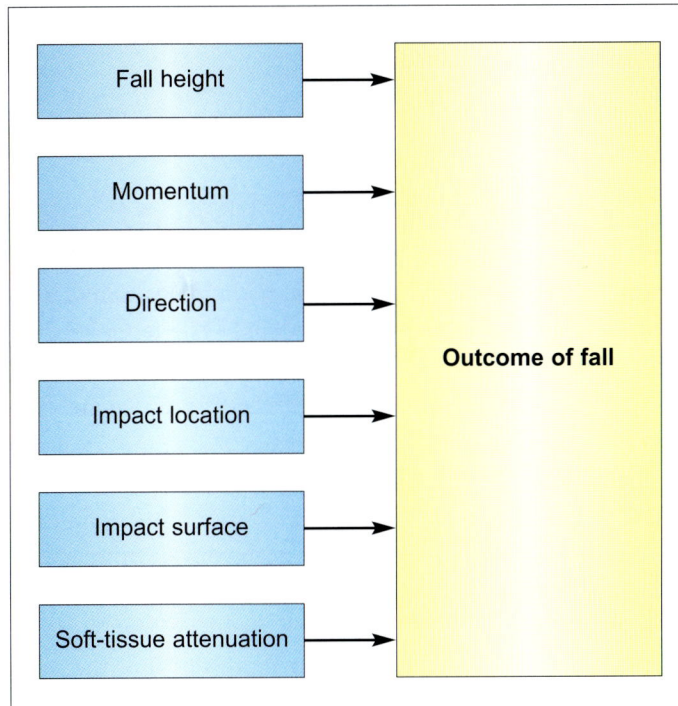

1.7 Factors that affect the impact of a fall and its outcome.

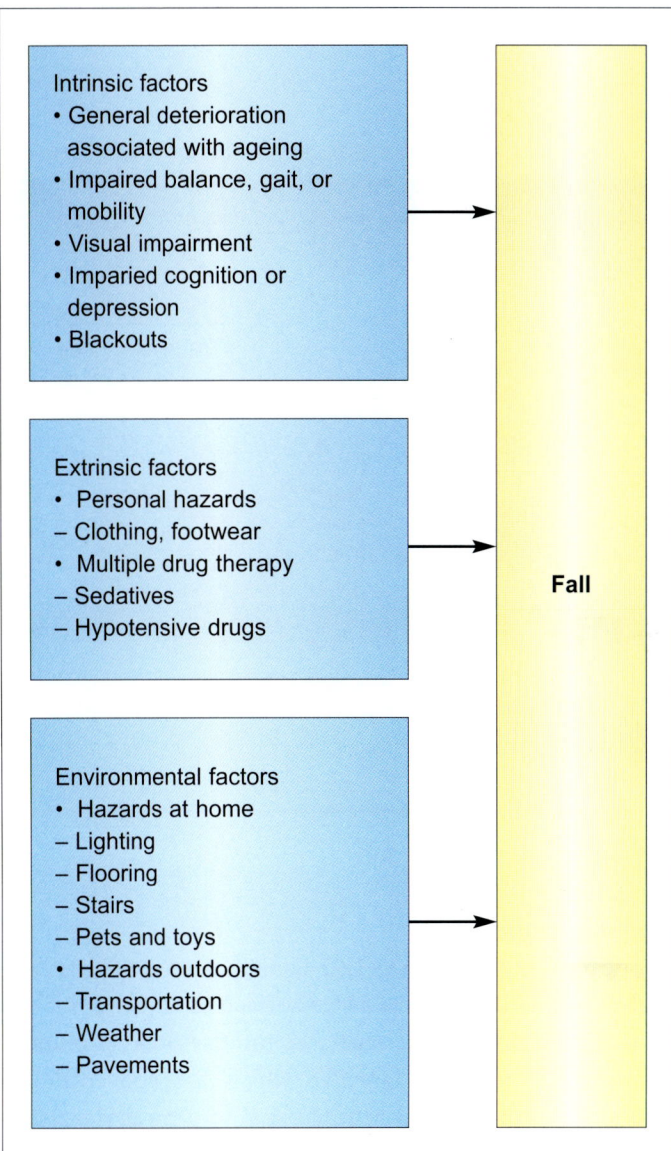

1.6 Factors that are associated with falls; several may be present.

arrangement (shape, geometry, and microarchitecture), its composition (intrinsic properties of bone materials), and its turnover (rate and balance of formation and resorption) are all such determinants of its ability to perform mechanical functions and to resist fracture.

Bone structure
Bones can be conveniently divided into flat bones such as the scapula, skull, and pelvis, and tubular bones which include the limb bones and vertebral bodies. The dense outer surface or cortex is composed of compact bone and the centre or medulla is braced by narrow plates or trabeculae, a construction which gives maximum strength for minimum weight (**1.8**). In the interstices of the medulla lies the bone marrow, where bone cells are in close contact with haemopoietic cells.

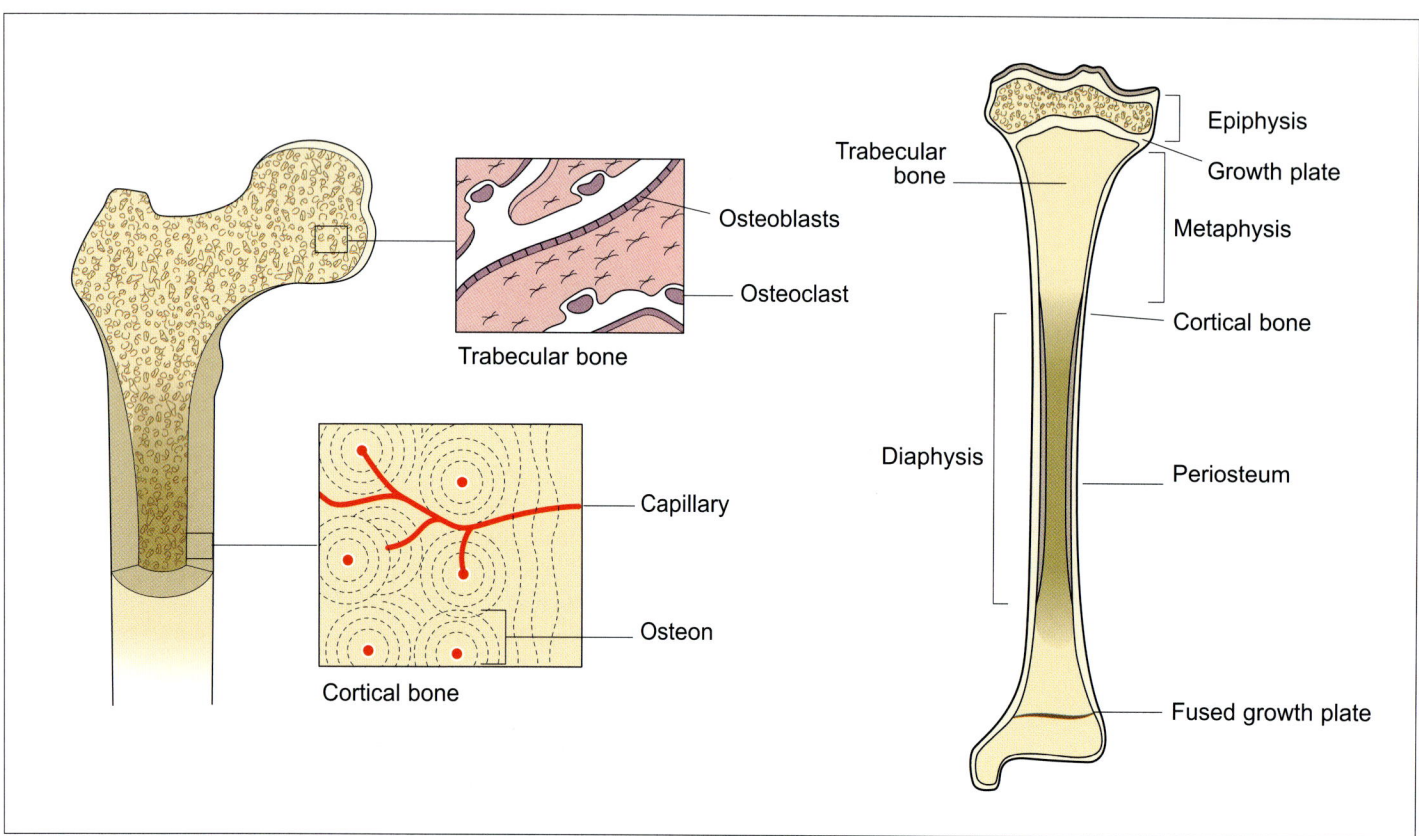

1.8 Gross structure of bone.

Cortical bone

Cortical (compact) bone (**1.9**) constitutes 75–80% of the skeletal mass. It forms the outer surface of all bone but the majority is found in the shafts of tubular bone. Compact bone is composed of lamellae which are concentrically arranged around a small central canal to form a Haversian system or osteon. Between the lamellae are osteocytes lying in lacunae which are connected with each other and with the central canal by fine canaliculi. Osteocytes lie no more than 300 μm from a blood vessel; the average cross-sectional diameter of a Haversian system is 500 μm. The Haversian systems, which may be up to 5 mm long, run parallel to the long axis of the bone, branching and communicating with each other. There are also interstitial lamellae between the Haversian systems, and circumferential lamellae which encircle the inner and outer surface of the bone.

Periosteal vessels penetrate compact bone through nutrient canals to supply the marrow, and branches of these form the intracortical vessels which lie, along with the venules, within the Haversian canals. The interconnecting canaliculi between the osteocytes allow for rapid movement of fluid for their nutrition and humoral intercommunication.

Haversian systems are formed either by the deposition of new bone on the endosteal or periosteal surfaces of cortical bone (primary osteons) or by osteoclasts cutting tunnels (cutting cones) into bone with subsequent deposition of new bone by osteoblasts (secondary osteons). The latter process is found in bone that is remodelling itself, and the outer limit of a secondary osteon can be identified by a cement line which separates it from adjacent bone.

Trabecular bone

Trabecular bone (**1.10**) is a rigid meshwork of mineralized bone which forms the greater part of each vertebral body and the epiphyses of the long bones, and is present at other sites such as the iliac crest. It contributes 20% of the total skeletal mass, but 65–70% of the total bone surface. Complete struts are called trabeculae, but incomplete spicules are also seen. The trabeculae usually lie so as to resist deformational stresses (either from weight bearing or from muscle activity) and their number, size, and distribution are related to these forces. The vertical trabeculae are usually thicker but strength is given by the cross-bracing horizontal trabeculae. Trabecular bone provides a large surface area and is the most metabolically active part of the skeleton, with a high rate of turnover and a blood supply that is much greater than that of compact bone. It acts as a calcium reservoir.

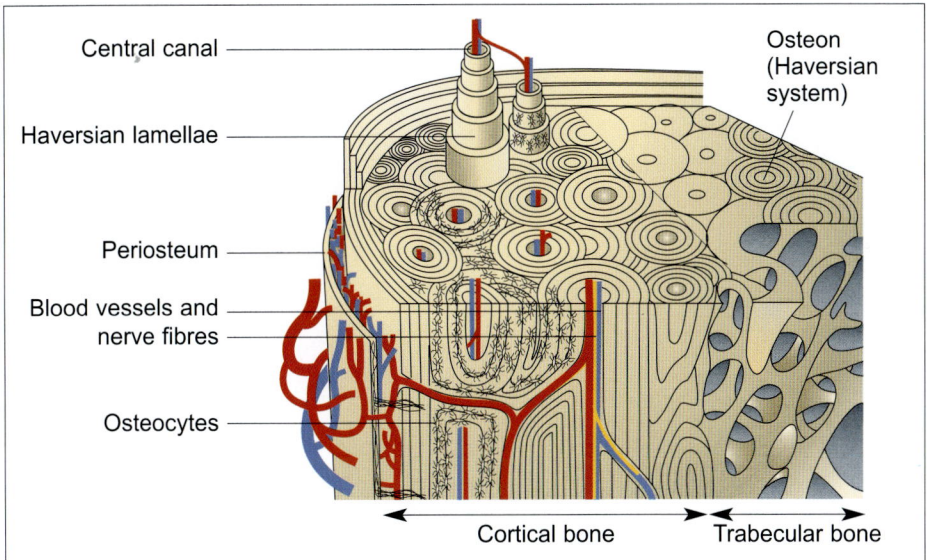

1.9 Normal cortical bone.

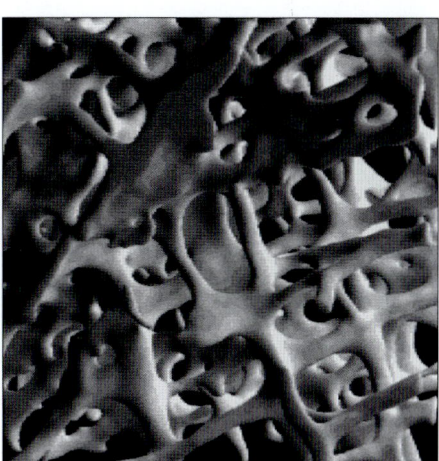

1.10 Normal trabecular bone of the iliac crest. (From Hildebrand T, *et al.* (1999). Direct three-dimentional morphometric analysis of human cancellous bone: microstructural data from spine, femur, iliac crest and calcaneus. *J Bone Mineral Res* **14**:1167–74.)

Trabeculae have a lamella arrangement but less often contain osteocytes. Growth occurs on their surfaces which are covered by a layer of osteoid (that is, unmineralized matrix), which is produced and subsequently mineralized by surface osteoblasts. Occasional osteoclasts lie on their surfaces in shallow pits known as Howships's lacunae.

Distribution of different types of bone

The proportions of cortical and trabecular bone differ at different sites in the skeleton (**1.11**). Trabecular bone is predominant in the vertebrae and femoral head, but cortical bone predominates at the distal radius and femoral neck. The intertrochanteric area of the femur is 50% cortical and 50% trabecular bone. This distribution and differential loss of cortical and trabecular bone in different scenarios accounts in part for the occurrence of different fractures in different situations: cortical bone loss predisposes to peripheral fractures such as of the hip and wrist, whereas trabecular loss predisposes to vertebral fractures.

Bone composition

The fundamental constituents of bone are the cells and the extracellular matix.

Bone cells
Osteoblasts

Osteoblasts are responsible for producing bone matrix constituents, chiefly collagen and noncollagenous matrix proteins that form osteoid (**1.12**, **1.13**). They control mineralization of bone. They originate from bone marrow stromal or connective tissue mesenchymal stem cells which

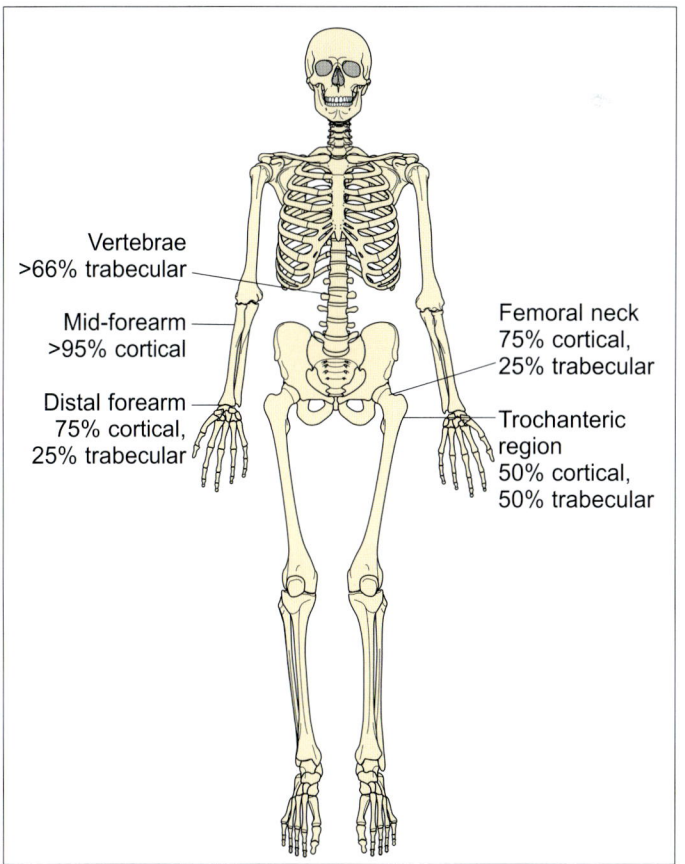

1.11 The distribution of trabecular and cortical bone throughout the skeleton.

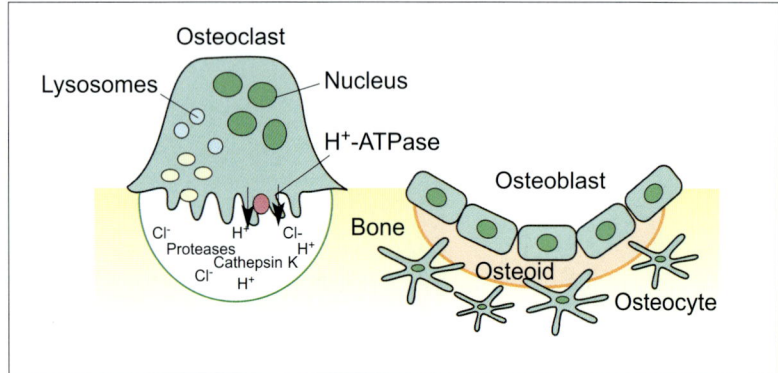

1.12 Bone cells.

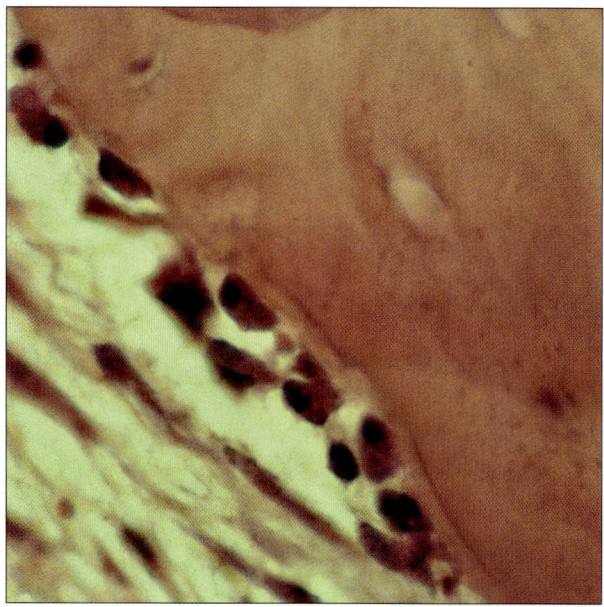

1.13 Osteoblasts with osteoid.

1.14 Osteoblast formation.

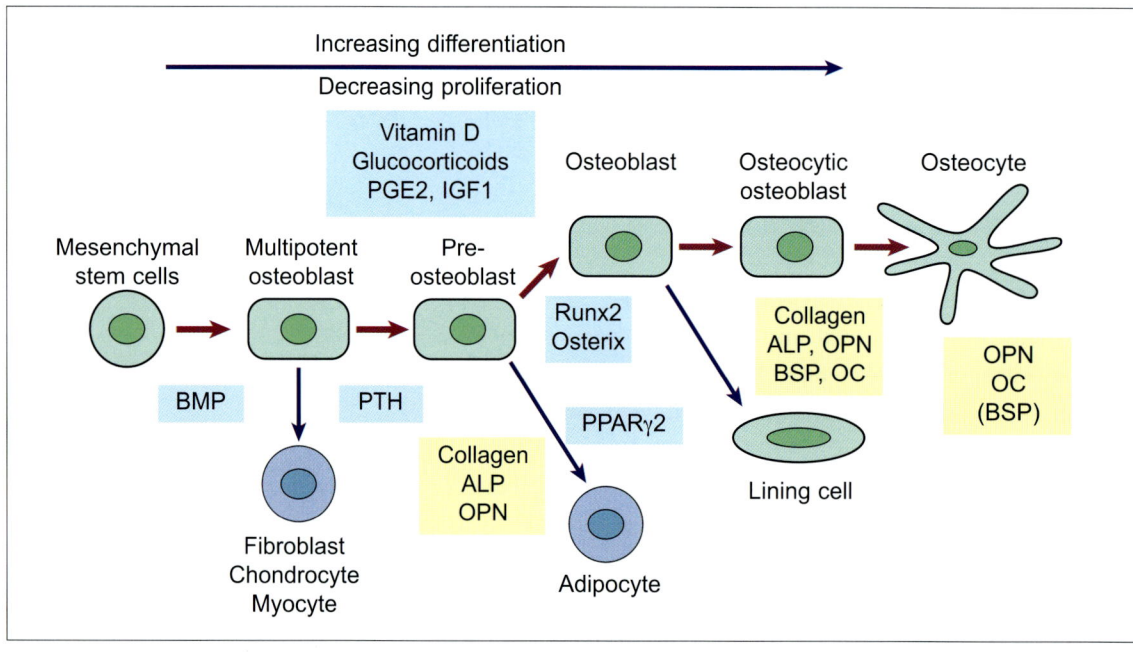

proliferate and differentiate into preosteoblasts and then mature osteoblasts, after being subject to different stimulations of local growth factors and transcription factors (**1.14**). Osteoblasts are found in clusters of up to about 400 cells at a bone-forming site. Surface osteoblast or lining cells line inactive trabecular surfaces. Activated osteoblasts line the layer of bone matrix they are making, the osteoid surface, prior to calcification. Their cellular structure reflects their high synthetic and secretory activity with a well-developed rough endoplasmic reticulum and large Golgi complex and a number of more or less bone-specific proteins, collagen type I in particular, are secreted. The plasma membrane of the osteoblast is rich in alkaline

phosphatase (ALP) and the ALP activity increases early in the mineralization phase. Osteoclasts have cell surface receptors for hormones including parathyroid hormone, vitamin D, and oestrogen, but also cytokine receptors. There is a close linkage between osteoblast and osteoclast activation, and cells of osteoblast lineage secrete cytokines that participate in osteoclastogensesis. Osteoblasts express cytokines on their surface including RANK ligand (RANKL) which, through interaction with RANK, promotes bone resorption. Osteoprotegerin is also secreted by osteoblasts, which is a decoy RANK receptor that can inhibit osteoclast formation.

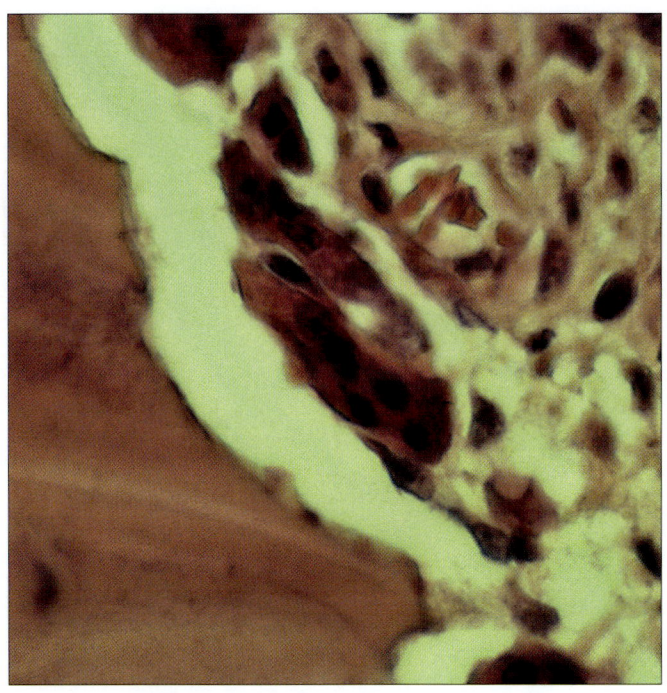

1.15 Osteoclasts.

After forming bone, some osteoblasts are embedded in the mineralized matrix and become osteocytes, some remain on the surface and become bone-lining cells, whereas others will undergo apoptosis (programmed cell death).

Osteocytes

Osteocytes are embedded deep within bone in small lacunae, having originated as osteoblasts and becoming trapped in the matrix they produced. They have numerous long cell processes which are in contact with other osteocytes and lining cells on the bone surface. They are surrounded by the periosteocytic space which is filled with extracellular fluid. Osteocytes have a role in maintaining extracellular calcium concentration. They may also act as mechanoreceptors and in the local activation of bone remodelling.

Osteoclasts

Osteoclasts are responsible for bone resorption. They are giant, multinucleated cells usually found in contact with calcified bone surface within lacunae that result from their resorptive activity (**1.15**). An activated resorption site may contain from one to five osteoclasts. Osteoclasts have a different origin from osteoblasts. They are derived from hematopoetic stem cells and are related to macrophages (**1.16**). Mature osteoclasts are formed by the fusion of osteoclast precursors. Osteoclast differentiation is promoted by the interaction of RANK expressed on osteoclasts and RANKL. They have abundant Golgi complexes, mitochondria, and transport vesicles containing lysosomal enzymes. Osteoclasts form sealed bone-resorbing compartments next to the bone surface, with a ruffled border formed by deep foldings of the plasma membrane facing the bone matrix. They undergo apoptosis after they have finished resorbing bone.

1.16 Osteoclast formation.

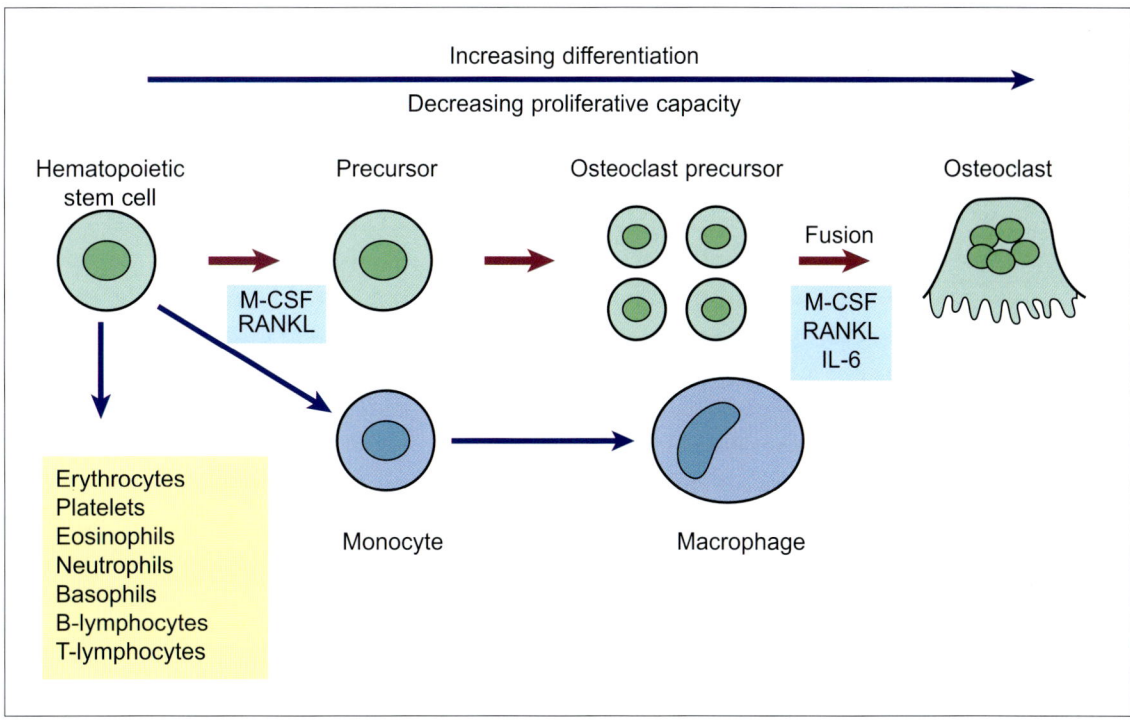

Table 1.2 Composition of bone

Bone mineral:
• Calcium
• Phosphorous (as hydroxyapatite $Ca_{10}(PO4)_6(OH)_2$)

Bone collagen – 90% of bone matrix:
• 13 genetically distinct types
• Type I collagen is the major component of bone

Non-collagenous proteins – 10% of matrix:
• Bone gla protein (osteocalcin)
• Matrix gla protein
• Osteonectin
• Proteoglycans – decorin, bone sialoprotein
• Cell attachment proteins – fibronectin, osteopontin, thrombospondin
• Regulatory growth factors – TGF, BMPs

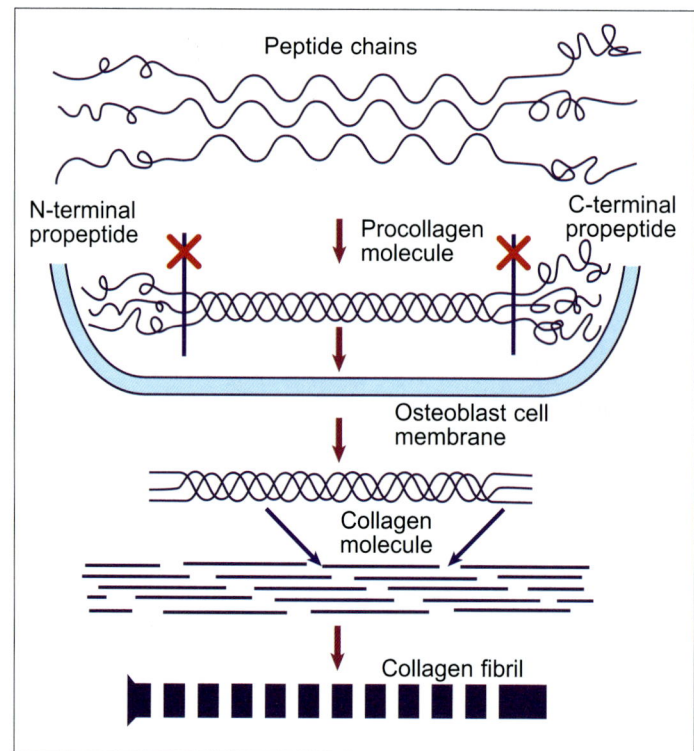

1.17 Schematic illustration of collagen formation.

Bone matrix and mineral

The extracellular matix is a 'composite' in materials science terms, a matrix comprised of collagen and ground substance that is mineralized. Crystals of hydroxyapatite are precipitated on the collagen fibres. The mineral phase gives compressive strength and rigidity, but it is the fibrous organic matrix that gives bone its resistance to tractional and torsional forces. The mineral phase accounts for up to 70% of adult bone.

Collagen forms 90% of bone matrix, of which type 1 is the major component. Noncollagenous proteins form the ground substance, primarily glycoproteins and proteoglycans, but there are other matrix proteins present in small amounts that have important although not fully characterized roles (*Table 1.2*). Most but not all of these noncollagenous proteins are synthesised by bone cells.

Type I collagen is formed in bone from the combination of two α-1 and one α-2 collagen polypeptides containing hydroxylated proline and lysine residues (**1.17**). It is secreted as procollagen from the osteoblast, when the amino-terminal and carboxy-terminal regions are cleaved. Type I collagen is helical; the nonhelical domains at the amino- and carboxy-termini are known as the N-telopeptide and C-telopeptide regions. The structure of type I collagen is stabilized by side chains of hydroxylysine residues which condense to form

pyridinium rings so that pyridinium cross-links are formed, connecting three different collagen molecules. These cross-links are described as pyridinoline or deoxypyridinoline cross-links, depending on the combination of hydroxylysine and lysine side residues[3,4]. The cross-linking is specific for each of the N- and C-terminal telopeptide regions, and is also relatively bone-specific[5]. The orientation of the collagen fibres alternates from layer to layer in adult bone, which gives the typical lamellar structure seen by polarizing light or electron microscopy.

Bone growth

Tubular bones grow in length by ossification at the metaphysis at cartilage growth plates (endochondral ossification). The cortex grows in diameter by subperiosteal deposition accompanied by endosteal resorption. This process leads to enlargement of the marrow cavity. Flat bones develop by intramembranous bone formation. An ossifying growth plate can be divided into functional zones. Chondrocytes initially proliferate and then actively synthesize matrix, the cells having an internal arrangement typical of secretory cells. Next, the cells hypertrophy, compressing the surrounding matrix. In the next zone calcification is found, initially with small isolated clusters of

1.18 Schematic drawing of bone turnover.

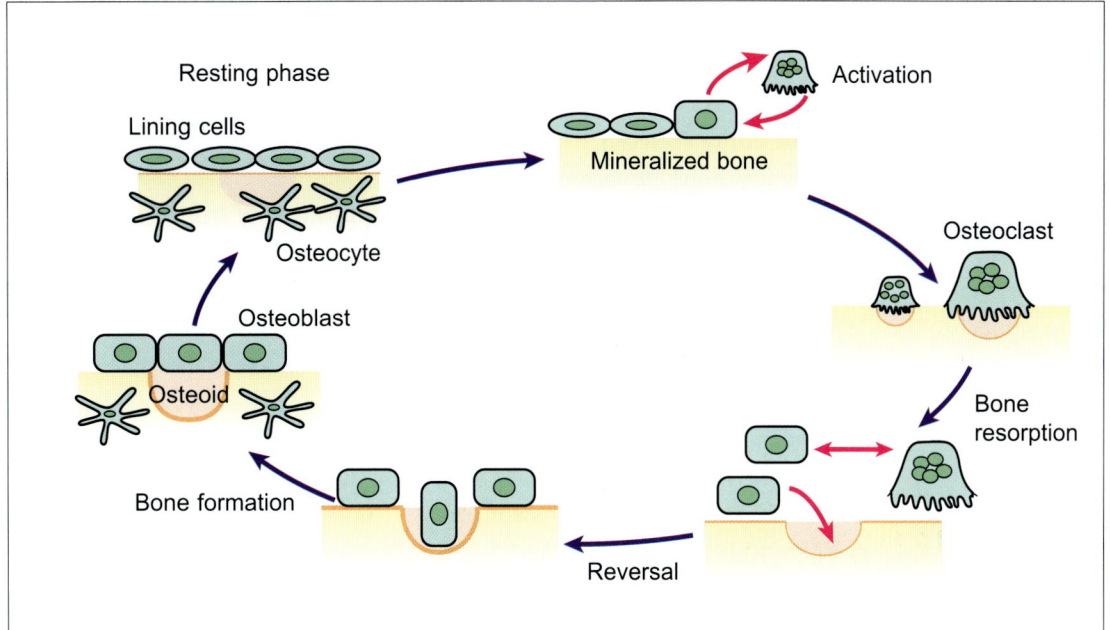

crystals which coalesce to an almost solid mass at the cartilage–bone junction. Capillary buds, osteoprogenitor cells, and osteoclasts then penetrate and resorb this somewhat amorphous mineralized matrix and is replaced by new bone formed by the osteoblasts.

Bone turnover and remodelling

Bone may seem inert but is a dynamic tissue and continually turns over throughout life. Maintenance of bone integrity relies on a closely controlled balance between osteoblastic bone formation and osteoclastic bone resorption. The initial phase of growth of the skeleton during childhood and adolescence is associated with increasing bone density and rigidity (**1.1**). This is followed by a phase through adulthood when there is a close coupling between formation and resorption and the bone mass is stable, but turnover allows continual renewal and repair of the skeleton. In later life there is an imbalance with a net loss of bone mass from both the trabecular and cortical compartments, which may lead to osteoporosis.

Bone turnover, or remodelling, occurs in discrete packets or remodelling units and at any given time about a million of these units are active[6,7]. Each packet is anatomically and chronologically separated. The normal remodelling sequence takes 100–200 days. There are cellular control mechanisms responsible that are only partially understood. The sequence is initial activation of osteoclast precursors followed by osteoclastic bone resorption (**1.18**). There is then a reversal, with subsequent osteoblastic bone formation

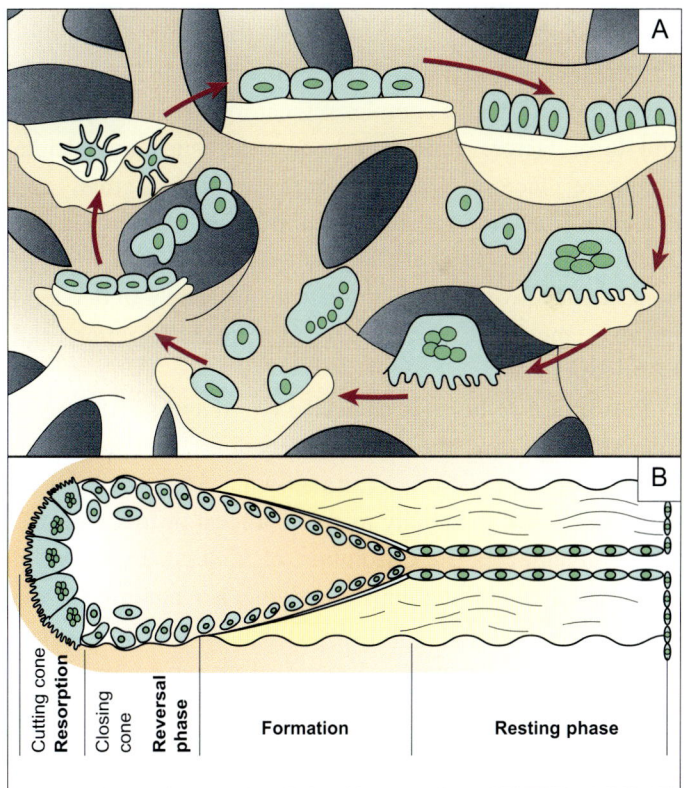

1.19 Bone remodelling. **A**: trabecular bone; **B**: cortical bone.

to repair the defect. This is followed by a resting phase before the cycle begins again. The remodelling cycle follows the same principles in both trabecula and cortical bone (**1.19**). However, in trabecular bone it is on the surface of trabeculae, but in cortical bone a tunnel is cut out by a cutting cone followed by a closing zone which results in the characteristic structure of the Haversian system. Bone remodelling is a slow process and it has been estimated that it takes 10 years to renew the entire skeleton.

Cortical bone and trabecular bone do not change with age in the same way. Trabecular bone is more active metabolically and the bone remodelling cells are in closer proximity to cells of the bone marrow and are probably more subject to the osteotropic cytokines that they produce. The effect of the greater metabolic activity is obviated by an earlier loss of trabecular bone and, in women, a more pronounced loss of trabecular bone of the vertebra after menopause. Cells in cortical bone are more distant to such cells and are more controlled by systemic osteotropic hormones such as parathyroid hormone (PTH) and 1, 25-dihydroxyvitamin D.

Mechanisms and control of bone turnover and remodelling

The balance between bone resorption and bone formation is maintained through a complex regulatory system of systemic and local factors acting on bone cells, such as calcium regulating factors, sex hormones, growth factors, and cytokine. Furthermore, the capability of the bone cells and the number of active cells will determine the production of bone matrix proteins, while other incompletely understood intrinsic mechanisms will determine mineralization and microstructure.

Resorption of bone at a specific site may be induced by microdamage, but the initiating event in the process of osteoclastic activation is unknown. After activation, osteoclasts have the ability to create a local decrease of pH, which precipitates the dissolution of mineral. Exposure of the matrix allows proteolytic enzymes to commence the degradation of the collagenous structure. The signals responsible for termination of bone resorption and initiation of bone formation (coupling) are not well understood; however, evidence suggests that liberation of matrix-embedded insulin-like growth factor system components (IGF-I and IGF-II and their binding proteins) may induce this shift. Other putative coupling factors include cytokines, of which interleukin-1 (IL-1), IL-6, IL-11, TGFβ and TNFα, appear to be most closely involved in the regulation of bone turnover.

Members of another of these systems are clearly important regulators of bone resorption; the osteoprotegerin (OPG) and RANK are members of the TNF receptor family and are receptors for RANK. It has been suggested that OPG acts as an inhibitor of the osteoclastic differentiation, by blocking the ligand-binding of RANK, an osteoclast differentiating factor (**1.20**).

Markers of bone turnover

During bone turnover, surplus products synthesized by the osteoblasts during bone formation or fragments released during bone resorption are found in blood and urine. The levels of these can be used as markers of bone formation, resorption, and rate of turnover (*Table 1.3*, **1.17**, **1.21**). Osteoblast-associated proteins are differentially expressed during bone formation and could ideally provide information on the formation process. However, when systemically assessed the sensitivity is insufficient. The bone specific iso-enzyme of ALP increases early during mineralization. Osteocalcin, the most abundant noncollagenous protein, increases when mineralization is in progression and in differentiated osteoblast when also bone sialo protein is expressed. Breakdown of bone tissue liberates collagen fragments and the terminal ends

---

Table 1.3 Markers of bone turnover

Bone formation
Serum
- Osteocalcin
- Bone-specific alkaline phosphatase
- Type I collagen C- and N-propeptide (PICP and PINP)

Bone resorption
Serum
- Free pyridinoline and deoxypyridinoline
- Pyridinoline cross-linking telopeptides (C- and N-telopeptides, CTx, NTx, ICTP)
- Tartrate-resistant acid phosphatase 5b
- Bone sialoprotein

Urine
- Pyridinoline crosslinks (pyridinoline and deoxypyridinoline)
- Pyridinoline cross-linking telopeptides (C- and N-telopeptides, CTx, NTx, ICTP)
- Osteocalcin fragments
- Hydroxyproline
- Calcium

1.20 Control of bone turnover. **A**: the interaction RANK/RANKL stimulates osteoclast differentiation leading to increased bone resorption.
B: osteoprotegerin is produced by osteoblast lineage cells and inhibits osteoclast differentiation by competitive binding to RANKL, the osteoclast differentiating and activation receptor.

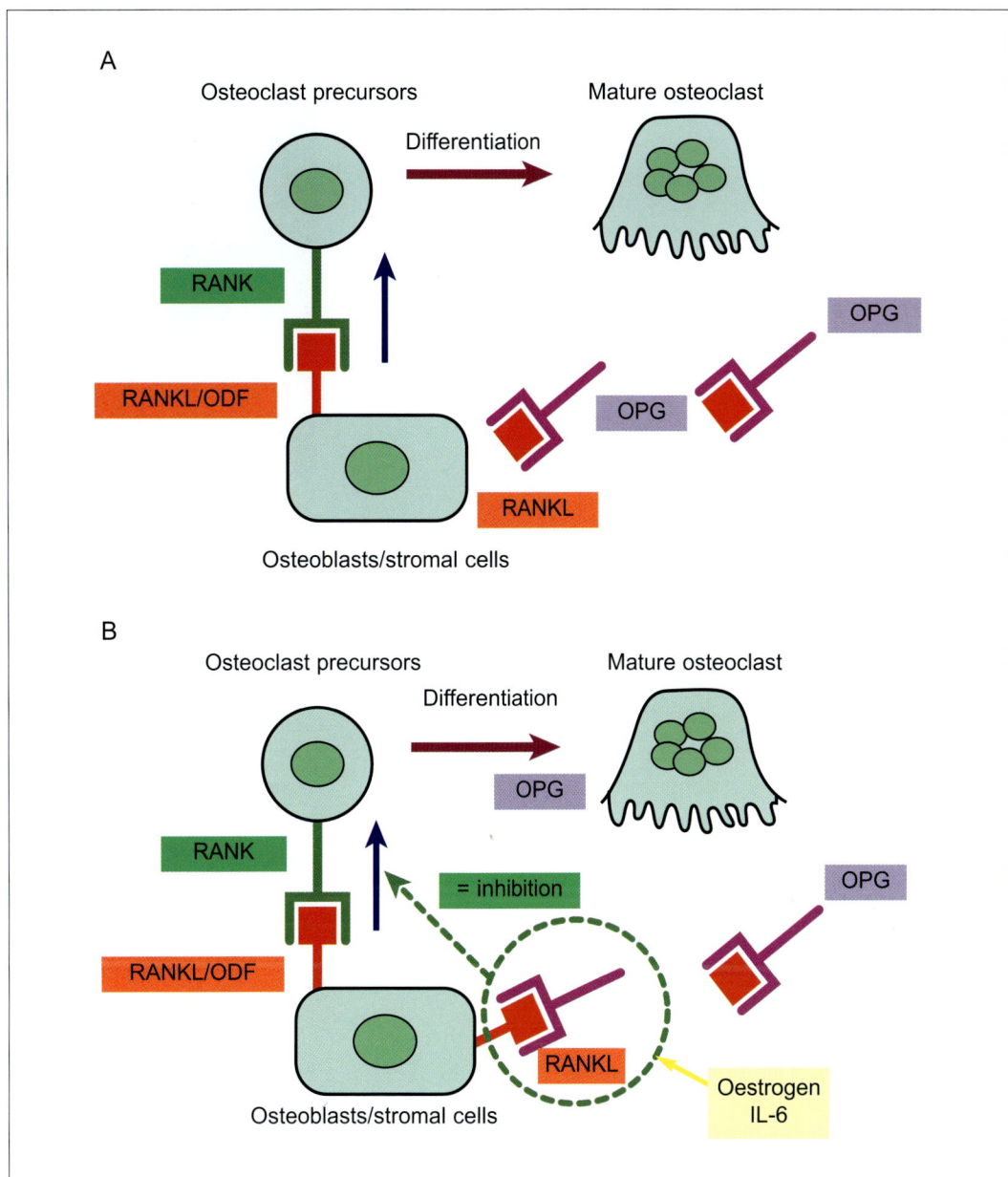

1.21 Collagen-related markers of bone turnover. NTx: N-telopeptide cross-links; CTx: C-telopeptide cross-links; ICTP: type I collagen pyridinoline cross-linked carboxyterminal telopeptide. (Adapted from Nishi Y, Atley L, Eyre DE, *et al*. (1999) Determination of bone markers in pycnodysostosis: effects of cathepsin K deficiency on bone matrix degradation. *J Bone Mineral Res* **14**(11):1902–1908.)

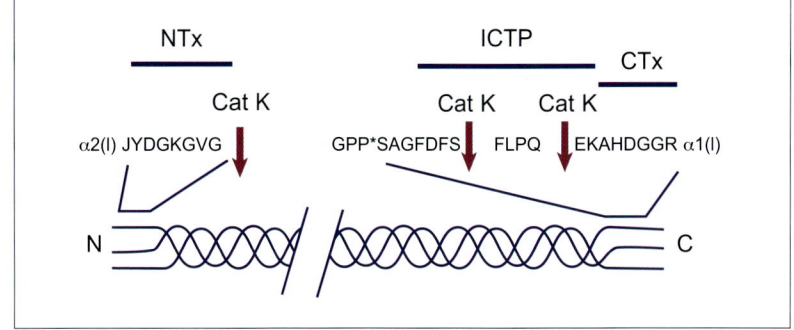

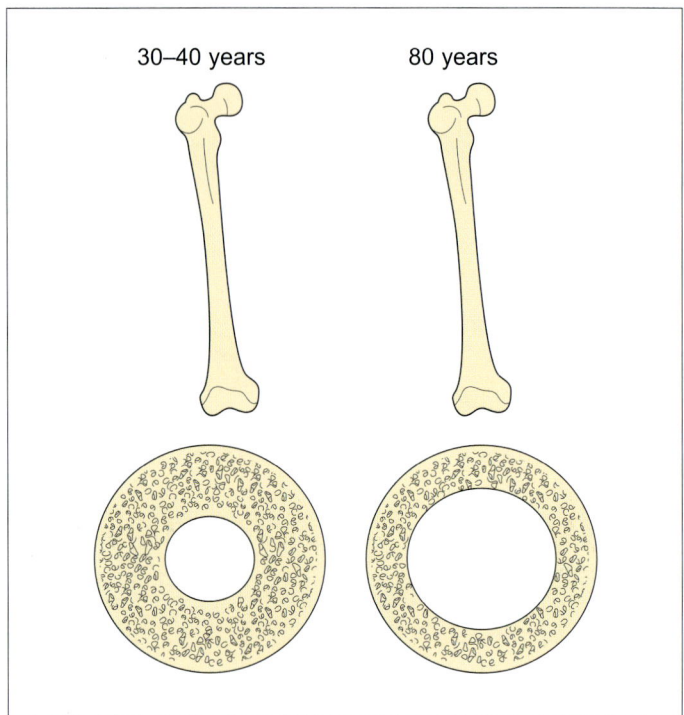

1.22 In cortical bone there is endosteal resorption with periosteal bone formation, leading to an age-related increase in the diameter of long bones and a decrease in cortical thickness. This process may be greater in men.

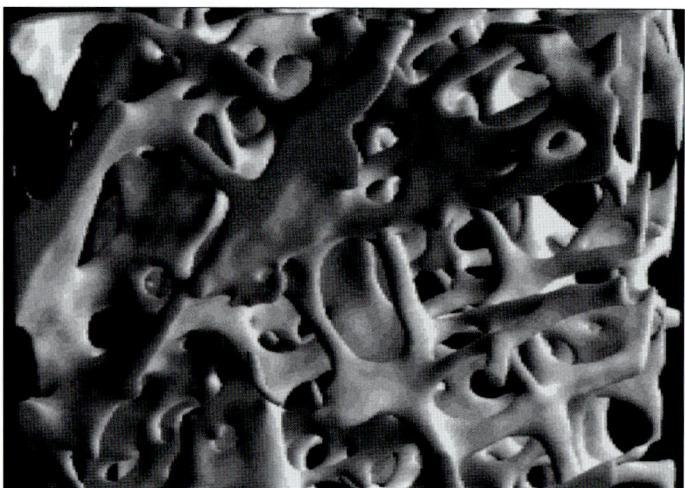

1.23 Changes in trabecular bone: there is thinning of trabeculae and loss of connectivity. (From Hildebrand T, *et al*. (1999). Direct three-dimentional morphometric analysis of human cancellous bone: microstructural data from spine, femur, iliac crest and calcaneus. *J Bone Mineral Res* 14:1167–74.)

(telopeptides) of bone collagen as well as pyridinium residues may be used as markers of bone resorption. Degradation of bone also requires production of lysosomal enzymes of which many are also produced by other cell types. However, a variant of tartrate resistant acid phosphatase is a relatively osteoclast-specific product and an indicator of bone resorption. For discussion of the utility of bone metabolic markers see Chapter 2.

Changes in microarchitecture

The turnover of bone will lead to local changes in microarchitecture. Cortical bone is removed mostly by endosteal resorption and resorption within the Haversian canals, resulting in increased porosity of the bone. Periosteal bone formation continues throughout life, with a consequent age-related increase in diameter of the bone but there is also a decrease in cortical thickness (**1.22**). The trabeculae in the vertebrae of young women are typically orientated with horizontal trabeculae positioned at frequent intervals between vertical trabeculae in a dense three dimensional matrix. The loss that occurs with ageing produces a general thinning of the trabeculae. This occurs in trabeculae orientated in the vertical plane as well as trabeculae orientated in the horizontal plane. The vertical trabeculae tend to be relatively conserved, while the thinning is more pronounced in the horizontal trabeculae (**1.23**). As bone loss proceeds, the progressive thinning of the horizontal trabeculae can lead to perforations, microfractures (**1.24**), and loss of trabecular connectivity (**1.25**) with reduction in the overall strength of the bone to resist the loading forces exerted by gravity and physical activity. This leads to increased susceptibility to fracture, particularly vertebral fracture[8].

Bone size and geometry

Bone size (i.e. mass) and its shape (i.e. distribution of mass, geometry) also have important roles in the biomechanical behaviour of bone and its ability to resist trauma (**1.26**). Large bones are stronger than smaller bones, and a decreased cross-sectional area of the radius is a risk factor for wrist fractures in girls and postmenopausal women. Large vertebrae will have greater end-plate areas resulting in lower spine-pressure values and small vertebrae are more likely to fracture. Geometry is important for the strength of the femoral neck. The hip axis length, from the lateral surface of the trochanter to the inner surface of the pelvis (**1.27**), varies and a short hip axis length gives a stronger structure for any given bone density.

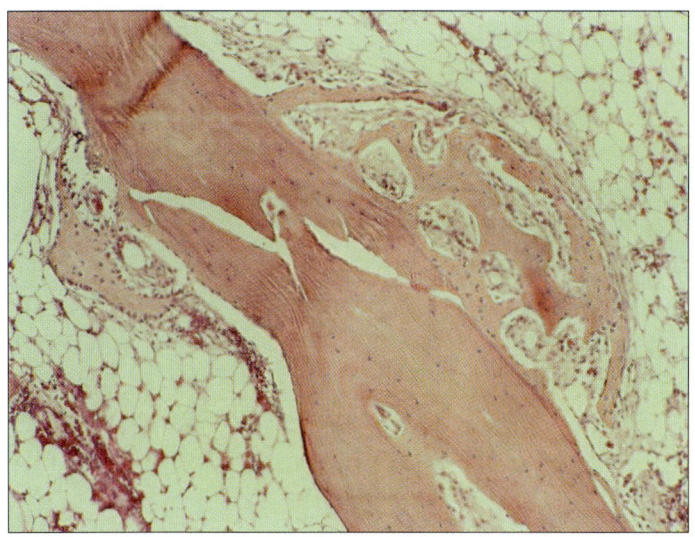

1.24 A microfracture of a trabeculum with surrounding callous formation.

1.25 The thinning and perforation of the horizontal trabeculae leads to loss of connectivity between the vertical trabeculae with reduction in strength.

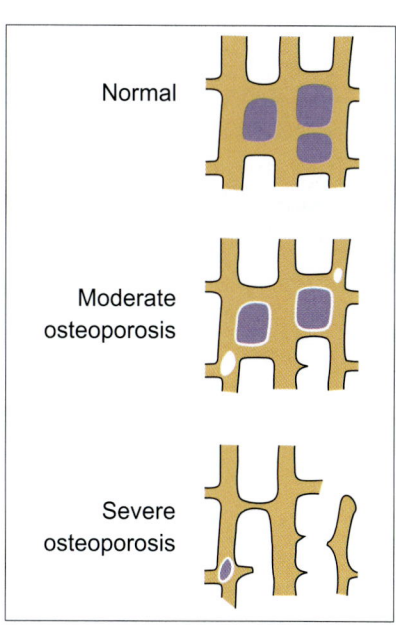

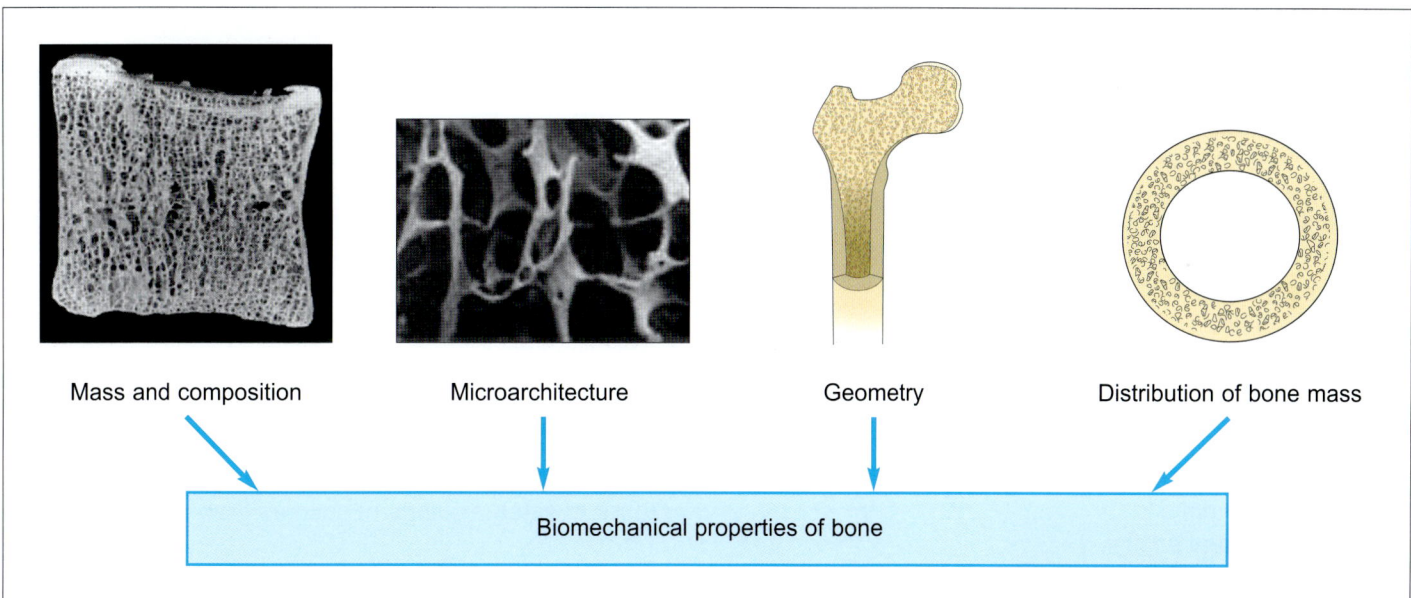

1.26 Bone structure and strength.

Falls

Fracture of long bones usually relates to trauma. The commonest cause of that trauma is a fall.

Falls become increasingly common with ageing. About 30% of individuals over 65 years fall each year, increasing to 50% of adults over 80 years, most commonly amongst residents of long-term care institutions. Most older people fall indoors where also the majority of hip fractures occur. The likelihood of an elderly person falling is increased if he

1.27 Hip axis length can be estimated from the DEXA measurement using a specific algorithm.

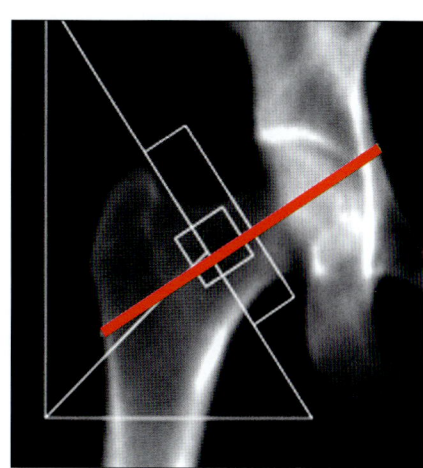

or she has fallen already. Although not all falls result in fracture, many result in impaired health, hospitalization, and permanent disability.

There are a wide range of intrinsic, extrinsic, and environmental factors that can result in a fall (*Table 1.4*, **1.6**). There will be a specific intrinsic treatable cause of the fall in 10% of cases; an identifiable environmental cause in a further 10%, but the cause of most falls is multifactorial and associated with general ill health, more specifically to sensory and musculoskeletal decline with lower limb weakness, unsteadiness, and loss of protective mechanisms.

Impact of falls

Not all falls result in a fracture. Different fractures predominate at different ages, due to to age-related differences in bone strength in different parts of the skeleton and also the impact associated with the fall (**1.7**). The impact is a consequence of the height from which the fall occurred and, in addition, the momentum and direction are important. Osteoporotic fractures are usually defined as being associated with a low energy fall from a standing height. However, fractures in the elderly often occur when

---

Table 1.4 Cause of falls in the elderly

Personal intrinsic factors
General deterioration associated with ageing
- Poor postural control
- Defective proprioception
- Reduced walking speed
- Weakness of lower limbs
- Slow reaction time
- Various comorbidities

Balance, gait or mobility problems
- Joint disease
- Cerebrovascular disease
- Peripheral neuropathy
- Parkinson's disease
- Alcohol

Visual impairment
- Impaired visual acuity
- Cataracts
- Glaucoma
- Retinal degeneration

Impaired cognition or depression
- Alzheimer's disease
- Cerebrovascular disease

'Blackouts'
- Hypoglycaemia
- Postural hypotension
- Cardiac arrhythmia
- TIA, acute onset cerebrovascular attack
- Epilepsy
- Drop attacks VBI

Personal extrinsic factors
Personal hazards
- Inappropriate footwear
- Clothing

Drug therapy
- Sedatives
- Hypotensive drugs

Environmental factors
Hazards at home
- Bad lighting
- Steep stairs
- Slippery floors
- Loose rugs
- Tripping over pets, grandchildren's toys
- Lack of safety equipment such as grab rails

Hazards outdoors
- Transportation
- Uneven pavements
- Bad weather

the person falls down some steps or from standing on a chair; bone fragility is clearly an important contributory factor to these fractures. Distal forearm fractures occur in younger people when the momentum is such that a fall will result in the person landing on their outstretched hand, whereas an older person moving more slowly is more likely to fall to one side onto their hip. The actual location of impact, its surface, and soft tissues to attenuate the impact as well as the person's protective responses are all important in determining whether the fall results in fracture. The 'soft tissues' may relate to body fat or to the flooring. Understanding all these factors is important when developing strategies to prevent fractures.

Fractures associated with osteoporosis

Fracture is the clinical manifestation of osteoporosis and typical sites are the vertebrae, distal forearm, and hip. There is also an age-related increase risk of fractures of the humerus, pelvis, ribs, clavicle, and scapula (**1.28**). Fractures with minimal trauma can also occur for other reasons and these must be always considered (*Table 1.5*).

Vertebral fractures

The vertebral column is the central core of the skeleton. It consists of 24 vertebrae adjoined by intervertebral discs and stabilized by intervertebral joints (facet joints) and ligaments (**1.29**). The ribs originate from the thoracic vertebra. The vertebra are mainly made of trabecular bone covered by a relatively thin cortical layer. The normal vertebra has equal height at the anterior edge, central part, and the posterior part. As changes in shape of a vertebra can be developmental or due to a fracture, it cannot always be known when it occurred and it is often therefore described as a vertebral deformity and not as a fracture. The deformation because of osteoporosis results in wedging (anterior depression), end-plate compression (central depression), or a total depression, i.e. crush fracture (**1.30**). Osteoporotic fractures rarely protrude into the spinal canal to cause neurological deficits.

Deformation of a vertebra occurs when the load exceeds the bone strength (**1.31**). The degree of deformity is mainly dependent on the microstructural integrity of the trabecular network, and is related to a lesser extent to the thin cortices of the vertebrae. The degree of deformation is therefore related to the degree of bone loss. Vertebral fractures are most commonly located at the lower thoracic spine (Th

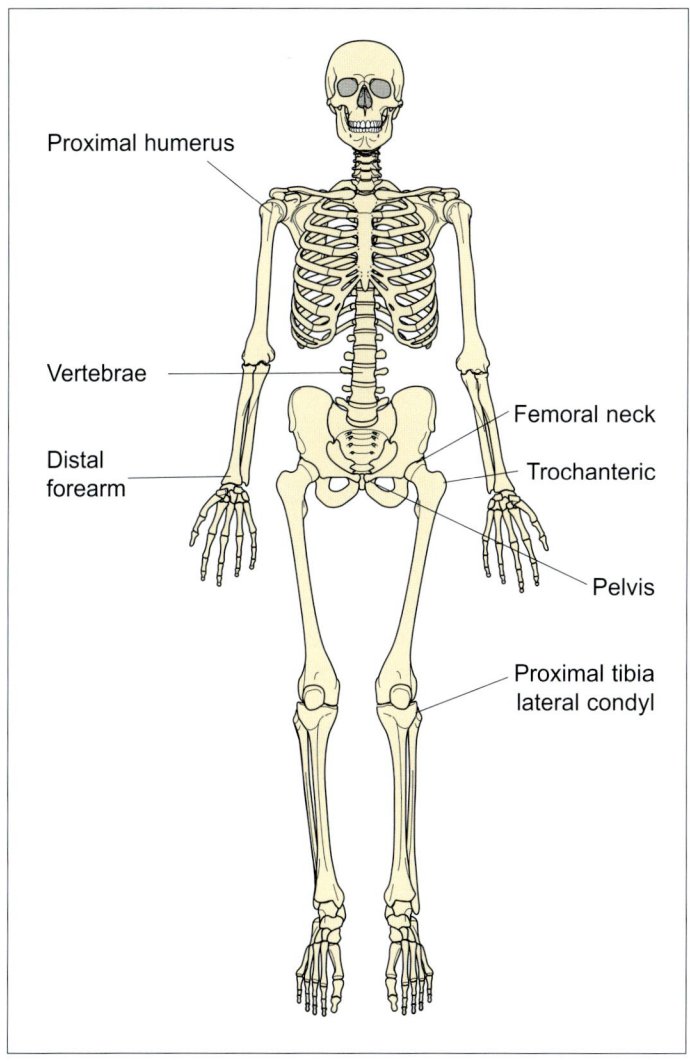

Proximal humerus

Vertebrae

Distal forearm

Femoral neck

Trochanteric

Pelvis

Proximal tibia lateral condyl

1.28 Typical sites of osteoporotic fracture.

Table 1.5 Causes of fracture

- Osteoporosis
- Primary malignancy including myeloma
- Metastatic malignancy – breast, prostate, lung, and renal most common
- Osteomalacia
- Paget's disease
- Osteomyelitis
- Traumatic vertebral fracture earlier in life
- Scheuermann's osteochondritis of the spine

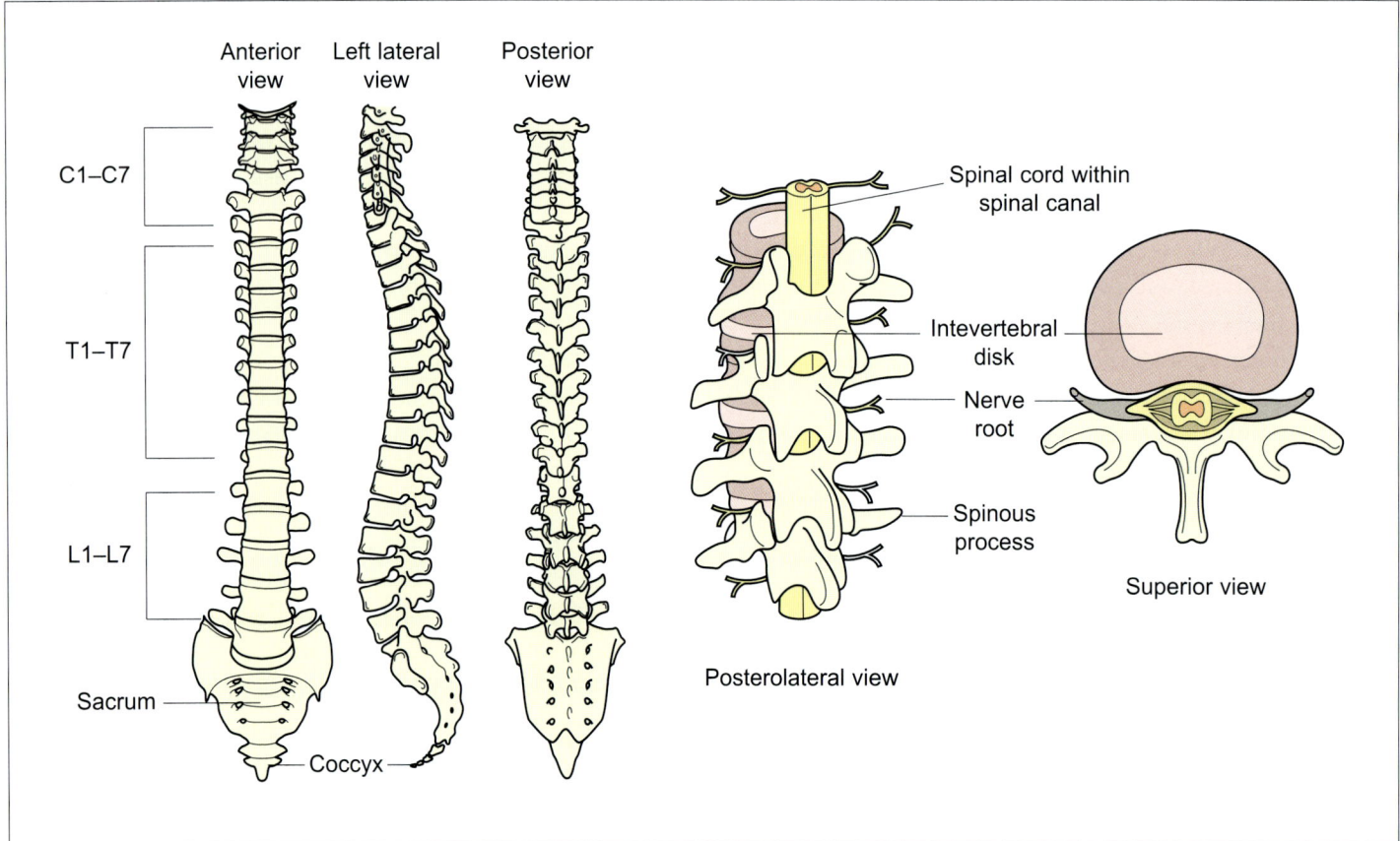

1.29 Structure of the vertebral column.

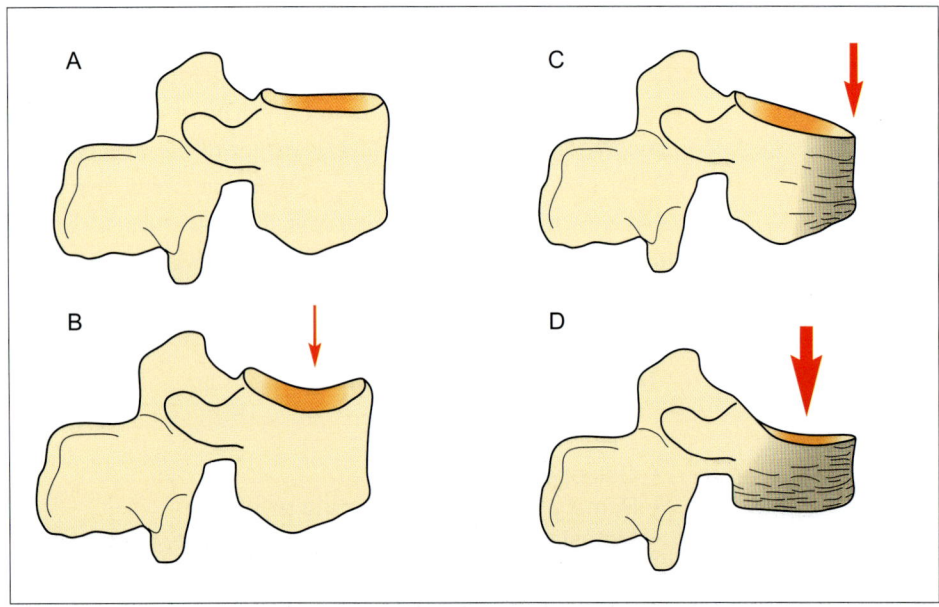

1.30 Vertebral deformities. **A**: normal; **B**: end-plate collapse; **C**: wedge fracture; **D**: crush fracture.

1.31 This lumbar vertebra (arrow) has a wedge-shaped deformity with height loss of the anterior border.

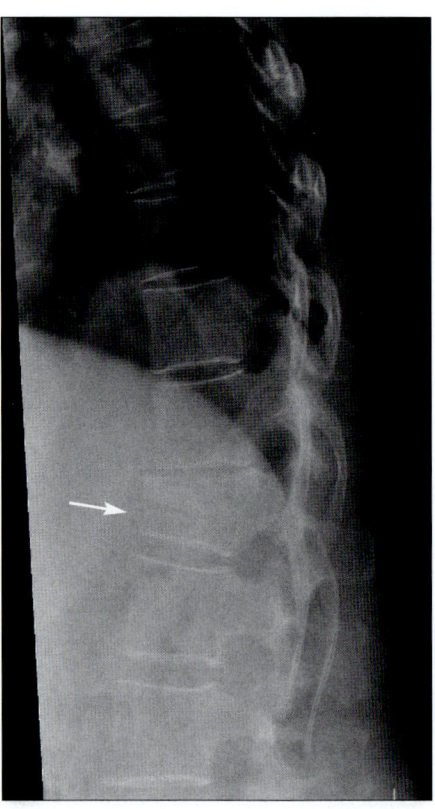

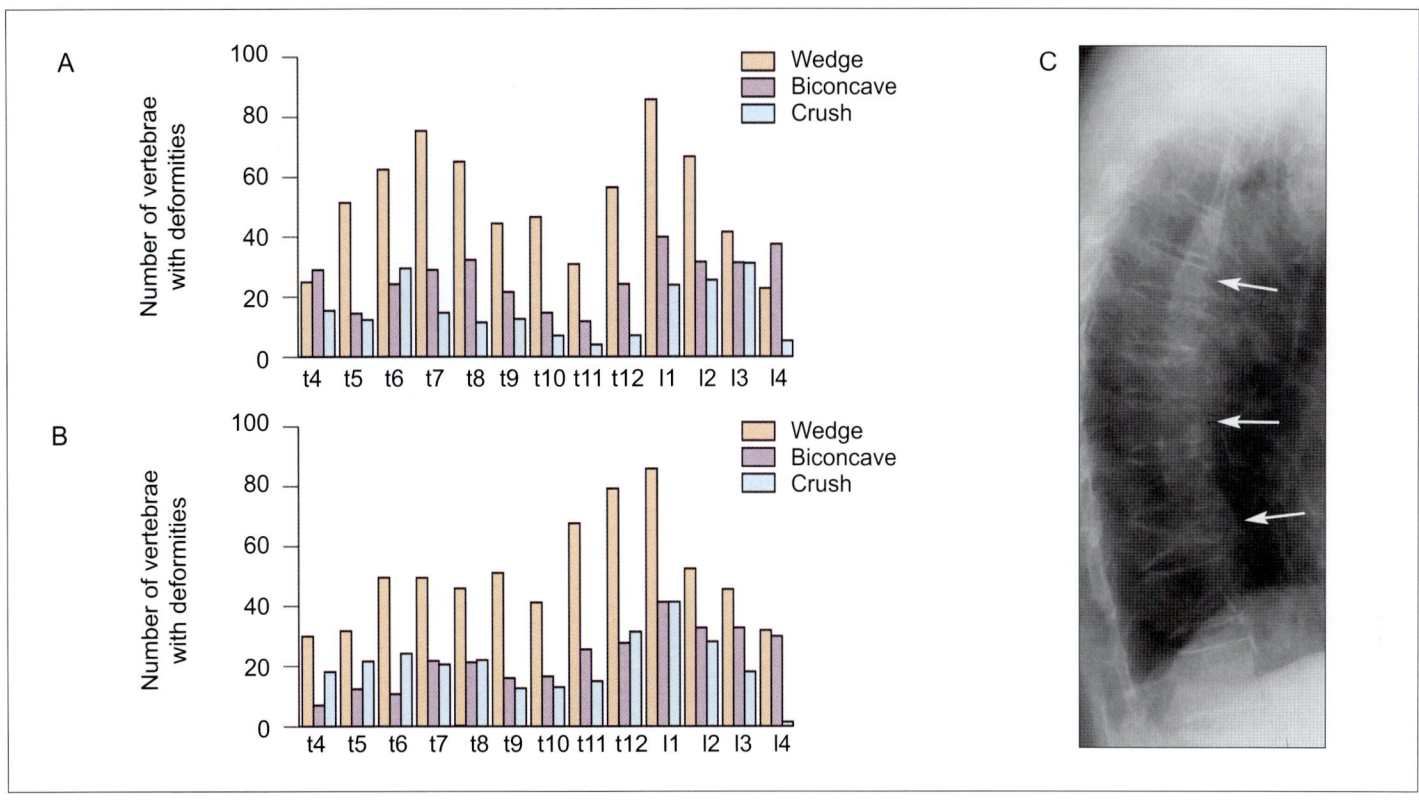

1.32 Vertebral fractures are most commonly located at the lower thoracic spine (Th 11–12) and upper lumbar spine (L1) in both men (**A**) and women (**B**). This is also shown in an X-ray (**C**). (Adapted from Ismail AA, Cooper C, Felsenberg D, *et al.* (1999). Number and type of vertebral deformities: epidemiological characteristics and relation to back pain and height loss. European Vertebral Osteoporosis Study Group. *Osteoporos Int* **9**(3):206–213.)

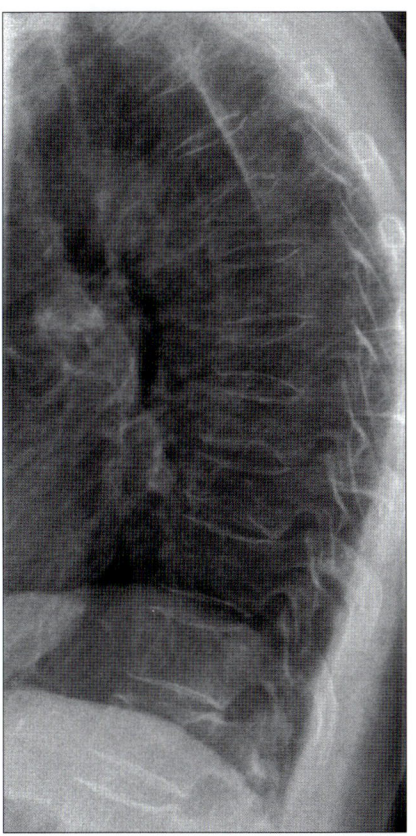

11–12) and upper lumbar spine (L1) and rarely above the level of Th 5[9] (**1.32**). Vertebral fractures are most often an incidental finding. Only about one-third present clinically, and then it is often with sudden onset of severe disabling back pain. Multiple fractures may be unknown to the person who just notices their decreasing body height.

End-stage vertebral osteoporosis results from multiple vertebral fractures at both the thoracic and lumbar spine (**1.33**). This leads to kyphosis, loss of height (up to 20 cm), restricted lung capacity, impaired swallowing, stomach, and the gut function, disturbed sleep, and problems with walking. The rib cage reaches inside the pelvic rim. Recent fractures can be demonstrated by increased uptake on bone scintigraphy (**1.34**) or by intraosseous oedema which can be visualized using magnetic resonance techniques (**1.35**).

1.33 Multiple vertebral fractures at both the thoracic and lumbar spine, resulting in kyphosis and loss of height (up to 20 cm). The rib cage reaches inside the pelvic rim.

Upper extremity fractures

The distal radius or Colles' fracture is one of the most common fractures (**1.36–1.38**) and, in women, is regarded as an indicator for osteoporosis and future fracture risk because it occurs at a relatively early age (see Chapters 2 and 3). The fracture is located at the vulnerable site at the distal end of radius where trabecular bone dominates and where the cortical bone is thinner towards the radio-carpal joint. The fracture occurs when a person falls or stumbles forward, reaching out with the hand to break the fall. Other fractures of the upper extremity occur following low-energy trauma (**1.36**). Fractures of the proximal humerus increase with age in both men and women and are the third most common fracture in persons over the age of 65 years (**1.39, 1.40**). They typically occur when the person is unable to reach out fully to counteract a fall and instead they fall slightly to the side and hit the shoulder region. The person is usually generally fit and living at home. Fractures related to osteoporosis also occur at the elbow (**1.41**).

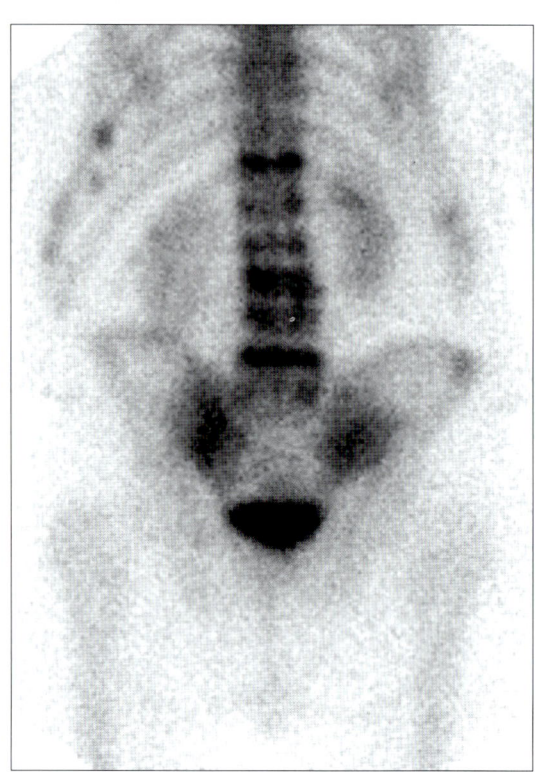

1.34 Scintigraphy of vertebral fracture.

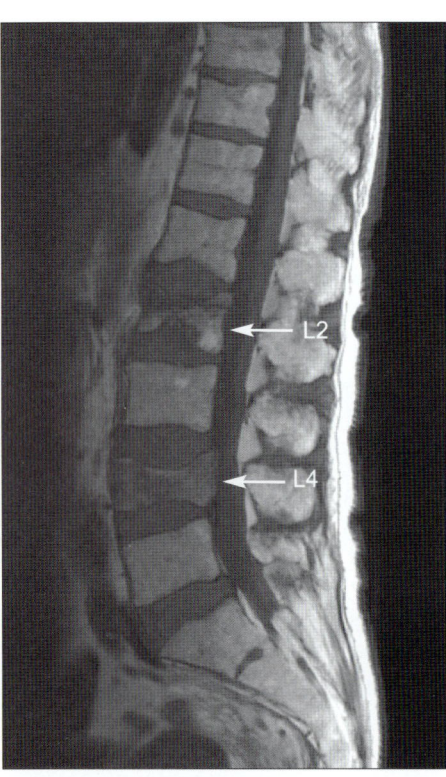

1.35 Vertebral fractures induce intraosseous oedema which can be visualized using magnetic resonance techniques. The signal is altered in L2 and L4 as a sign of recent fracture, not yet healed. Vertebral fractures are commonly stable and rarely compromise the spinal space.

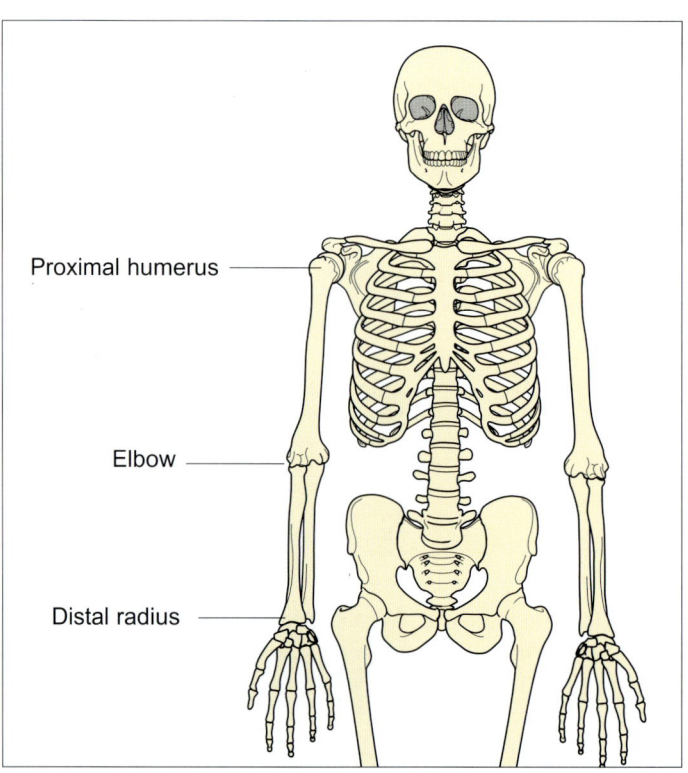

1.36 Common sites of fractures of the upper extremities. The relative distribution of the most common fractures in women: distal radius fracture 15–20% and proximal humerus fracture <5%.

1.37 Distal radius fracture in an 84-year-old woman. The fracture is severely displaced with dorsal angulation and axial compression. In addition, the head of the ulna is fractured, as is the styloid process. The axial compression causes prominence of the ulnar head, a finding that patients later often find disturbing.

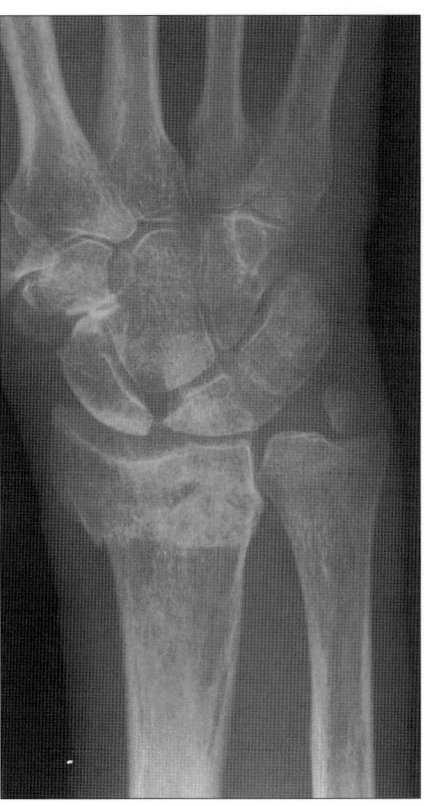

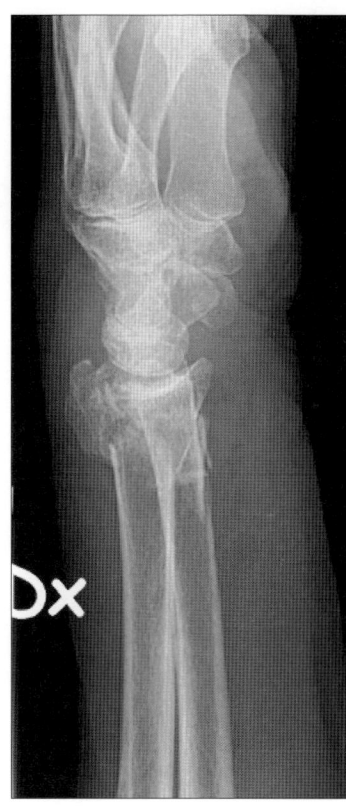

1.38 The side view is necessary to evaluate the dorsal displacement Colles's fracture.

1.39 Fractures of the upper arm (proximal humerus) commonly occur at the surgical neck, another region rich in trabecular bone and thin cortical bone. This fracture is caused by a fall towards an outstretched arm. The majority of fractures are not significantly displaced and are thereby stable, as seen here.

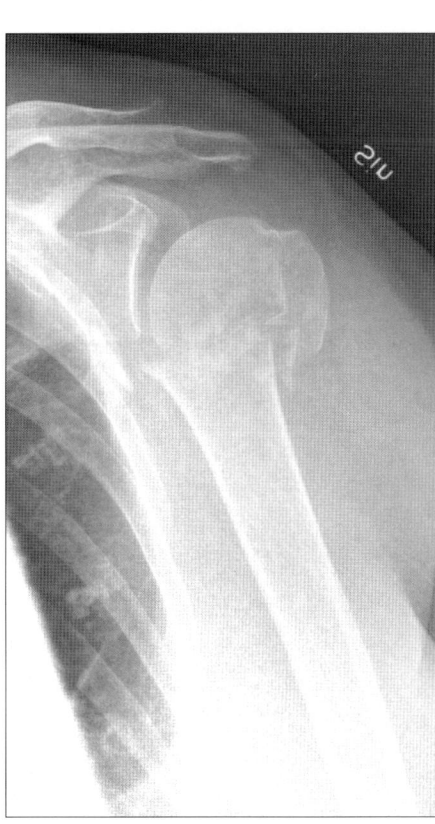

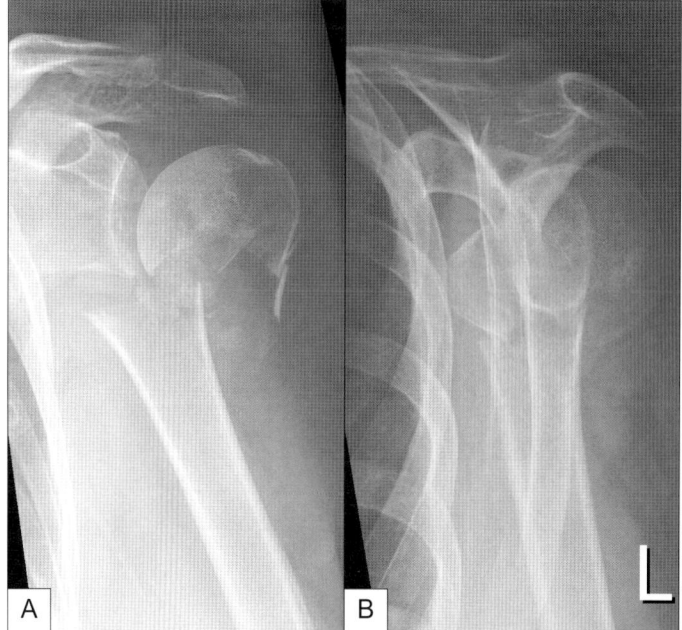

1.40 A, **B:** A fracture of the proximal humerus where the head of the humerus is multifragmented and has very little contact with the humeral shaft. This fracture requires surgical treatment.

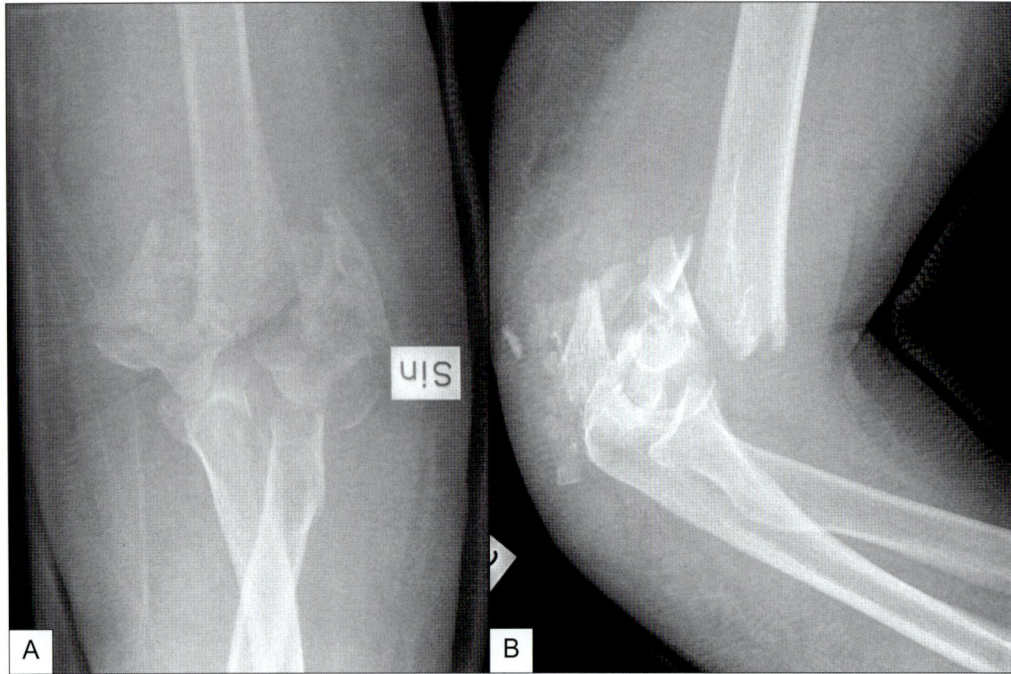

1.41 A, B: With severe osteoporosis, fracture of the elbow can be very detrimental. The fracture can be extremely fragmented (bag-of-bones) and unstable, as in this 84-year-old woman. These fractures are often impossible to reduce or stabilize.

Lower extremity fractures

Many different types of fracture may occur in the lower extremity after low-energy trauma (**1.42**). Fractures of the hip are most common. These involve the femoral neck (cervical, 47%) or the trochanter (53%), which is mainly trabecular bone (**1.43–1.47**). Fractures of the proximal femur just below the trochanter are called subtrochanteric and are more severe or difficult to treat optimally. The typical age in Europe to sustain a hip fracture is 80 years and many individuals are frail with comorbidities and are already unable to live independently.

Pelvic fractures constitute less than 1% of fractures and are common only in the very elderly and usually occur in the pubic rami (**1.48**). Fracture of the lateral condyl of the proximal tibia is associated with osteoporosis (**1.49**).

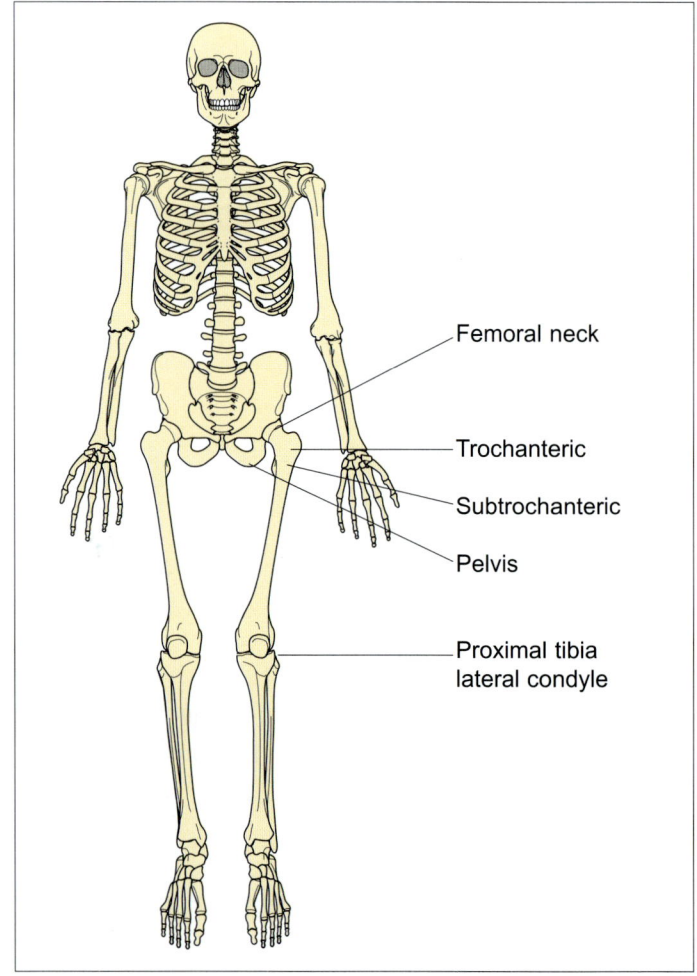

Femoral neck

Trochanteric

Subtrochanteric

Pelvis

Proximal tibia lateral condyle

1.42 Common sites of fractures of the lower extremities.

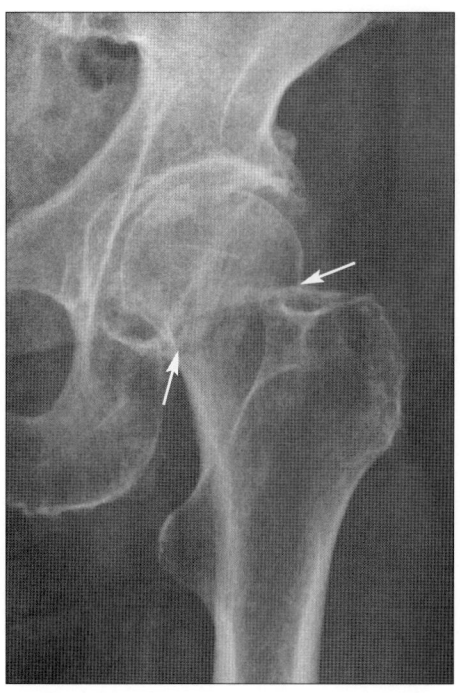

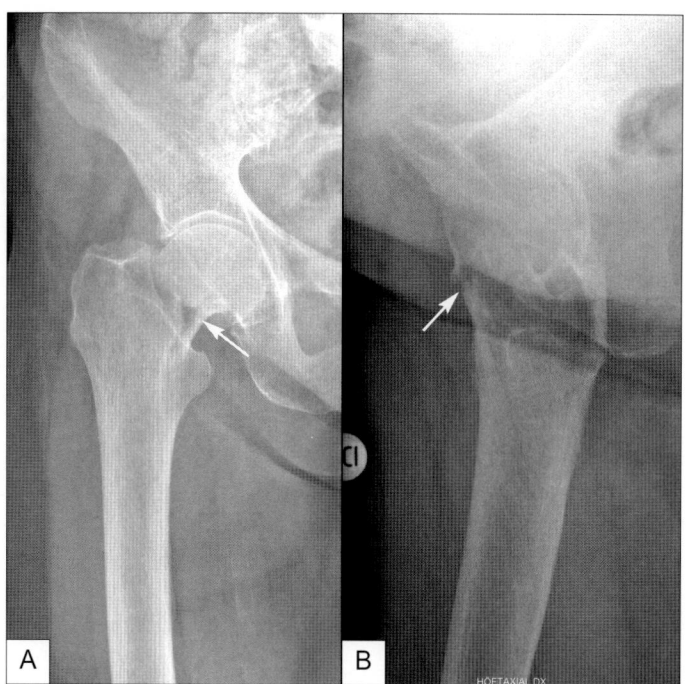

1.43 Fractures (arrows) of the femoral neck (cervical) may be graded according to displacement. The mildly displaced fractures (Garden I) have a more favourable outcome with regard to healing. Impaired healing is caused by disruption of the vascular supply from the circumflex artery.

1.44 This fracture of the femoral neck has a greater degree of displacement. Displacement must be evaluated in two planes, anterior-poterior (**A**) and lateral (**B**). Notice also the thin cortices of the femoral shaft in this 89-year-old woman. Arrows indicate the fracture.

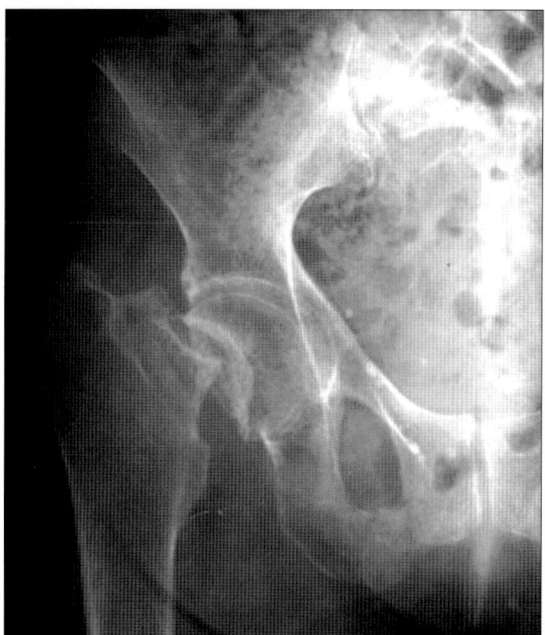

1.45 A severely displaced femoral neck fracture. The patient has previously had a pelvic fracture of the pubic ramus.

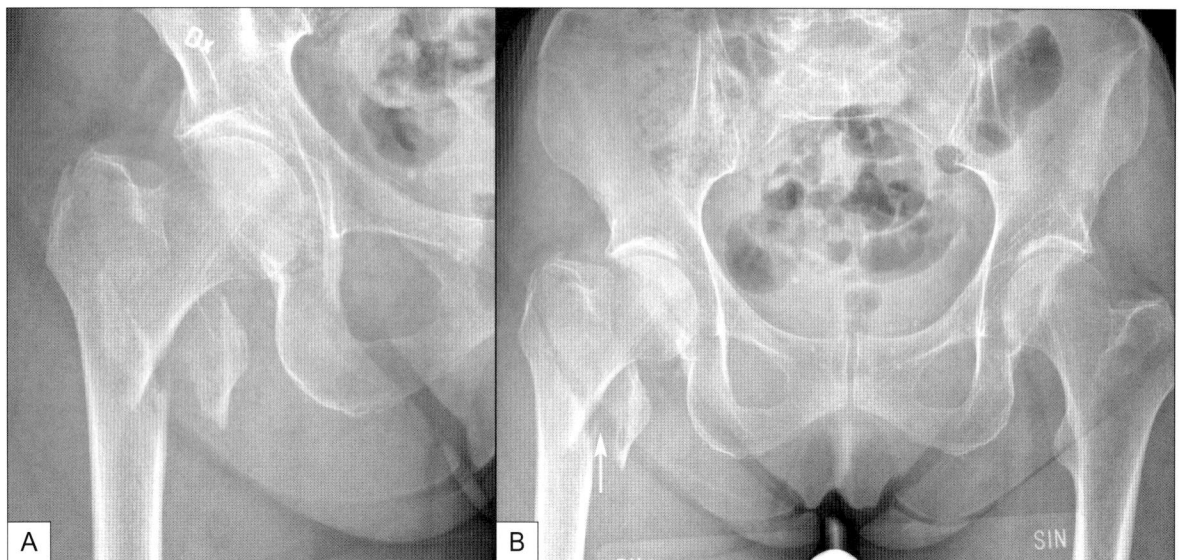

1.46 A: A trochanteric fracture mainly involves trabecular bone and it may be multifragmented (as in this case), a factor of major importance for obtaining stability after reduction. Note that this fracture involves the lesser trochanter. **B:** A pelvic view should always be included in the assessment of a hip patient.

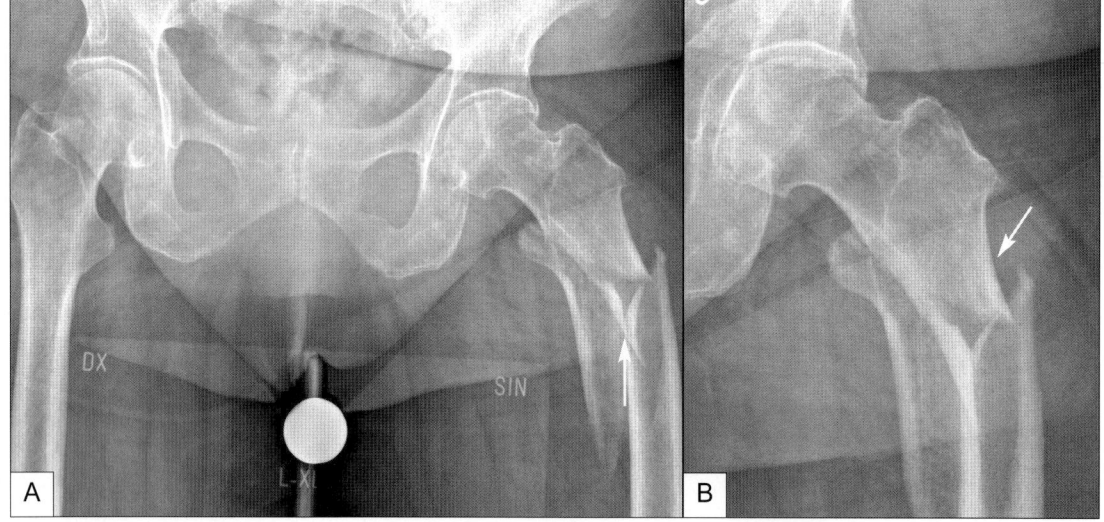

1.47 A, B: A fracture of the proximal femoral diaphysis is often described as subtrochanteric. This is a spiral fracture with a large intermediate fragment on the medio-dorsal side, including the lesser trochanter.

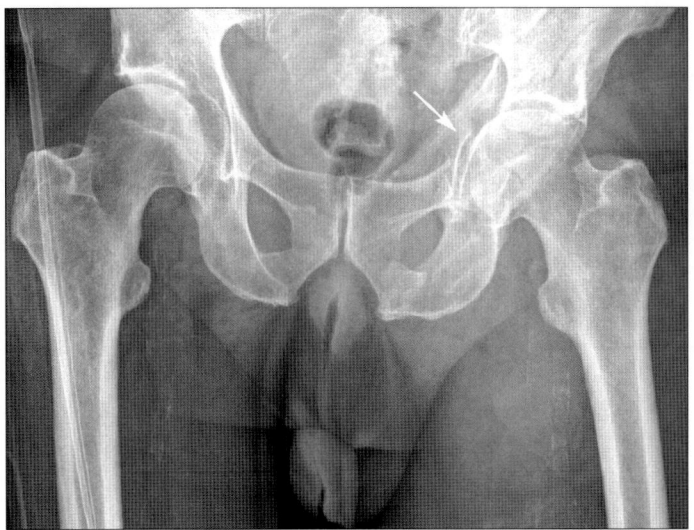

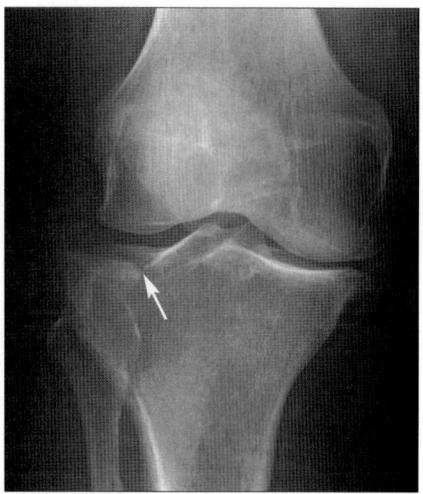

1.49 Fracture of the lateral condyl of the proximal tibia is associated with osteoporosis. In younger persons, the cruciate and collateral ligaments are injured instead and joint stability must be tested in these patients. The fracture is intra-articular with a depression of the joint surface and therefore requires surgical reduction.

1.48 The pelvic fracture related to osteoporosis is most often located at either or both of the inferior or superior rami. The patients clinically present with similar signs and symptoms as those with hip fracture. Acetabular fractures, that in the most severe cases cause protrusion of the femoral head into the pelvis (arrow), are rare after low-energy trauma.

Other causes of fracture

Fractures may arise for reasons other then osteoporosis and trauma and the possibility of primary and secondary bone cancer must always be considered (**1.50–1.52**). This includes myeloma. Nonmalignant lesions such as cysts (**1.53**) can also present as a fracture following minimal trauma. Bone conditions such as osteomalacia (**1.54**) and Paget's disease (**1.55**) may also present with fracture.

1.50 A, **B:** Breast cancer is the most common cause of metastatic bone disease in women, while in men it is prostate cancer. Neurological deficits from osteoporotic fractures are uncommon and, when present, particularly in the elderly, malignancy should always be ruled out. Bone metastases of the spine are preferably visualized and evaluated by MRI (**B**) as it provides information on both the skeletal and nonskeletal involvement. In this case L1 (arrow) has a generally higher signal similar to that of an osteoporotic fracture, but in addition virtually all vertebral bodies are infiltrated by malignant cells (the dark areas), whereas the spinal space is intact.

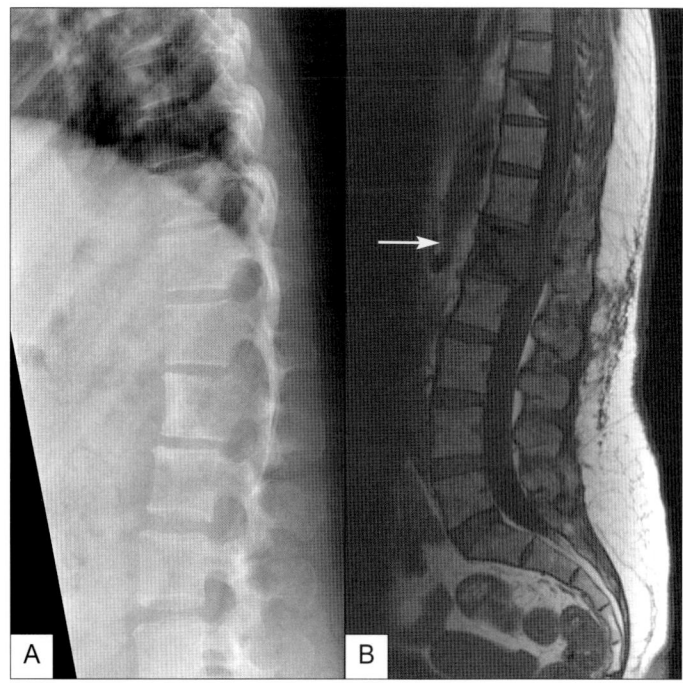

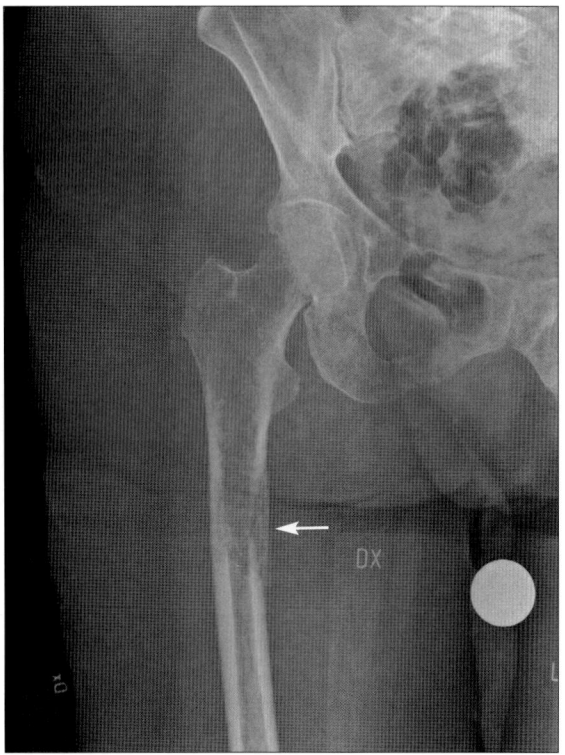

1.51 Metastases of the long bones are not as frequent as in the spine. Metastases of the long bone are mostly seen in the proximal femur/hip and the proximal humerus, both regions rich in metabolically active trabecular bone. Metastases are either osteolytic or sclerotic in nature. Osteolytic metastases in the long bones (arrow) leads to cortical thinning and high fracture risk without prior trauma.

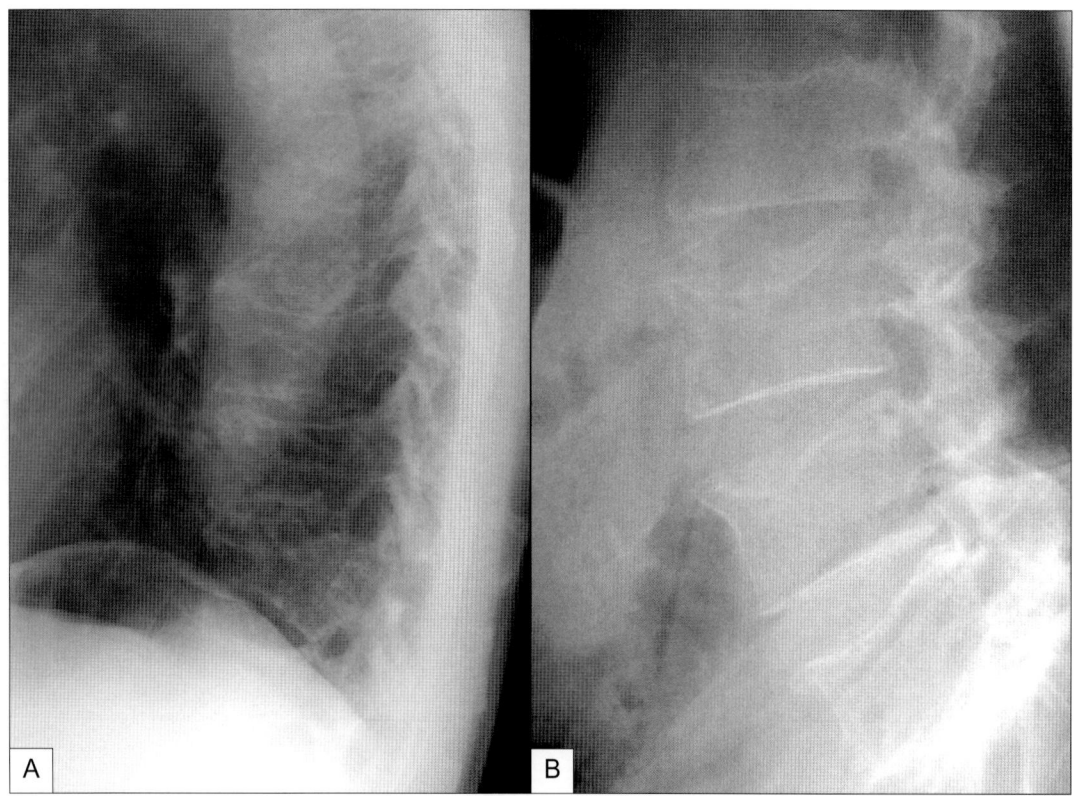

1.52 A, B: A 71-year-old man with widespread myeloma resulting in vertebral deformities.

1.53 Bone cysts are most often benign and are accidentally found, particularly in the small bones of the hands and feet. In children, solitary cyst have a predilection for the proximal humerus and are associated with fractures after minor trauma. The cyst heals with the fracture.
A: Bone cyst (arrow) in a young person that was identified because of a fracture from a minor trauma
B: Bone cyst in the proximal femur (arrow) in a patient presenting with a dull ache in the groin (MRI).

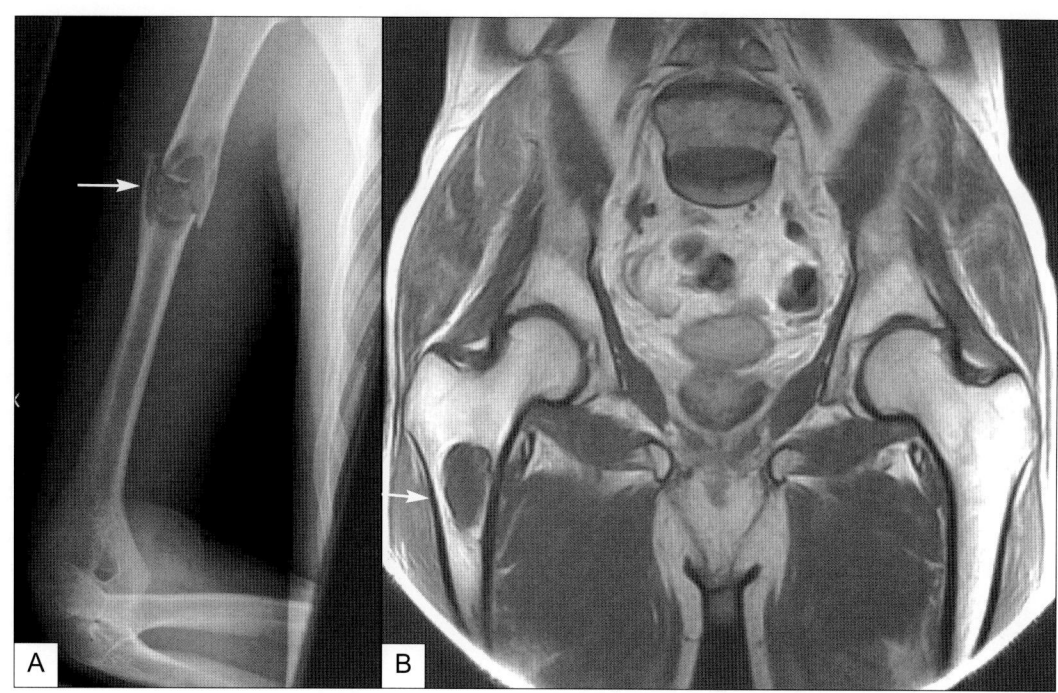

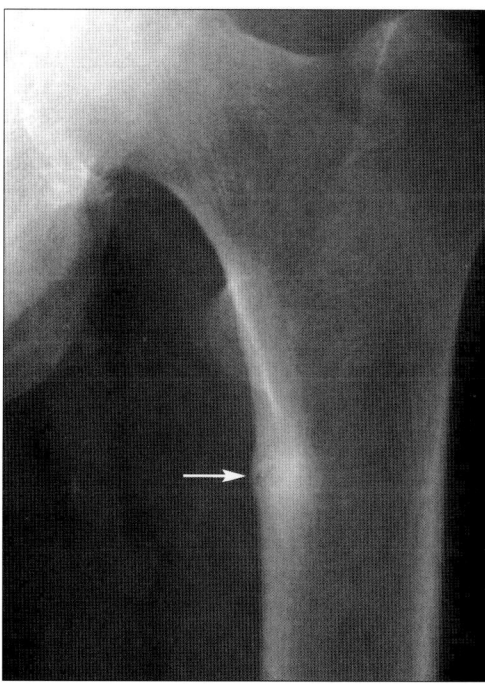

1.54 Pseudofracture (Looser's zones) (arrow) of the medial aspect of the proximal femur in osteomalacia.

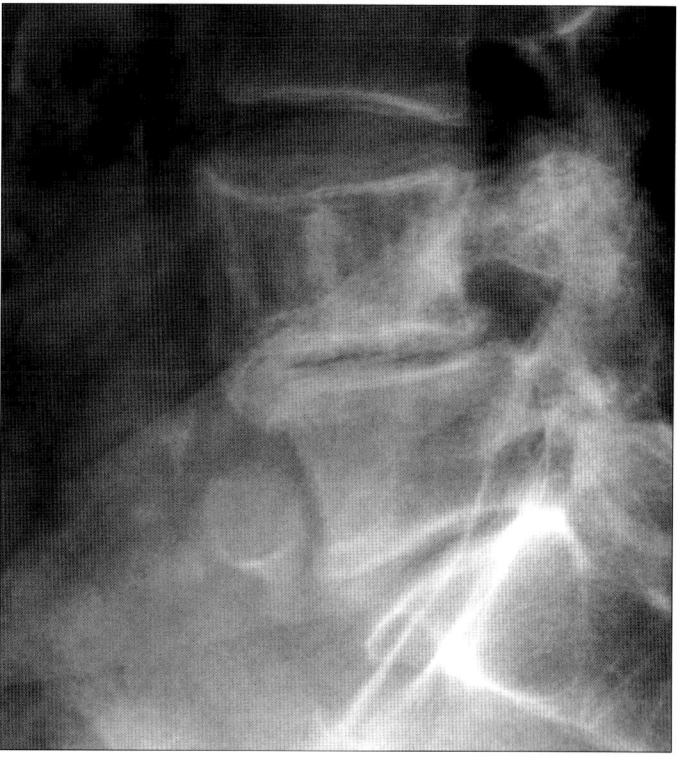

1.55 Paget's disease of bone affecting the fourth lumbar vertebra with typical disorganization of bone structure.

References

1 World Health Organisation (1994). Assessment of fracture risk and its application to screening for postmenopausal osteoporosis: report of a World Health Organization Study Group. *WHO Technical Report Series* **843**. World Health Organization, Geneva.

2 NIH Consensus Conference (2001). Osteoporosis prevention, diagnosis, and therapy. NIH Consensus Statement Online 2000 March 27–29;**17**(1):1–36 available at URL http://consensus.nih.gov/2000/2000Osteoporosis111html.htm.

3 Eyre DR, Paz MA, Gallop PM (1984). Cross-linking in collagen and elastin. *Ann Rev Biochem* **53**:717–748.

4 Horgan DJ, King NL, Kurth LB, Kuypers R (1990). Collagen cross-links and their relationship to the thermal properties of calf tendons. *Arch Biochem Biophys* **281**(1):21–26.

5 Garnero P, Sornay-Rendu E, Claustrat B, Delmas PD (2000). Biochemical markers of bone turnover, endogenous hormones, and the risk of fractures in postmenopausal women: the OFELY study. *J Bone Mineral Res* **15**(8):1526–1536.

6 Frost HM (1969). Tetracycline-based histological analysis of bone remodelling. *Calcif Tissue Res* **3**(3):211–237.

7 Parfitt AM (1984). The cellular basis of bone remodelling: the quantum concept re-examined in light of recent advances in the cell biology of bone. *Calcif Tissue Int* **36**(Suppl. 1):S37–S45.

8 Mosekilde L (1993). Vertebral structure and strength *in vivo* and *in vitro*. *Calcif Tissue Int* **53**(Suppl. 1):S121–S125.

9 Ismail AA, Cooper C, Felsenberg D, *et al.* (1999). Number and type of vertebral deformities: epidemiological characteristics and relation to back pain and height loss. European Vertebral Osteoporosis Study Group. *Osteoporos Int* **9**(3):206–213.

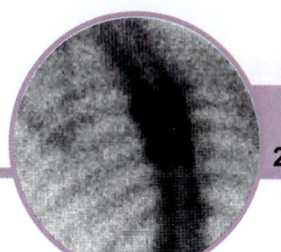

Chapter 2

Epidemiology, risk, and risk factors

Introduction

Osteoporosis is defined in terms of bone quality, bone mass, bone architecture, and fracture risk. The epidemiology of osteoporosis therefore relates to all these and to their outcomes. Clinically, osteoporosis is recognized by the occurrence of fractures following low-energy trauma, the best documented of these being hip, vertebral, and distal forearm fractures. The definition has been previously considered (*Table 1.1*).

The incidence of osteoporosis is best measured indirectly as the incidence of fractures that are attributable to the condition. Prevalence is best measured by the frequency of reduced bone mineral density (BMD) or numbers of those with vertebral deformity. The risk of sustaining a fracture related to osteoporosis can be considered for the future lifetime from the age that the risk increases – that is from 50 years. Alternatively, risk can be considered as the probability of sustaining a fracture during a meaningful period and 10 years is considered more appropriate when deciding whether or not to intervene to reduce that risk.

Epidemiology of osteoporosis

There is a normal distribution of bone density across the population for any age and either sex (**2.1**). Bone strength declines and the risk of fracture increases with reduced bone density. Normal bone density is defined as being -1 standard deviation or greater than the mean at 30–40 years (peak bone mass). Bone density between -1 SD and -2.5 SD of peak bone mass (T-score) has been defined by the WHO as osteopenia, and equal or below 2.5 SD of peak bone mass as osteoporosis[1].

As bone density declines with ageing, the number at any age with osteoporosis will increase (**2.2**)[2]. It is estimated that 54% of postmenopausal white women in the northern USA have osteopenia, and a further 30% have osteoporosis in at least one skeletal site. In the UK, it is estimated that around 23% of women aged 50 years or more have osteoporosis as defined by WHO. For the diagnosis of osteoporosis, it has been recommended by the International Osteoporosis Foundation to measure BMD by dual energy X-ray absorptiometry (DXA) at the hip, and by this definition the

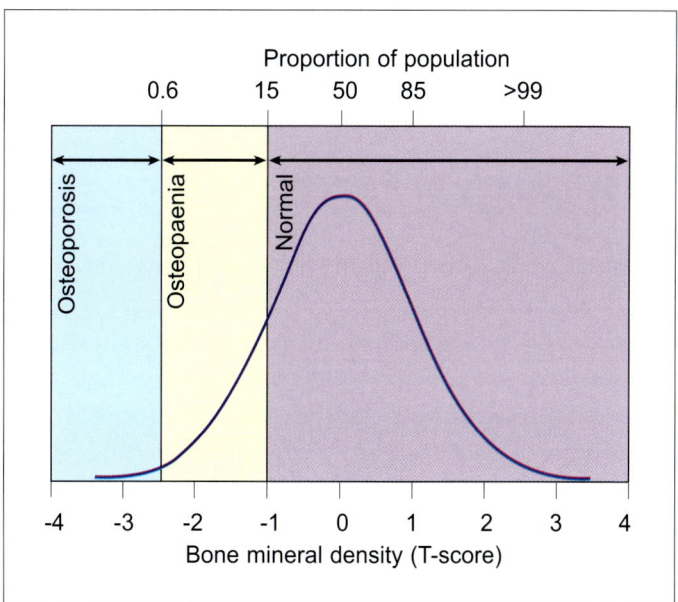

2.1 Distribution of bone density in healthy women aged 30–40 years. (Adapted from WHO (2003). Prevention and Management of Osteoporosis. *WHO Technical Report Series* No. **921**. World Health Organization, Geneva.)

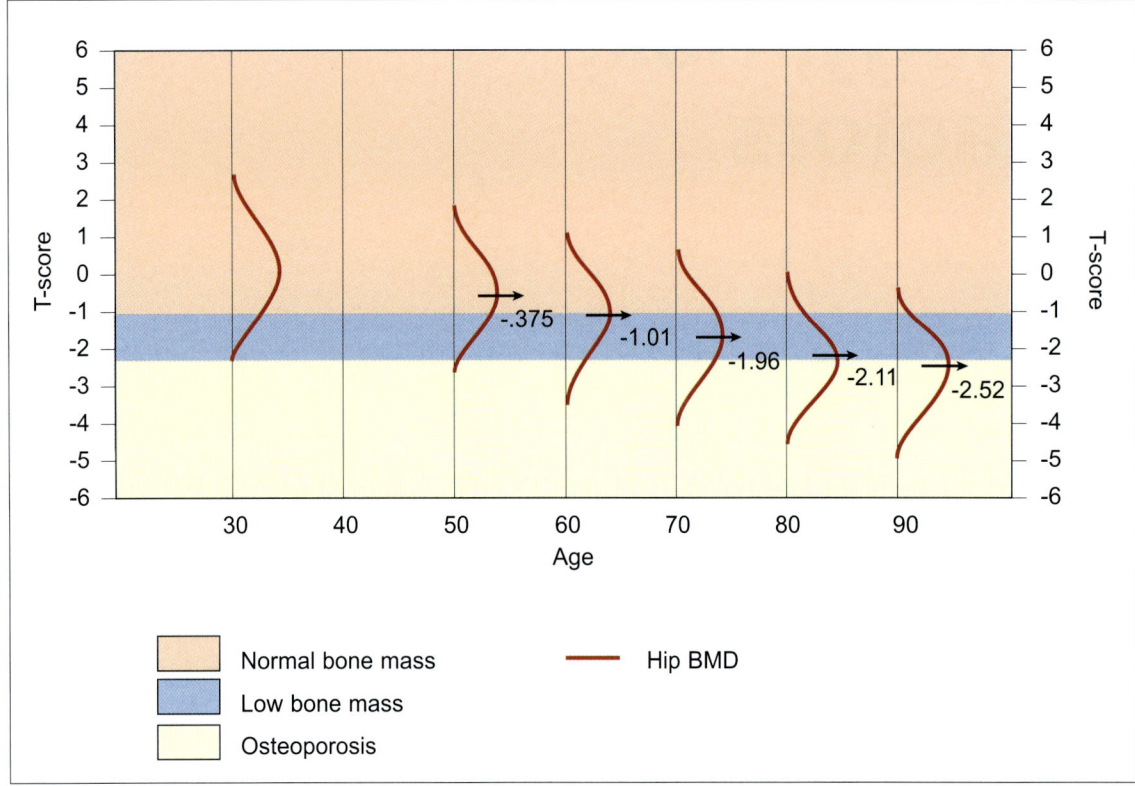

2.2 The distribution of bone density at increasing ages. (Adapted from Kanis J, *et al.* (1994). The diagnosis of osteoporosis. *J Bone Mineral Res* **9**(8):1137–1141.)

general prevalence of osteoporosis rises from 5% in women at the age of 50 years to 50% at the age of 85, and in men the comparable figures are 2.4% and 20%[3]. The dramatic increase from midlife into older age in the percent of women who have osteoporosis in Sweden is demonstrated in Figure **2.3**. This is set against the trend of longevity with women aged 80 having a life expectancy of over 8 years.

Epidemiology of fracture

Fractures occur most frequently in adolescents and young adults and, in later life, increase from age 50 years (**2.4**). At 75 years, over 40% of women will have sustained a fracture[4]. In adolescents and young adults they are more frequent in males than females when they are usually associated with major trauma such as road traffic accidents and sports injuries. The sites of fracture are usually long bones, most commonly the forearm[5]. In later life, fractures are more common in females than males and follow low-energy trauma, most commonly falls. The majority of these fractures in those aged over 50 years are the result of underlying osteoporosis.

The fractures that are most strongly associated with age and osteoporosis are of the distal forearm (Colles' fracture),

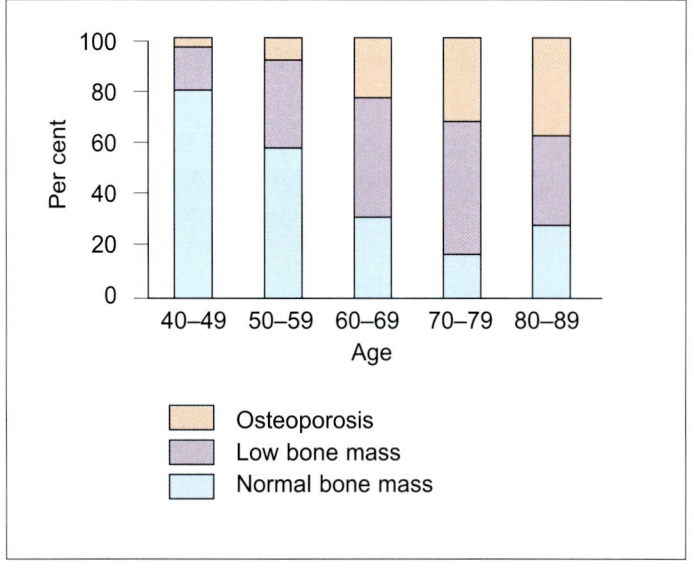

2.3 The percentage of women in Sweden with normal bone mass, low bone mass, and osteoporosis in the hip at increasing ages. (Adapted from SBU (1995). Measurement of bone mineral density. *SBU Report* **127**. Swedish Council of Technology Assessment in Health Care, Stockholm.)

the proximal femur, and of the vertebrae (**2.5**). These sites are predominantly trabecular bone. The incidence rates of proximal humeral, rib, clavicle, and scapula also rise with

2.4 Incidence of fractures in the UK. (Adapted from Donaldson LJ, *et al.* (1990). Incidence of fractures in a geographically defined population. *J Epidemiol Community Health* **44**(3):241–245.)

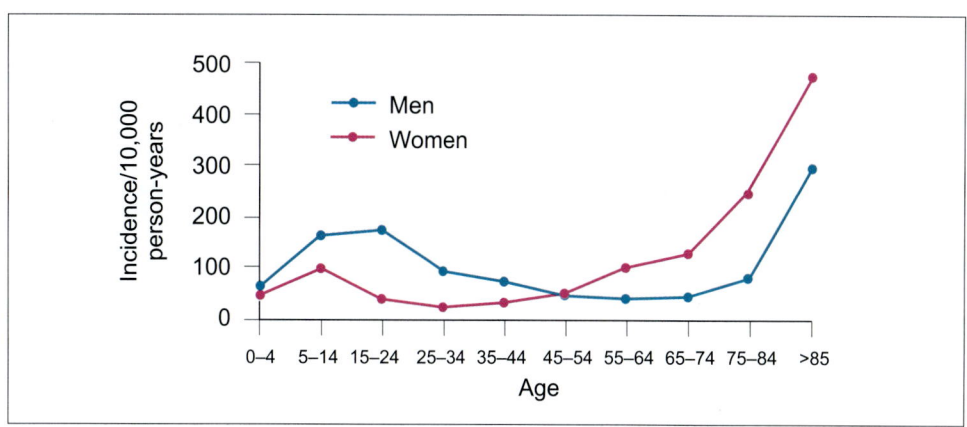

2.5 Incidence of the major age-related fractures in men and women. (Adapted from Cooper C, Melton LJ (1992). Epidemiology of osteoporosis. *Trends Endocrinol Metab* **314**:224–229.)

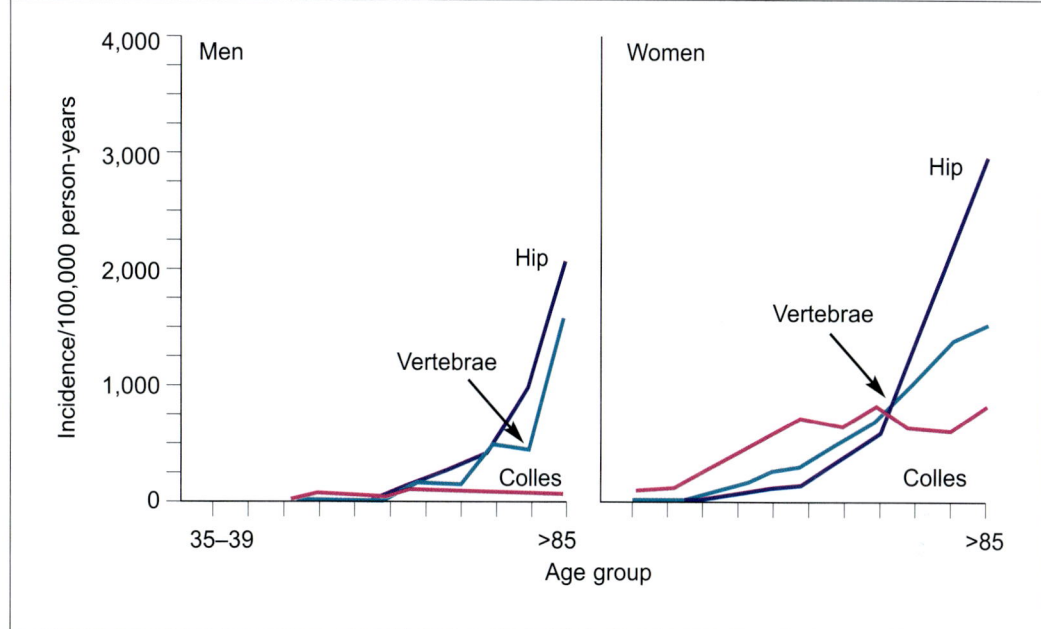

age and are greater in women than in men. About 80% of proximal humeral fractures occur in individuals aged 35 years and over, three-quarters occurring in women.

Vertebral fractures

The incidence and prevalence of radiological vertebral deformities increase with age. One in eight men and women over 50 years in Europe are estimated as having vertebral deformity from a large epidemiological study conducted across 18 European countries[6]. Vertebral deformity is describing a radiological finding (see Chapter 1) and it is not possible to say with certainty when and how it arose. This term is used in epidemiological studies. If it appears that the deformity is related to a fracture, then that term is used.

Vertebral deformities are more prevalent in males than females aged 50–59 years and there is a less dramatic age-related increase in males which is seen from 70 years (**2.6**).

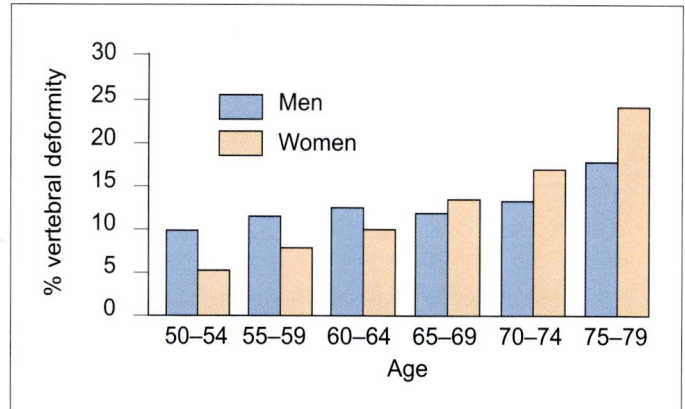

2.6 Age distribution of vertebral fractures. (Adapted from O'Neill TW, *et al.* (1996). The prevalence of vertebral deformity in European men and women: the European Vertebral Osteoporosis Study. *J Bone Mineral Res* **11**(7):1010–1018.)

It is likely that many vertebral deformities in younger men are developmental and have occurred during growth and that they do not represent fractures. The prevalence of vertebral deformities increases in females from age 50 years. The number of vertebral deformities present in any individual also increases with age. These age-related vertebral deformities most likely represent fractures and relate to osteoporosis. The majority of vertebral fractures result of compressive loading associated with activities such as lifting or changing positions, but can also be discovered incidentally. Only one-third of new vertebral fractures relates to falls.

The prevalence of vertebral fracture varies between populations with a demonstrated threefold difference across Europe and up to twofold difference within European countries in the European Vertebral Osteoporosis Study (EVOS)[6]. It is difficult to know the true incidence of vertebral fractures as only one-third present clinically. A prospective radiological study in Europe of men and women aged 50–79 years found an age-adjusted incidence of vertebral deformities of 1% per year among women and 0.6% per year among men[7].

Distal forearm fracture

Most distal forearm fractures (see Chapter 1) occur in women, the age-adjusted female to male ratio being 4:1 (**2.7**). There is a rapid rise in incidence after the menopause which plateaus at about 65 years, but overall around 50% occur in women aged 65 years and older. At 75 years, almost 20% of women have sustained a distal forearm fracture[4]. The incidence in men changes little between 20 and 80 years. A multicentre study in the UK found annual incidences of 9 and 37 per 10,000 men and women over 35 years respectively[8].

Hip fracture

The incidence of hip fractures increases exponentially with age (**2.8**). Ninety percent occur in people over 50 years of age and the average age of sustaining a hip fracture in developed countries is 80 years. The estimated rates in westernized countries are 33/100,000 person-years in women aged aged 50–54 years, rising to over 1808/100,000 person-years in women 80 years and older, with rates in men of 28 and almost 900, respectively[9] (*Table 2.1*). However, the female preponderance of hip fractures is not common to all populations. The age-specific incidence varies between countries (**2.9**). Worldwide, there were estimated to be 1.31

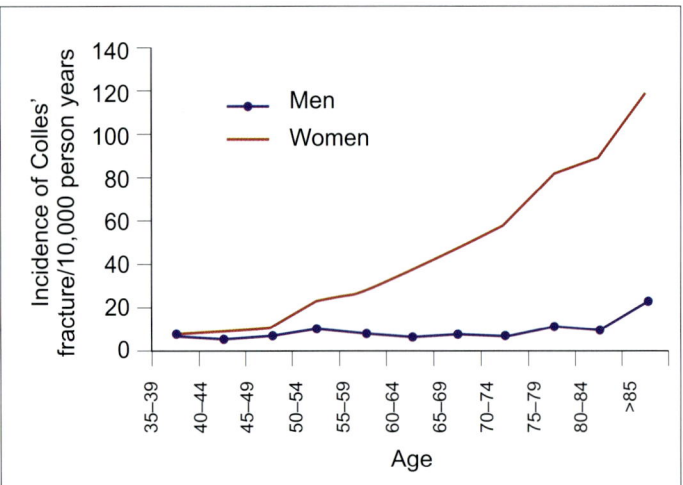

2.7 Age distribution of distal forearm fractures. (Adapted from O'Neill TW, *et al.* (2001). Incidence of distal forearm fracture in British men and women. *Osteoporos Int* **12**(7):555–558.)

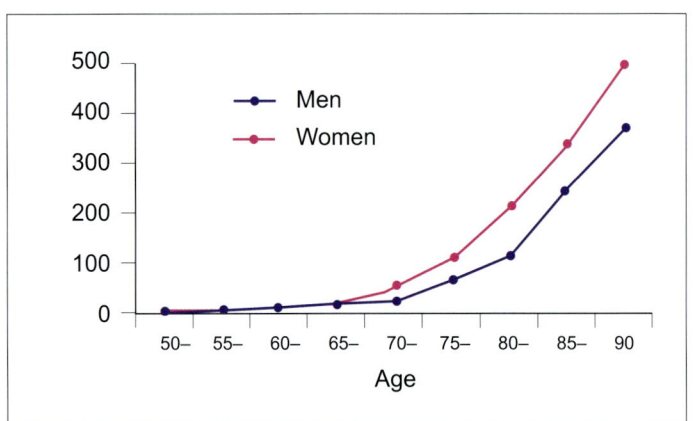

2.8 Age distribution of hip fractures. (Adapted from Rogmark C, *et al.* (1999). Incidence of hip fractures in Malmö, Sweden, 1992–1995. A trend-break. *Acta Orthop Scand* **70**(1):19–22.)

million hip fractures in 1990, about 909,000 in women and 405,000 in men[10]. Fracture rates vary in different countries (*Table 2.1*), being highest in North America and Europe, particularly in Scandinavia. The risk of osteoporotic fractures is lower in nonwhite than white populations. Incidence rates are extremely low in African countries and intermediate among Asian populations. Rates vary in regions and in Asia the rates for hip facture are twofold higher in Hong Kong than in Korea, with intermediate are reported from Malaysia, Thailand, and mainland China.

Table 2.1 Incidence of hip fracture (rates/100,000) in 1990 by age, sex, and region

| | Men: age (years) | | | | | | | Women: age (years) | | | | | | |
Region	50–54	55–59	60–64	65–69	70–74	75–79	80+	50–54	55–59	60–64	65–69	70–74	75–79	80+
W. Europe	28	33	67	103	203	331	880	33	54	115	184	362	657	1808
S. Europe	10	16	34	55	81	190	534	11	21	47	100	170	380	1075
E. Europe	38	38	88	88	194	194	475	58	58	155	155	426	426	1251
N. Europe	58	66	97	198	382	682	1864	74	78	190	327	612	1294	2997
N. America	33	33	81	123	119	338	1230	60	60	117	252	437	850	2296
Oceania	20	34	63	92	180	445	1157	31	63	112	204	358	899	2476
Asia	19.5	19.5	36.5	46.5	102	150	364	14	14	38	74.5	155.5	252	562.5
Africa	6	10	14	27	8	0	116	4	12	17	12	16	50	80
Latin America	25	40	40	106	106	327	327	19.5	50	50	162.5	162.5	622	622
World	22.5	24.5	47.3	68.7	119.1	219.4	630.2	23.9	28.4	69.1	121.6	239.8	457.7	1289.3

(Adapted from Gullberg B *et al.* (1997). Worldwide projections for hip fracture. *Osteoporos Int* **7**:407–413.)

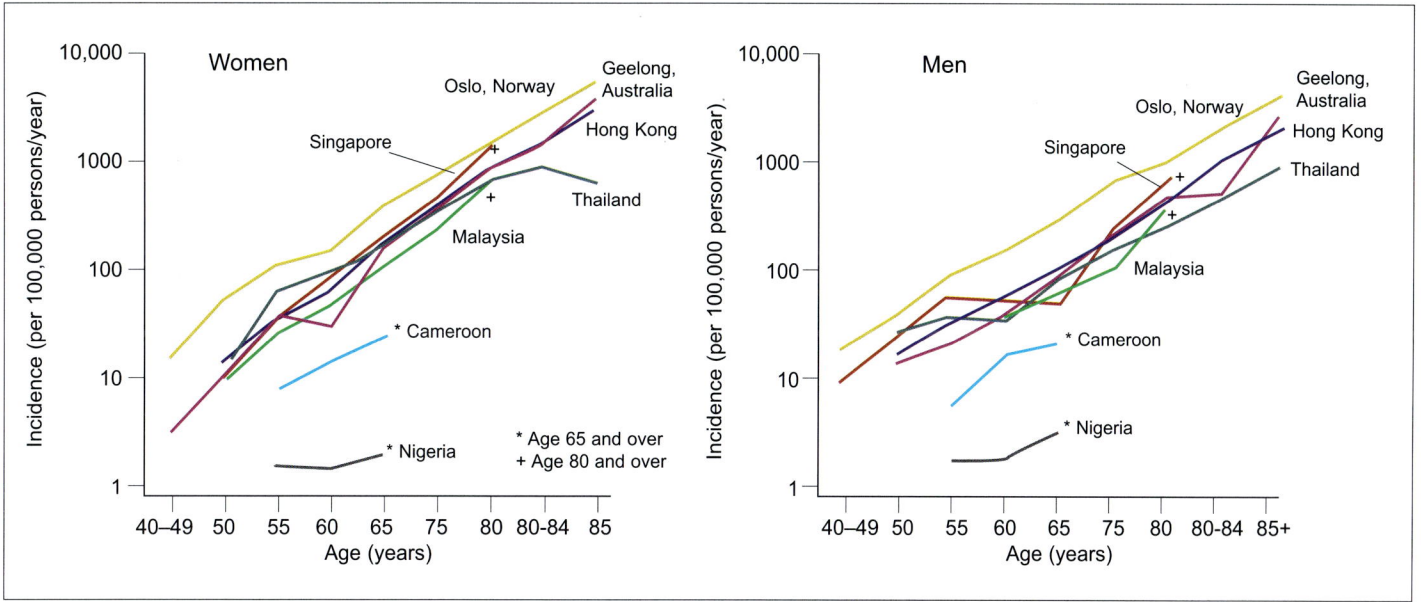

2.9 The age-specific incidence of hip fractures in different countries. (Adapted from Zebaze RM, Seeman E (2003). Epidemiology of hip and wrist fractures in Cameroon, Africa. *Osteoporos Int* **14**(4):301–305.)

Other fractures

Fractures are more common with ageing at other sites, in particular the proximal humerus and pelvis. Fractures of the humerus are estimated to account for approximately 8% of all fractures sustained by adults[11] and, in persons over 40 years of age, three-quarters of these are of the proximal humerus[12]. Data suggest that fracture of the proximal humerus is the third most common fracture over age 65[11,13]. Fractures of the proximal humerus have shown a similar pattern of increase with age as other common fragility fractures[11] in both men and women, with women being somewhat older at the time of fracture, average around 70–74 years versus 65 years in men[13]. Pelvic fractures account for approximately 2% of all adult fractures[11]. Pelvic fractures in the elderly occur from minor trauma or from skeletal insufficiency. The majority of patients are women (up to 80%) and above the age of 80 years.

The lifetime risk of fracture is considerable. For a man or woman aged 50 years in the UK, the future lifetime risk of fracture is 20.7% and 53.2% respectively (*Table 2.2*)[11]. The lifetime risk of fractures from age 50 years of the forearm is 16.6% in women and 2.9% in men, whereas of the hip is 11.4% in women and 3.1% in men[11]. The risk of future fracture can also be expressed as a 10-year probability[11] (*Table 2.3*), which has the advantage that it is an expression of absolute risk over a more meaningful period to when considering possible intervention. It makes it clear that the greatest potential gain from any intervention is at older ages when the absolute risk is highest. The 10-year probability will increase with increasing relative risk[14] (*Table 2.4*). As a consequence, there is most to gain by treating older women with risk factors that increase the probability of them sustaining a fracture. Interventions then become cost-effective.

Table 2.2 Estimated lifetime risks of fractures (%) in the UK at various ages

Current age (years)	Any fractures	Radius/ulna	Femur/hip	Vertebra
Women				
50	53.2	16.6	11.4	3.1
60	45.5	14.0	11.6	2.9
70	36.9	10.4	12.1	2.6
80	28.6	6.9	12.3	1.9
Men				
50	20.7	2.9	3.1	1.2
60	14.7	2.0	3.1	1.1
70	11.4	1.4	3.3	1.0
80	9.6	1.1	3.7	0.8

(Adapted from van Staa TP, *et al.* (2001). Epidemiology of fractures in England and Wales. *Bone* **29**:517–22.)

Table 2.3 Estimated 10-year risks (%) of fractures in the UK at various ages

Current age (years)	Any fractures	Radius/ulna	Femur/hip	Vertebra
Women				
50	9.8	3.2	0.3	0.3
60	13.3	4.9	1.1	0.6
70	17.0	5.6	3.4	1.3
80	21.7	5.5	8.7	1.6
Men				
50	7.1	1.1	0.2	0.2
60	5.7	0.9	0.4	0.3
70	6.2	0.9	1.4	0.5
80	8.0	0.9	2.9	0.7

(Adapted from van Staa TP, *et al.* (2001). Epidemiology of fractures in England and Wales. *Bone* **29**:517–22.)

Table 2.4 Probability of fracture during the next 10 years in men and women from Sweden (according to age and risk relative to the average population)

Age (years)	Relative risk hip, clinical spine, humeral, or Colles' fracture	50	60	70	80
		10-year probability of fracture (%)			
Men	1	3.3	4.7	7.0	12.6
	2	6.5	9.1	13.5	23.1
	3	9.6	13.3	19.4	13.9
	4	12.6	17.3	24.9	39.3
Women	1	5.8	9.6	16.1	21.5
	2	11.3	18.2	29.4	37.4
	3	16.5	26.0	40.0	49.2
	4	21.4	33.1	49.5	58.1

(Adapted from Kanis JA, *et al.* (2002). Ten-year risk of osteoporotic fracture and the effect of risk factors on screening strategies. *Bone* **30**:251–58.)

Epidemiology of fracture – future trends

The number of hip fractures is increasing throughout the world. From an estimated 1.26 million in 1990, the projected number is 2.6 million by 2025 and 4.5 million worldwide by 2050[9]. It is estimated that the percentage increase will be greater in men (310%) than women (240%). The increase will be in Europe (**2.10**) and all populations across the globe (**2.11**). The predicted increases in hip fractures in westernized populations is because of increased survival and growing numbers of very elderly who will be inherently at greater risk of fracture. However, it is predicted that there will be most dramatic changes in Asian populations in particular, and it has been estimated that from 26% of all hip fractures occurring in Asia in 1990, that this will rise to 37% in 2025 and to 45% in 2050. This is already being seen in the more urbanized countries of Singapore and Hong Kong where age-adjusted hip fracture rates have been found to be similar to those in white Americans, whereas much lower rates were found in Malaysia and Thailand[15]. Other osteoporotic fractures are also predicted to increase. This is because of the increase in populations and predicted dramatic improvements in life expectancy in less developed countries, as well as changes in lifestyles that will increase individual risk of fracture. People are becoming less physically active and changes in transportation increase the risks of trauma.

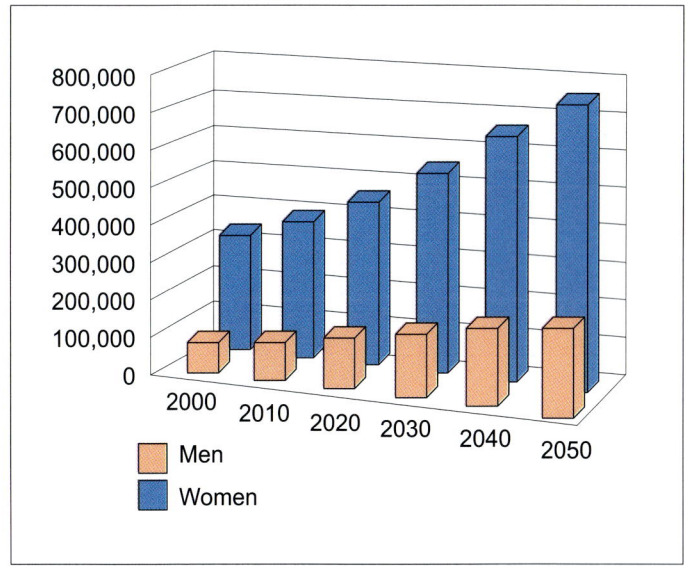

2.10 Projected number of yearly incident fractures in the European Community member states. (Adapted from European Communities (1998). *Report on Osteoporosis in the European Community: action for prevention.* European Communities, Luxembourg.)

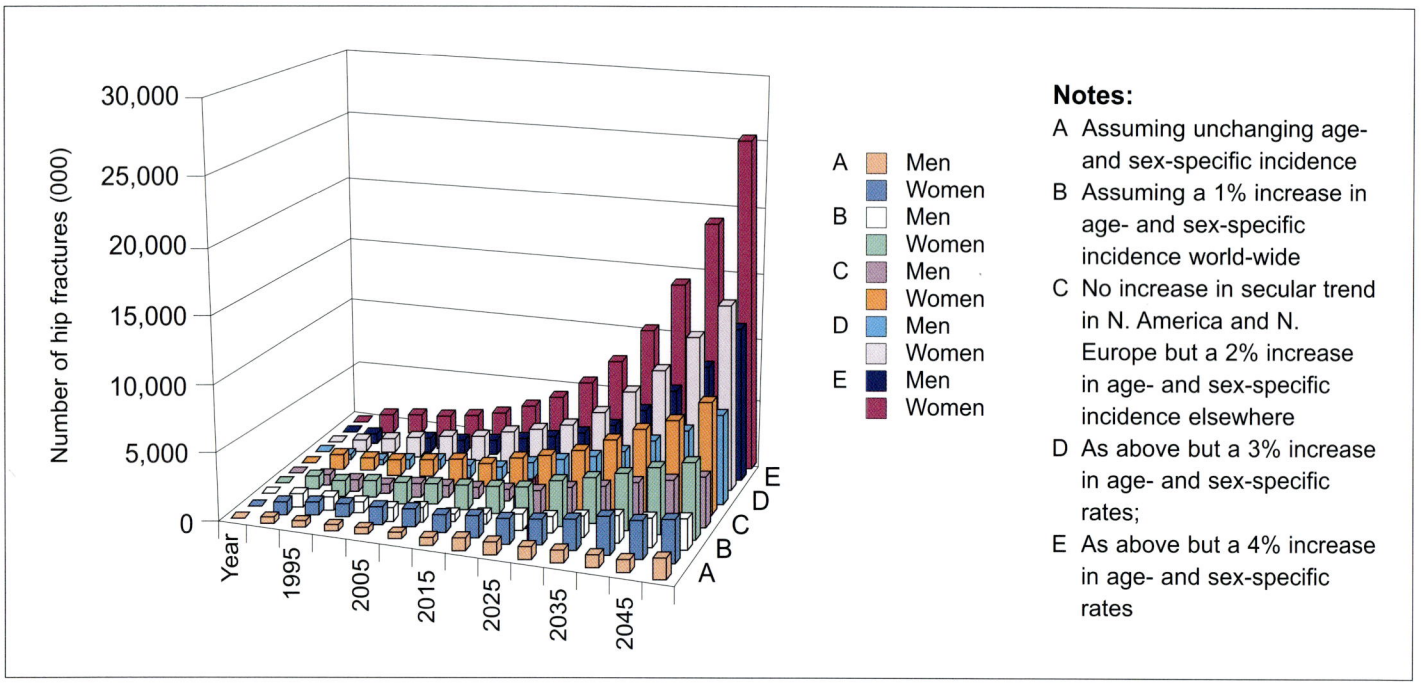

Notes:

A Assuming unchanging age- and sex-specific incidence

B Assuming a 1% increase in age- and sex-specific incidence world-wide

C No increase in secular trend in N. America and N. Europe but a 2% increase in age- and sex-specific incidence elsewhere

D As above but a 3% increase in age- and sex-specific rates;

E As above but a 4% increase in age- and sex-specific rates

2.11 Worldwide forecasts for hip fracture, 2050. (Adapted from Gullberg B, *et al.* (1997). Worldwide projections for hip fracture. *Osteoporos Int* **7**(5):407–413.)

Outcome after fracture – function, mortality

The clinical manifestation of osteoporosis is fracture following low-energy trauma, such as a fall from a standing height. Fracture of a long bone will result in pain and loss of mobility of the limb. Vertebral fracture presents acutely with pain in about one-third of cases. As a consequence, function is lost, activities are limited. and participation is restricted. The person may become isolated and also fearful of falling and sustaining another fracture, of which they are at increased risk.

The impact of osteoporosis and fracture can be represented in terms of the WHO International Classification of Functioning (**2.12**). This is a valuable model to evaluate the outcomes of osteoporosis and fracture. At the clinicopathological end of this classification, osteoporosis is characterized by loss of bone mass and architecture, and a fracture results in loss of integrity of the skeleton with pain. For the individual, a fracture not only results in pain and loss of function of that limb or structure,

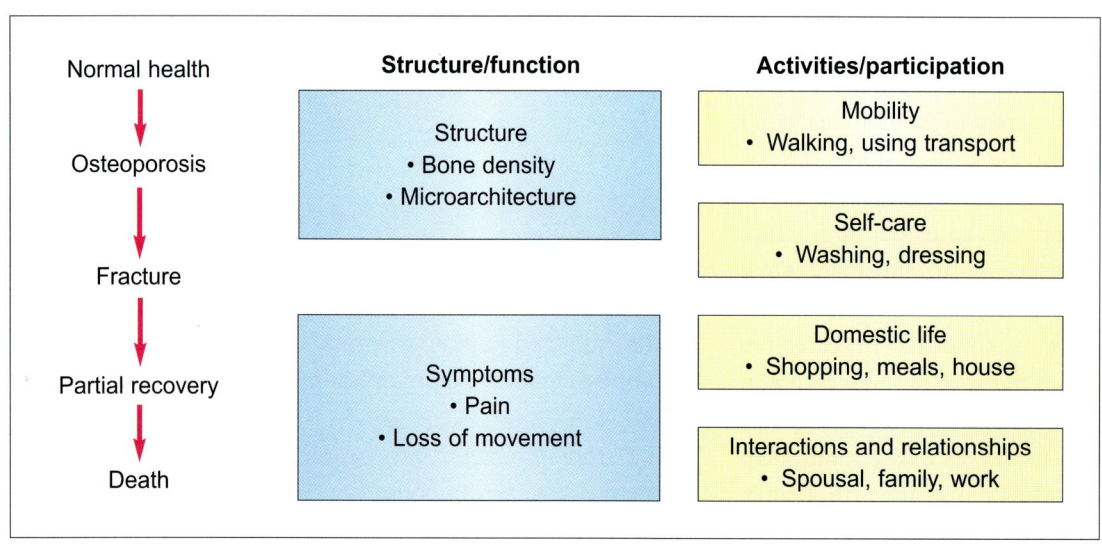

2.12 Impact of osteoporosis in terms of the WHO International Classification of Functioning.

2.13 Vertebral fractures and quality of life. (Adapted from Hall SE, *et al.* (1999). A case-control study of quality of life and functional impairment in women with long-standing vertebral osteoporotic fracture. *Osteoporos Int* **9**(6):508–515.)

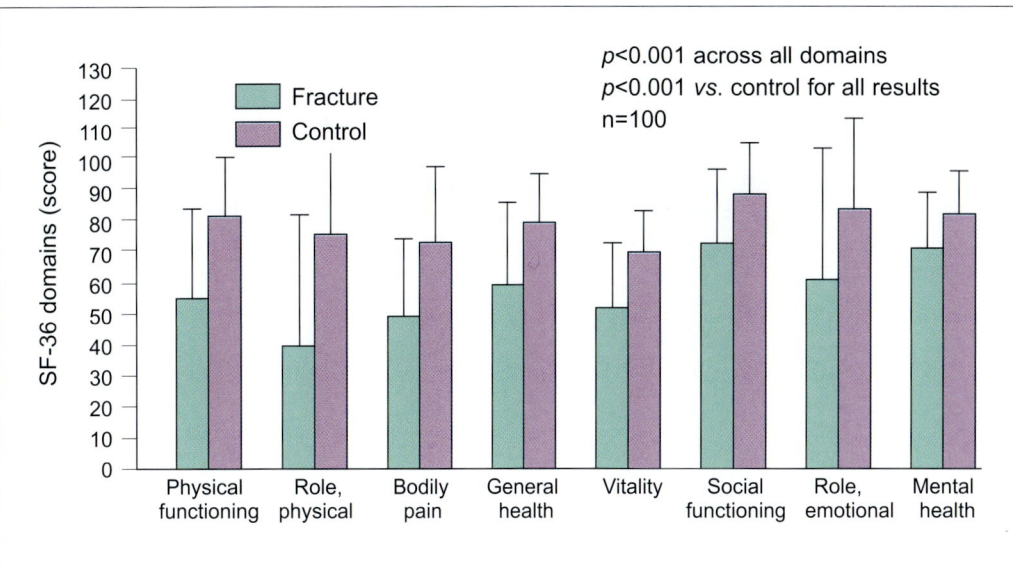

but will result in limitation of a wide range of activities, such as walking, and this will restrict their participation within society such as going out with friends. These physical difficulties associated with osteoporosis result in increased dependence and the enormous indirect costs of the condition. Many fractures result in hospitalization, but this will depend not only on the severity of the fracture and the impact on the individual but also on the local system of healthcare and social support.

Vertebral fractures

Vertebral fracture is associated with acute back pain in only one-third of fractures, but new vertebral fractures, including those that do not come to immediate clinical attention, are associated with clinically important increases in back pain and functional limitations (**2.13**).

Each additional new fracture is associated with further pain and limitation of activities with restriction of participation. The pain associated with an acute fracture can be severe for a couple of weeks and up to one-fifth are hospitalized and some will require subsequent long-term care. Fractures of the lower thoracic and upper lumbar spine are associated with more pain. Pain and disability worsen with each new vertebral fracture, with an increasing total number of vertebral fractures and with worsening of spinal deformity (**2.14**).

With increasing number of vertebral deformities there is loss of height and kyphosis (**2.15**). The abdomen becomes protuberant with increased skin folds and often intertrigo (**2.16**). The ribs may painfully impinge on the pelvic brim when stooping. There may be reflux oesophagitis and stress

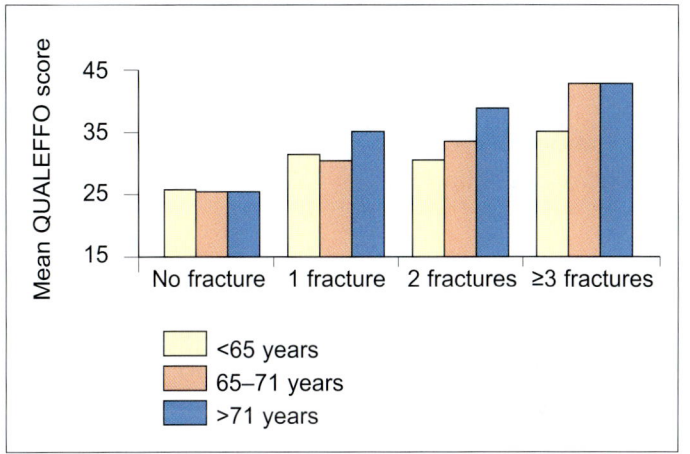

2.14 Impact of age and number of vertebral fractures. (Adapted from Oleksik A, *et al.* (2000). Health-related quality of life in postmenopausal women with low BMD with or without prevalent vertebral fractures. *J Bone Mineral Res* **15**(7):1384–1392.)

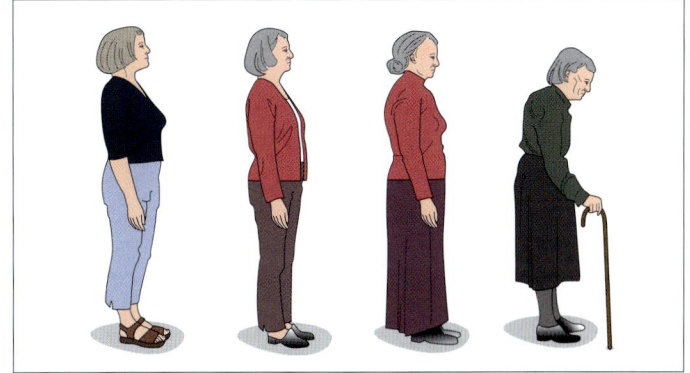

2.15 Progressive loss of height associated with vertebral deformities.

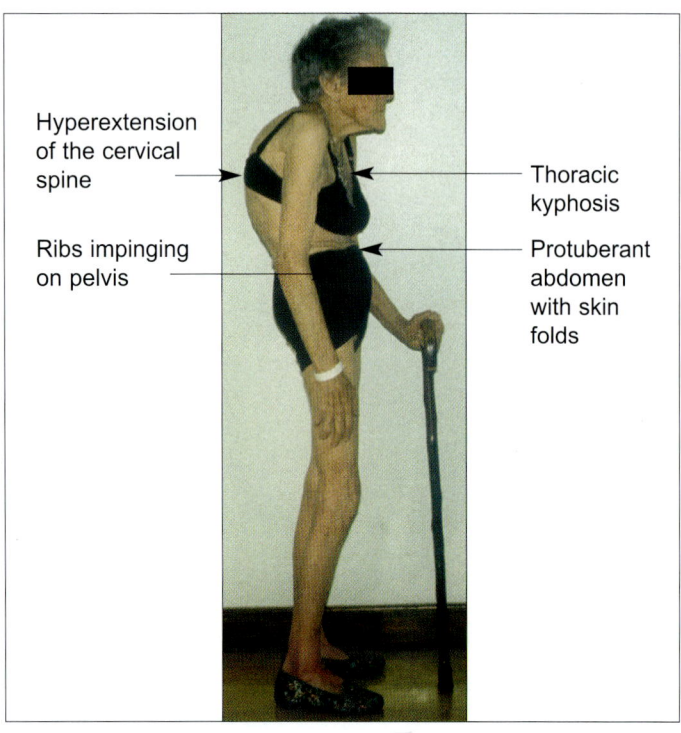

2.16 The clinical problems associated with vertebral osteoporosis and fracture.

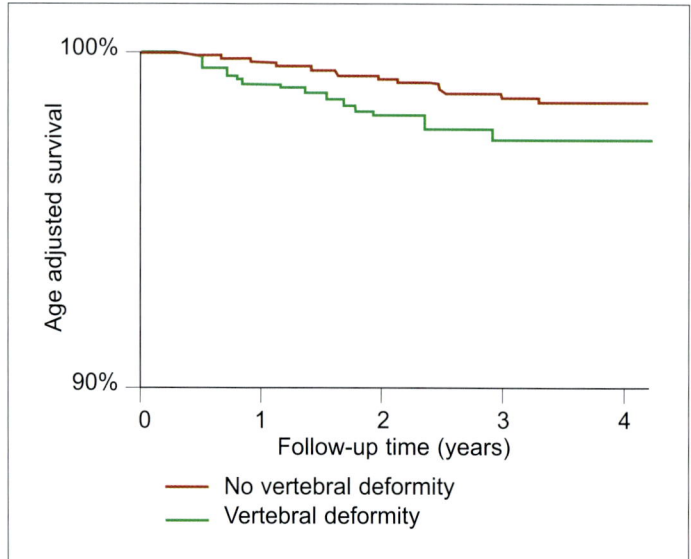

2.17 There is an increased mortality associated with vertebral deformities. Age-adjusted Kaplan Meier survival curves in women. (Adapted from Ismail AA, *et al.* (1998). Mortality associated with vertebral deformity in men and women: results from the European Prospective Osteoporosis Study (EPOS). *Osteoporos Int* 8(3):291–297.)

incontinence. All aspects of quality of life are affected and this is not just related to pain. Comorbidity is common at this advanced age and contributes to the impact on quality of life. Vertebral fractures are also associated with a gradual increase in mortality (**2.17**), in contrast to hip fractures in which the excess mortality is greatest shortly after the fracture. This increasing mortality associated with vertebral fractures may in fact be explained by confounders that relate independently to bone density and to mortality, in particular advanced age, comorbidities, and general frailty.

Distal forearm fracture

Fracture of the distal forearm can have a major effect on what the person can do (*Table 2.5*). In a survey in the UK, one in five men and women were admitted to hospital, more often men than women (23.4% *vs.* 18.6%). Below age 50 years, 22.6% of those with fracture required admission. Above 50 years the proportion admitted rose gradually with age: 14.5% at age 50–59 years, 15.9% at age 60–69 years, 17.6% at age 70–79 years, and 26% at age 80 years and over[8]. Many do not return to their prefracture status, with long-term limitation of function and some develop algodystrophy (reflex sympathetic dystrophy).

Hip fracture

The average age of sustaining a hip fracture is 80 years in western Europe, and many are frail with comorbidities. The hip fracture results in pain, loss of mobility, and excess mortality (**2.18**). Nearly all are hospitalized, and most

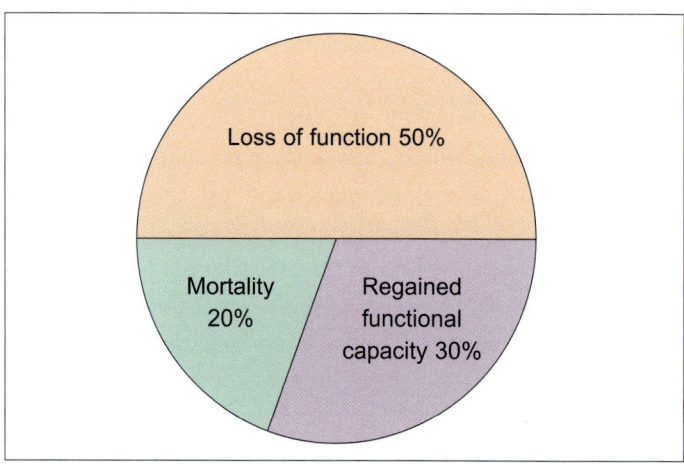

2.18 Outcome after hip fracture at 1 year. (Adapted from Sernbo I, Johnell O (1993). Consequences of a hip fracture: a prospective study over 1 year. *Osteoporos Int* 3(3):148–153.)

Table 2.5 Distal forearm fractures (Colles)

- 20% hospitalized
- Require 4–6 weeks in plaster
- Impaired function
- Algodystrophy

undergo surgical repair of the fracture or replacement of the joint. At 1 year, hip fracture is associated with 50% loss of function and only 30% have regained function[16]. Many lose their independence and require long-term care. Increasing age and comorbidity are important contributory factors to the occurrence of hip fractures and are determinants of outcome. The outcome is worse for those already in care when they sustain a fracture, but many of those who do return to their own homes do not return to their prefracture lifestyle.

One-year mortality has been found to be up to 40% in various studies. Excess mortality is greatest in the first 6 months (**2.19**), and in younger people[17]. Mortality is greater for those with coexisting illnesses and poor prefracture functional status. Major causes of death are pneumonia, pulmonary embolism, stroke, myocardial infarct, and cardiac failure.

Other fractures

Proximal humerus fractures mainly occur in people who are relatively fit. The immediate problems arise from the shoulder pain and restricted movement. Pain normally begins to subside after 2–4 weeks, but rehabilitation after a proximal humerus fracture often exceeds 3 months of training. The short- and long-term functional outcome is related to both fracture-related and patient-related factors. Age at the time of fracture, prefracture health, and functional status and the displacement of the fracture affect the functional outcome. Clinical status at 1 year is predictive of long-term outcome. More than half report some shoulder pain and functional limitation up to 13 years after fracture[18]. Comorbidities significantly affect the results regardless of fracture type. Fracture of the proximal humerus is also associated with increased mortality, most pronounced in men and during the 3 first years after fracture, with cardiovascular disease and malignancy being the commonest causes of death.

Older people sustaining pelvic fractures commonly have comorbidities and are frail. The prefracture functional status has implications for outcome. However, as previously noted, estimates of effect on dependency are related to the structure of health and social care and are not exactly comparable. In the study from the UK, up to 21 % of the patients were institutionalized prior to fracture[19], whereas the majority were living independently in the studies from France and the USA. At discharge, only half of the patients

2.19 Mortality following hip fracture is increased at all ages. This is greatest with the elderly, but the excess mortality is in younger people. There is a steep decrease in mortality in the first 6 months following the fracture. After reaching a nadir, mortality increases at a rate greater than that of the general population. (Adapted from Kanis JA, *et al.* (2003). The components of excess mortality after hip fracture. *Bone* **32**(5):468–473.)

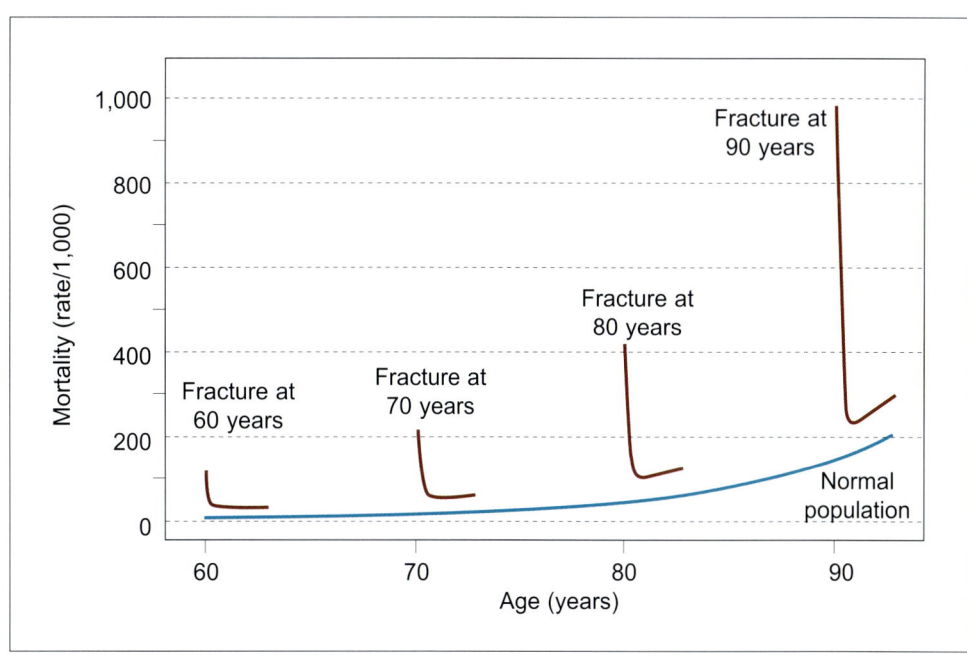

had regained self-sufficiency[20] and half had been transferred to care homes[19]. Most patients with pelvic fracture require hospitalization. In addition, a number of complicating conditions are common during and after hospitalization due to the frailty of many of the patients. Many do not regain their functional status. The 1-year mortality has been reported to be almost 30%.

Economic impact

The socio-economic impact of osteoporosis relates to fracture (**2.20**). Many fractures will result in hospitalization and surgery, and management is often complicated by intercurrent problems related to comorbidity. Many who sustain fractures are elderly with multiple health problems. Rehabilitation may therefore be prolonged. In the long term, many have limitation of activities and restricted participation, with the need for care and support from carers and from social services. Some require residential care, usually those who were only just coping independently before the fracture. Only about half of those people who sustain a hip fracture are discharged home as many require long-term rehabilitation or long-stay residential care after discharge from the acute hospital. Such acute and long-term needs account for the high direct and indirect costs associated with osteoporosis. In Sweden, the acute hospital costs of osteoporotic fractures were higher than for myocardial infarction, breast cancer, and prostate cancer combined[21]. However, the indirect costs related to support in the community are greater than the direct costs, although

these are more difficult to quantify. Additional costs may relate to the loss of support that the person who sustained the fracture had previously given others living with them. Loss of work productivity is usually not important because of the age at which most disabling osteoporotic fractures occur, although carers may be affected.

These costs have been estimated in various countries (*Tables 2.6, 2.7*). The costs related to hip fracture are best documented. Such costings do not often include the costs of therapies and the indirect costs are always difficult to estimate. Osteoporosis clearly has an enormous direct cost to health systems which will increase with the ageing of the population in all parts of the globe.

Hip fracture

Hip fractures are the most costly due to hospitalization, rehabilitation, and the large number needing long-term care and support. They are the most frequent cause of hospital admission due to fracture, accounting for over 60% in men and 70% in women and they account for about 70% of hospital-bed days due to fracture in Sweden[21]. In Canada, the cost of hip fracture has been estimated at US$22,292 during the first year, 58% related to the initial hospitalization and inpatient rehabilitation, but there was a wide variation depending on age and care setting before and after the fracture[22]. Hospital stays increase with age. Hip fractures in women are associated with the longest stays in hospital and only about 50% are discharged home.

Estimates of total cost of hip fractures in the USA have ranged from $24,000 to $33,500 (1995 $)[23]. In the UK, hip fractures were the most expensive, comprising 87% of the

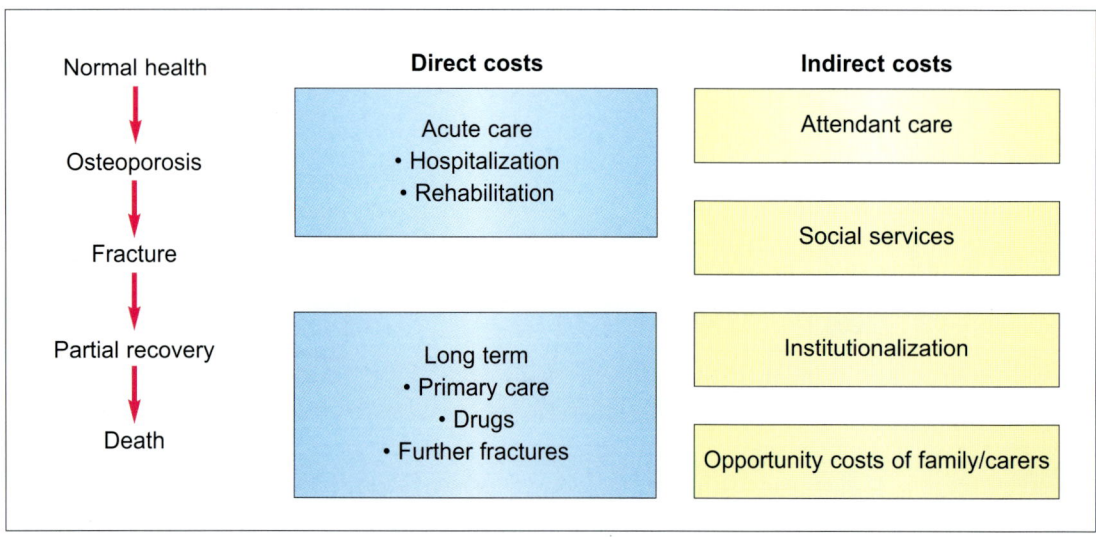

2.20 A model of the costs of osteoporosis and fracture at the different stages.

Table 2.6 The direct and indirect costs of osteoporotic fractures in the UK

Fracture type	Acute costs per patient (£)	Social care & long-stay costs per patient (£)	Follow-up costs per patient (£)	Drug costs per patient (£)	Total cost per fracture (£)
Hip	4808	7152	164	0	12,124
Wrist	368	0	100	0	468
Vertebra	96	0	321	62	479
Other	1200	0	138	0	1338

(Adapted from Dolan P, Torgerson DJ (1998). The cost of treating osteoporotic fractures in the United Kingdom female population. *Osteoporos Int* **8**:611–617.)

Table 2.7 Healthcare expenditures for the treatment of osteoporotic fractures in the United States in 1995

Type of service (millions $US)	Inpatient hospital	Emergency room	Outpatient doctor	Outpatient hospital	Other outpatient costs*	Nursing home	Total
Type of fracture							
Hip	5576	130	67	9	90	2811	8682
Other sites	3018	437	403	56	104	1064	5082
Forearm	183	55	93	8	4	41	385
Spine	575	20	13	3	10	126	746
All other sites	2259	362	297	45	91	899	3953
Total	8594	567	470	65	194	3875	13,764

*Includes healthcare, ambulance services, and medical equipment.

(Adapted from Ray NF, *et al.* (1997). Medical expenditures for the treatment of osteoporotic fractures in the United States in 1995: report from the National Osteoporosis Foundation. *J Bone Mineral Res* **12**:24–35.)

total costs of osteoporotic fractures in women, and 60% of their cost is indirect due to the need by many of long-term hospital and community care[24]. The acute hospital cost of a hip fracture was estimated at £4,808 in 1998 with a total cost per fracture at £12,124[24]. In the European Community, the total hospital costs of hip fracture in 1998 were estimated to be over 3.5 billion Euros, with estimated total care costs of over 9 billion Euros[25].

Distal forearm fracture
Direct costs of distal forearm fractures are less but they were the next most frequent fracture sustained by women after hip fracture to result in hospital admission in Sweden[21]. There are significant costs as one in five men and women who had sustained a distal forearm fracture were admitted to hospital in a UK study[8], with the proportion requiring admission increasing with age. The estimated average health care costs per fracture were estimated at £468 in the UK in 1998[24], with similar estimates in other countries.

Vertebral fracture
Vertebral fractures only present acutely in about one-third of cases, but were responsible for almost 70,000 hospital admissions in 1997 in the USA Nationwide Inpatient Sample, about one-quarter of the number due primarily to hip fracture. It is estimated that less than 10% require hospital admission. In Sweden, vertebral fractures were the third most frequent fracture in women and second most

frequent in men that resulted in admission in those over 50 years of age[21]. Hospitalization rates increase with age and comorbidity. There is a lack of data about costs of vertebral fractures and much depends on admission rates, but the total health care costs have been estimated at $1,200 per patient in 1997[26].

Risk factors for osteoporosis and for fracture

Some people are more at risk than others of becoming osteoporotic and sustaining a low-energy fracture. The determinants of this relate to the aetiology of osteoporosis and fracture (1.5–1.7). Determinants of bone strength, falls, and impact of falls are all important. Many of these determinants, or 'risk factors' which have been identified in epidemiological studies, may work in several ways (2.21); age is associated with reduced bone mass, changes in architecture, reduced bone turnover, increased risk of falling, and increased impact of a fall.

Risk factors are clinically important in identifying who is most likely to sustain a future fracture. Combinations of risk

Bone related / **Fall related**

Bone related		Fall related
• Bone mass	• Genetics	• Neuromuscular
• Geometry	• Maternal hip	• Cognitive
• Turnover	fracture	• Vision
• Architecture	• Previous	• Drugs
	fracture	
	• Weight	
	• Mobility	
	• Smoking	

2.21 Determinants of fracture may variably relate to bone mass, falls, or increase fracture risk for other reasons.

Table 2.8 Risk factors for osteoporosis and fracture

- Age
- Female
- Previous fracture after low-energy trauma
- Radiographic evidence of osteopenia, vertebral deformity, or both
- Loss of height, thoracic kyphosis (after radiographic confirmation of vertebral deformities)
- Low body weight (body mass index <19)
- Treatment with corticosteroids
- Family history of fractures owing to osteoporosis (maternal hip fracture)
- Reduced lifetime exposure to oestrogen (primary or secondary amenorrhoea, early natural or surgical menopause (<45 years))
- Disorders associated with osteoporosis (previous low bodyweight; rheumatoid arthritis; malabsorption syndromes, including chronic liver disease and inflammatory bowel disease; primary hyperparathyroidism; long term immobilization)
- Behavioural risk factors:
  – Low calcium intake (<700 mg/d)
  – Physical inactivity
  – Vitamin D deficiency (low exposure to sunlight)
  – Smoking (current)
  – Excessive alcohol consumption

(Adapted from Woolf AD, Akesson K (2003). Preventing fractures in elderly people. *BMJ* **327**(7406):89–95.)

Table 2.9 Risk factors for falls

Intrinsic factors
- General deterioration associated with ageing
- Problems with balance, gait, or mobility
- Visual impairment
- Impaired cognition or depression
- 'Blackouts'

Extrinsic factors
- Personal hazards: inappropriate footwear or clothing
- Multiple drug therapy: sedatives, hypotensive drugs

Environmental factors
- Hazards indoors or at home: bad lighting, steep stairs, lack of grab rails, slippery floors, loose rugs, pets, grandchildren's toys, cords for telephone and electrical appliances
- Hazards outdoors: uneven pavements, streets, paths, lack of safety equipment, snowy and icy conditions, traffic and public transportation

(Adapted from Woolf AD, Akesson K (2003). Preventing fractures in elderly people. *BMJ* **327**(7406):89–95.)

factors are more sensitive and are being used as indications for bone densitometry, to predict 10-year probability of fracture and to identify who will benefit most from an intervention. In addition, some risk factors are modifiable and will themselves be the target of the intervention, such as increased risk of falling due to osteoarthritis of the knee. Although it is not always clear whether the effect of the risk factor is through falling or bone strength, such as a previous history of fracture, it is useful to try to separate them out when planning how to prevent fracture in that individual. The risk factors that will help identify those at risk of osteoporosis and fracture or at risk of falling are given in *Tables 2.8* and *2.9*. The major risk factors of fracture are age, female gender, falling, low bone mass, and previous low-trauma fracture. There is an interaction between risk factors of fracture, and the presence of multiple factors in various combinations increases risk.

The increasing incidence of fracture with age has been already demonstrated, along with the increased incidence of fractures sustained by women compared to men. The risk of fracture increases with decreasing bone density, with an approximate twofold increased risk for each standard deviation difference in T-score. The association with fracture at any site is strongest for bone density measured at that site (*Table 2.10*). The probability of future fracture also increases independently with increasing age (*Table 2.11*, **2.22**)[27]. A women with osteoporosis (T-score -2.5) at 50 years has a probability of fracture in the next 10 years of

Table 2.10 Relative increase in risk of fracture (with 95% confidence interval) in women for each standard deviation decrease in bone mineral density below the age-adjusted mean

Site of measurement	Forearm fracture	Hip fracture	Vertebral fracture	All fractures
Distal radius	1.7 (1.4–2.0)	1.8 (1.4–2.2)	1.7 (1.4–2.1)	1.4 (1.3–1.6)
Femoral neck	1.4 (1.4–1.6)	2.6 (2.0–3.5)	1.8 (1.1–2.7)	1.6 (1.4–1.8)
Lumbar spine	1.5 (1.3–1.8)	1.6 (1.2–2.2)	1.7 (1.4–2.1)	1.5 (1.4–1.7)

(Adapted from Marshall D, *et al.* (1996). Meta-analysis of how well measures of bone mineral density predict occurrence of osteoporotic fractures. *BMJ* **312**:1254–1259.)

Table 2.11 Ten-year probability of fracture (%) at hip, spine (clinical spine fracture), proximal humerus, or distal forearm according to age and T-score at the femoral neck

Age (years)	T-score					
Women	+1	0	-1	-2	-3	-4
50	2.4	3.8	5.9	9.2	14.1	21.3
60	3.2	5.1	8.2	13.0	20.2	30.6
70	4.3	7.1	11.5	18.3	28.4	42.3
80	4.6	7.7	12.7	20.5	31.8	46.4
Men						
50	1.2	2.0	3.4	5.8	9.6	15.9
60	1.6	2.7	4.5	7.3	11.8	18.7
70	2.3	3.8	6.2	10.0	16.0	25.0
80	3.6	5.8	9.3	14.7	22.6	33.3

(Adapted from Kanis JA, *et al.* (2001). Ten-year probabilities of osteoporotic fractures according to BMD and diagnostic thresholds. *Osteoporos Int* **12**(12):989–995.)

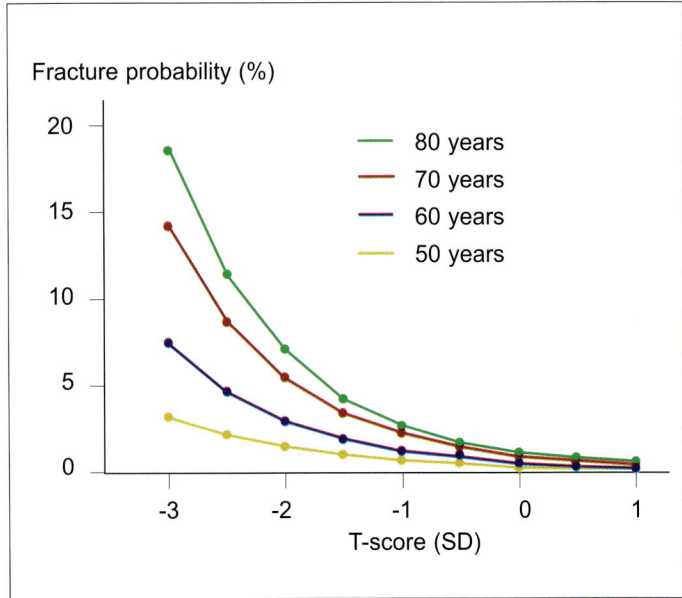

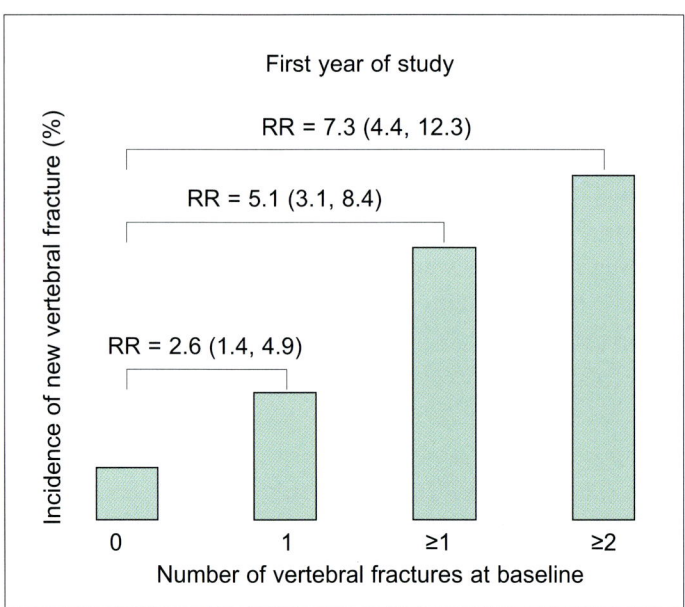

2.22 Hip bone density (T-score), age, and probability of hip fracture. For any given T-score the risk of fracture is higher with increasing age. (Adapted from Kanis JA, *et al.* (2001). Ten year probabilities of osteoporotic fractures according to BMD and diagnostic thresholds. *Osteoporos Int* **12**(12):989–995.)

2.23 Effect of prior vertebral fracture on risk of subsequent vertebral fracture (2,725 postmenopausal women randomized to placebo). (Adapted from Lindsay R, *et al.* (2001). Risk of new vertebral fracture in the year following a fracture. *JAMA* **285**(3):320–323.)

11.3%, but a 70-year-old woman with the same bone density has a 10-year probability of fracture of 22.8%, i.e. double the risk.

Previous fracture is a major risk factor for sustaining a further fracture. In a meta-analysis of several large cohorts, a previous fracture history was associated with a significantly increased risk of any fracture (relative risk [RR] 1.86, 95% confidence intervals [CI] 1.75–1.98) and hip fracture (RR 1.85, 95% CI 1.58–2.17), with low bone mass only accounting for a minority of this risk[28]. The presence of a vertebral fracture is a potent risk factor for the occurrence of future vertebral fractures, with a large prospective study[29] finding that one preexisting vertebral fracture at baseline

resulted in a 2.6-fold increase in the risk of having another fracture during the subsequent year (**2.23**). Having ≥1 or ≥2 baseline vertebral fractures increased this risk by fivefold and sevenfold, respectively. Almost 20% of women with a confirmed incident (new) fracture experienced a subsequent vertebral fracture within 1 year of the initial fracture.

Prevalent vertebral fractures also significantly increase by 2–4-fold the risk of future hip fracture, demonstrated over 3–4 years (**2.24**). Ismail *et al.* studied 6,788 women aged 50 years and over who were recruited from 31 European centers and followed for a median of 3 years. Prevalent vertebral vertebral deformities at the baseline radiograph were a strong predicitor of of incident hip fractures (RR 4.5;

Table 2.12 Fall-related factors and risk of hip fracture

Risk factors	Hip fractures/1000 women years
High fall risk + low BMD	28.5
Either high fall risk or low BMD alone	11.3
Low fall risk and low risk by BMD	5.4

BMD: bone mineral density. (Adapted from Dargent-Molina P, *et al.* (1996). Fall-related factors and risk of hip fracture: the EPIDOS prospective study. *Lancet* **348**(9021):145–149.)

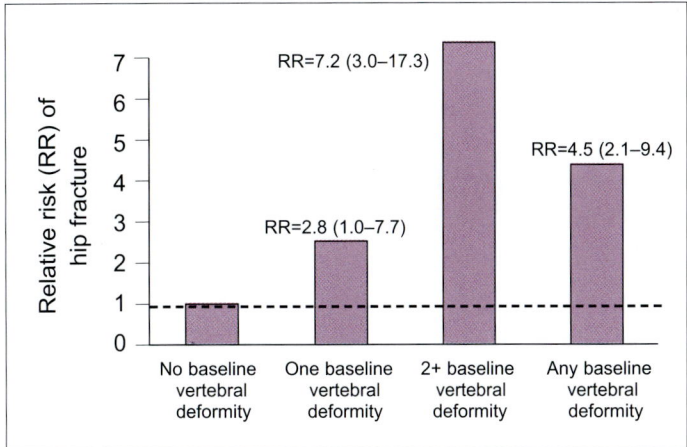

2.24 Risk of hip fracture following vertebral fracture. (Adapted from Ismail AA, *et al.* (2001). Prevalent vertebral deformity predicts incident hip though not distal forearm fracture: results from the European Prospective Osteoporosis Study. *Osteoporos Int* **12**(2):85–90.)

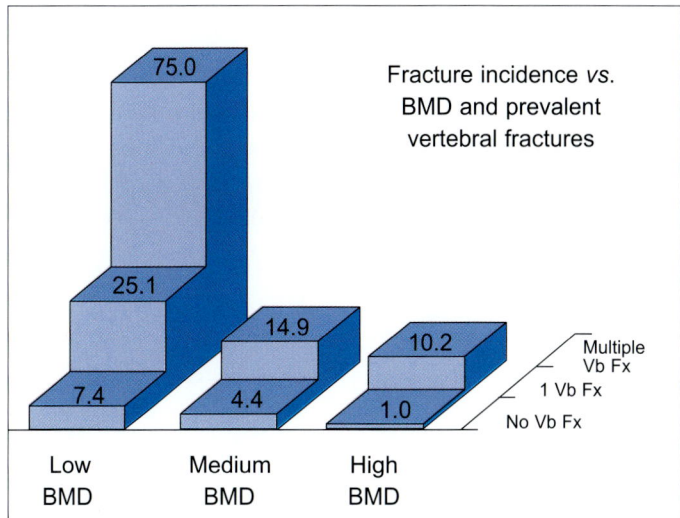

2.25 Combination of previous vertebral fracture and low bone density identifies those at most risk of subsequent fracture. (Adapted from Ross PD, *et al.* (1991). Pre-existing fractures and bone mass predict vertebral fracture incidence in women. *Ann Intern Med* **114**(11):919–923.)

2.26 Bone density and clinical risk factors in combination predict fracture: the annual risk of hip fracture according to the number of risk factors and the age-specific calcaneal bone density. (The risk factors were: age ≥80; maternal history of hip fracture; any fracture (except hip fracture) since the age of 50; fair, poor, or very poor health; previous hyperthyroidism; anticonvulsant therapy; current long-acting benzodiazepine therapy; current weight less than at the age of 25; height at the age of 25 ≥168 cm; caffeine intake more than the equivalent of two cups of coffee per day; on feet 4 hours a day; no walking for exercise; inability to rise from chair without using arms; lowest quartile (standard deviation >2.44) of depth perception; lowest quartile (0.70 unit) of contrast sensitivity; pulse rate >80 per minute). (Adapted from Cumming RG, *et al.* (1997). Calcium intake and fracture risk: results from the study of osteoporotic fractures. *Am J Epidemiol* **145**(10):926–934.)

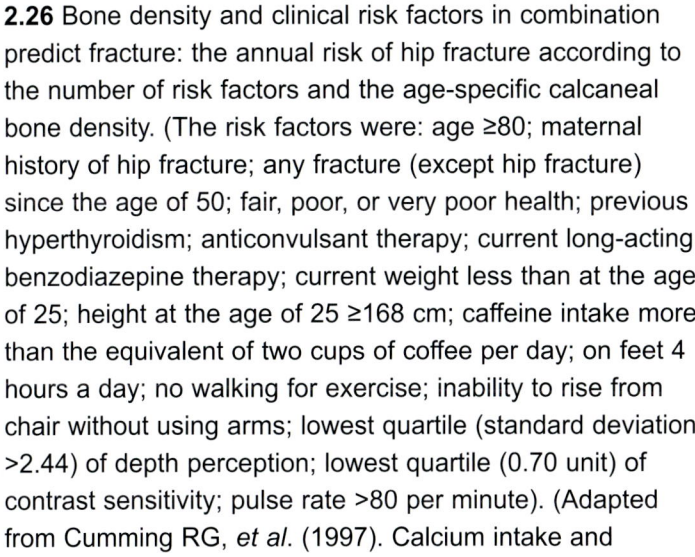

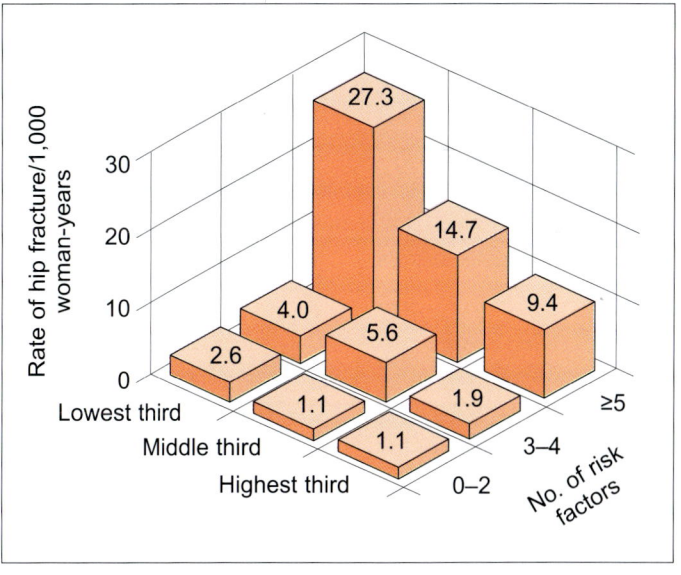

95% CI 2.1–9.4). The predictive risk increased with increasing number of prevalent deformities, particularly for subsequent hip fracture: for ≥2 deformities there was a relative risk of 7.2 (95% CI 3.0–17.3)[30]. Those at most risk of subsequent fracture may also be identified by previous vertebral fracture and low bone density (**2.25**)[31].

The incidence of hip fracture has been shown to be related to both bone density, measured at the heel, and to the numbers of risk factors identified in the Study of Osteoporotic Fractures (**2.26**)[32]. In a study of elderly women in residential homes in France, the risk of hip fracture was greatest in those with low bone density and at risk of falling (*Table 2.12*)[33]. This interaction between risk factors can be used in strategies to find for those at highest risk (see Chapter 3).

Falls and their impact

Fractures of the long bones of the appendicular skeleton usually follow a fall, and it is important to identify those at

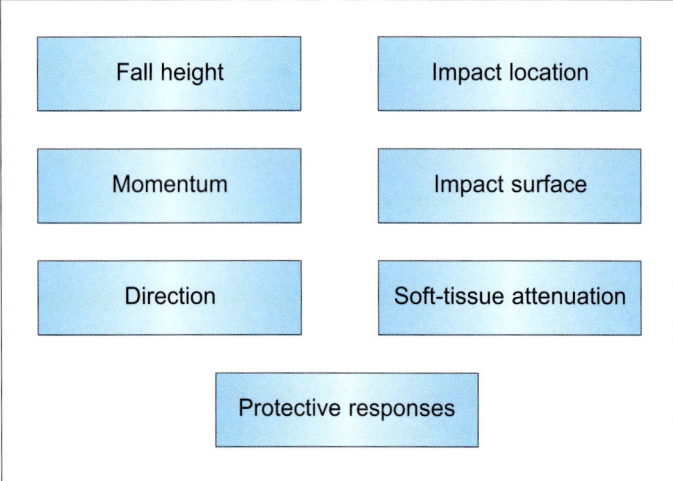

2.27 Factors affecting impact of falls.

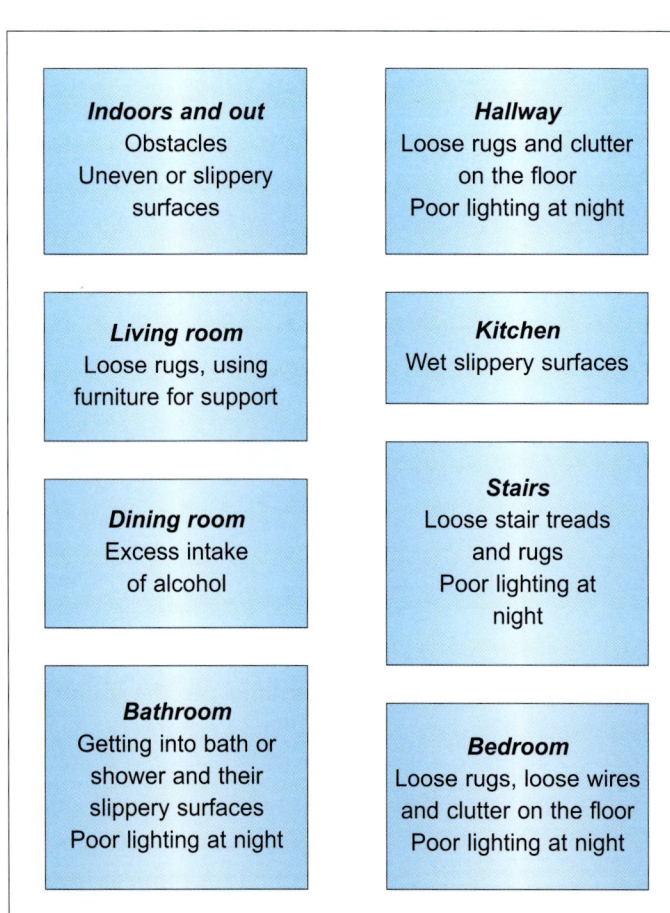

2.28 Home hazards.

greatest risk of falling and sustaining a fracture as a result. The physical impact of any fall will vary between individuals depending on factors such as momentum and soft tissue attenuation (**2.27**), and these have already been considered (**1.7**). Falls result from the external environment, such as uneven pavements, personal intrinsic factors such as impaired balance or poor vision, and from personal extrinsic factors such as poor footwear or hypnotic drugs (*Table 2.9*, **2.28**, **2.29**).

Bone turnover and fracture risk

Measurement of BMD is at present the method of choice in the evaluation of fracture risk. Methods utilising X-ray absorptiometry have adequate precision, but questions remain regarding accuracy since these methods do not capture all aspects of bone quality and of fracture risk. Bone quality is dependent on macro- and microstructure, matrix properties, and bone remodelling to acquire maximum strength. Increasing evidence suggest that the risk of osteoporosis and fracture is associated with increased bone

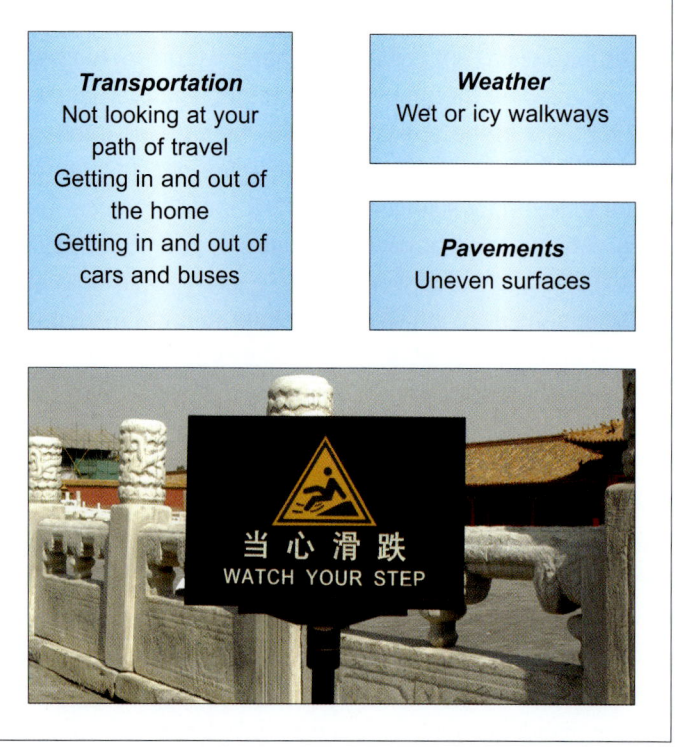

2.29 Street hazards.

turnover as measured by markers of resorption and formation, independently of BMD.

Products synthesized in excess by osteoblasts during bone formation or fragments released during bone resorption are used as markers of bone turnover when they are released and measurable in serum or urine. Assuming that bone turnover under normal circumstances remains at a fairly steady state, the ratio between bone formation markers and bone resorption markers give information on normal metabolic activity. In states of disease, alterations of marker levels should provide an insight into the metabolic disturbances in that particular bone disorder, but it needs to

be kept in mind that biochemical markers of bone turnover reflect the activity of the entire skeleton.

At present, the markers predominantly reflecting bone formation with acceptable specificity and sensitivity are osteocalcin, bone-specific alkaline phosphatase (ALP), and procollagen type I N-terminal propeptide. For evaluating bone resorption, pyridinoline (Pyr), deoxypyridinoline (Dpd) and the N- or C-terminal type I collagen telopeptides (NTx, CTx) are most used, while increasing data are also suggesting tartrate resistant acid phosphatase (TRAP 5b) has a place in the evaluation of fracture risk and potentially also monitoring of treatment[4] (*Table 1.3*, **2.30**).

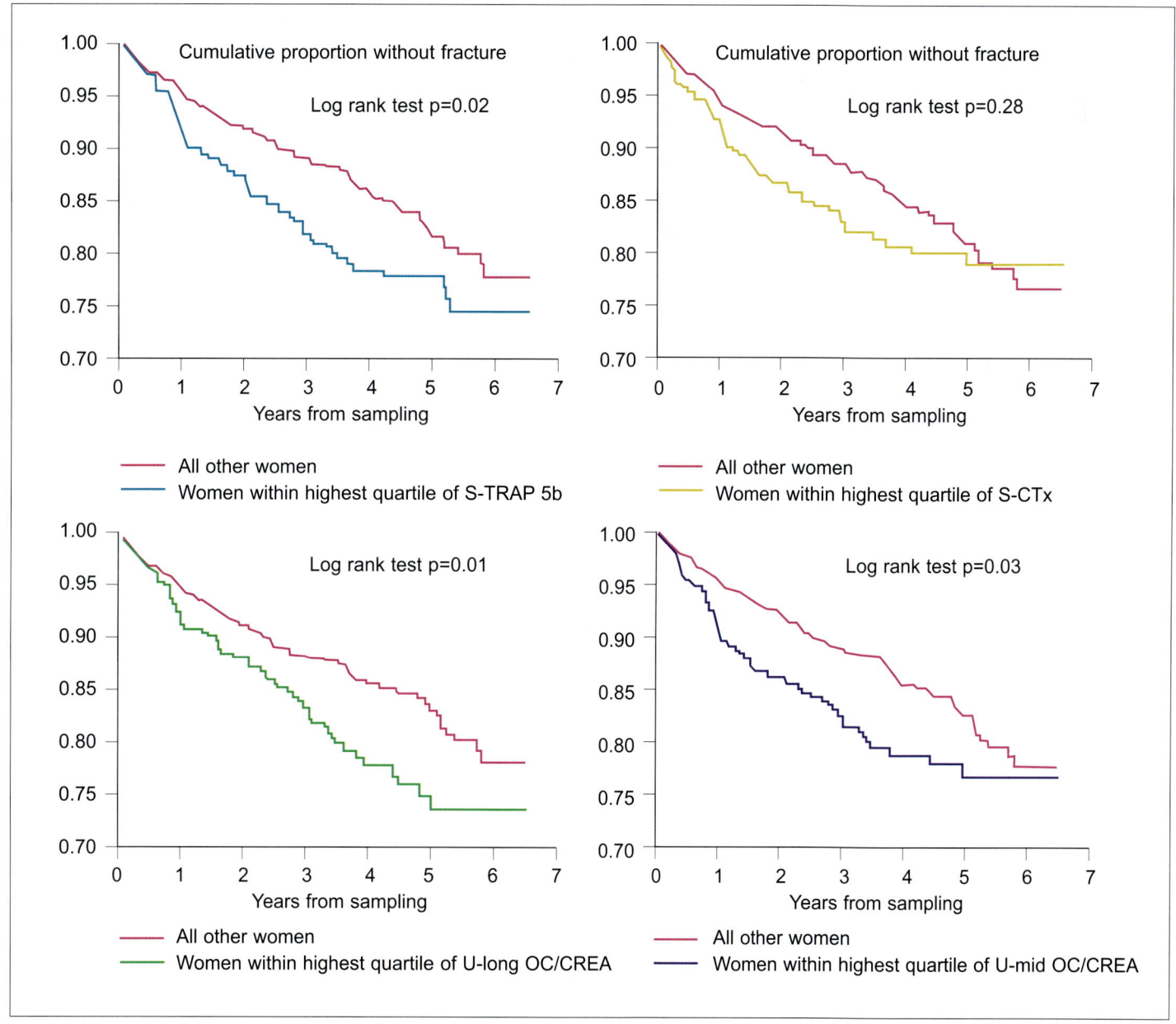

2.30 TRAP 5b and U-Oc seem particularly promising in predicting fracture in this prospective study with a 3–6.5 year follow-up. (Adapted from Gerdhem P, *et al.* (2004). Biochemical markers of bone metabolism and prediction of fracture in elderly women. *J Bone Mineral Res* **19**:386–393.)

Ideally, a biochemical marker should predict all types of fracture, or at least major fractures such as hip and vertebral fractures, and combinations of formation and resorption markers should provide additional aetiological insight. Most early studies evaluating bone markers in association with fracture were retrospective and suggest bone metabolic alterations between fracture patients and controls; however, because the fracture preceded the bone marker measurement, it is uncertain whether the difference in turnover was caused by the fracture or existed prior to the fracture[34]. Clearly a fracture in itself and the extended process of fracture healing initiate long-term changes of bone turnover lasting up to 1 year[35].

Evaluation of bone markers as a predictor of fracture in the individual patient is currently limited by variability from person-related causes and, to a lesser extent, from analytical variability. However, population-based studies have provided essential insight on the relationship between

fracture and alterations of bone turnover, and such prospective studies have shown consistent relationships between resorption markers, alone or in combination with BMD and fracture risk. In the EPIDOS study of postmenopausal women, urine free Dpd and CTx independently predicted hip fracture (odds ratio [OR] 1.9–2.5)[36]. The predictive ability is increased even further when high urinary CTx is combined with measurements of BMD to a more than fourfold fracture risk in women also with low bone mass (**2.31**)[37].

Soon after menopause, bone turnover increases, with a negative bone formation/bone resorption ratio. Early menopause is a well known risk factor for osteoporosis, as is high bone turnover in the early menopausal period with a doubled risk of sustaining vertebral or peripheral fractures during the first 15 years postmenopause, compared with women having normal early menopausal bone turnover[38].

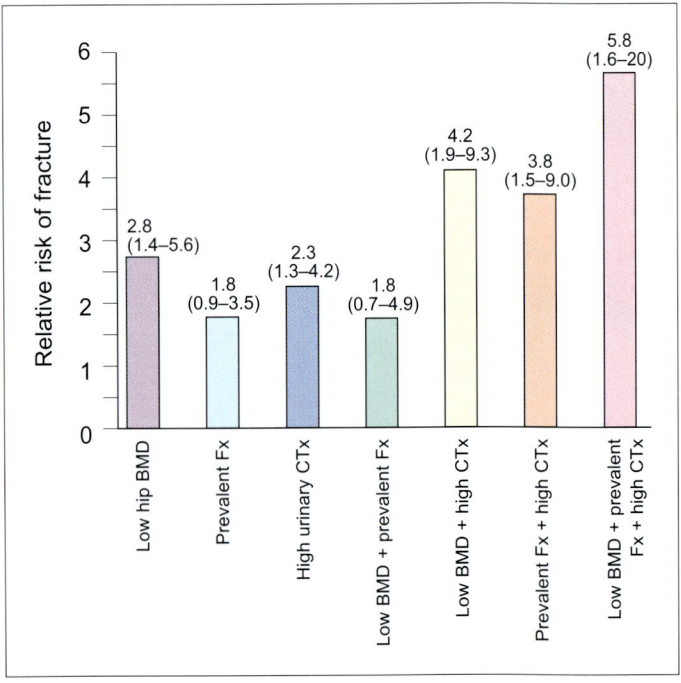

2.31 The combination of different independent predictors can be used to identify women with the highest risk of fracture. This is particularly evident when combining BMD, a history of previous fracture, and a bone resorption marker. (Adapted from Garnero P, *et al.* (2000). Biochemical markers of bone turnover, endogenous hormones, and the risk of fractures in postmenopausal women: the OFELY study. *J Bone Mineral Res* **15**:1526–1536.)

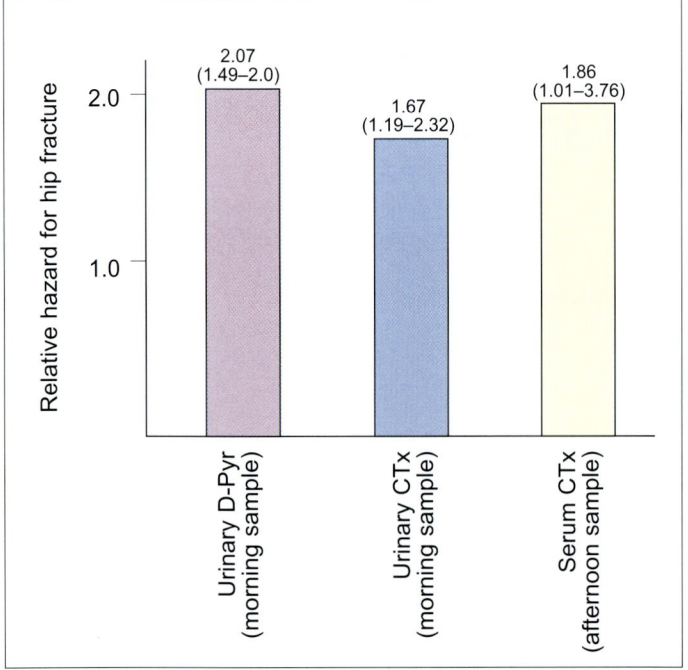

2.32 In this study, bone markers are shown to predict hip fracture in elderly women. Data in the study are based on the EPIDOS prospective study. (Adapted from Garnero P, *et al.* (1996). Markers of bone resorption predict hip fracture in elderly women: the EPIDOS Prospective Study. *J Bone Mineral Res* **11**(10):1531–1538.)

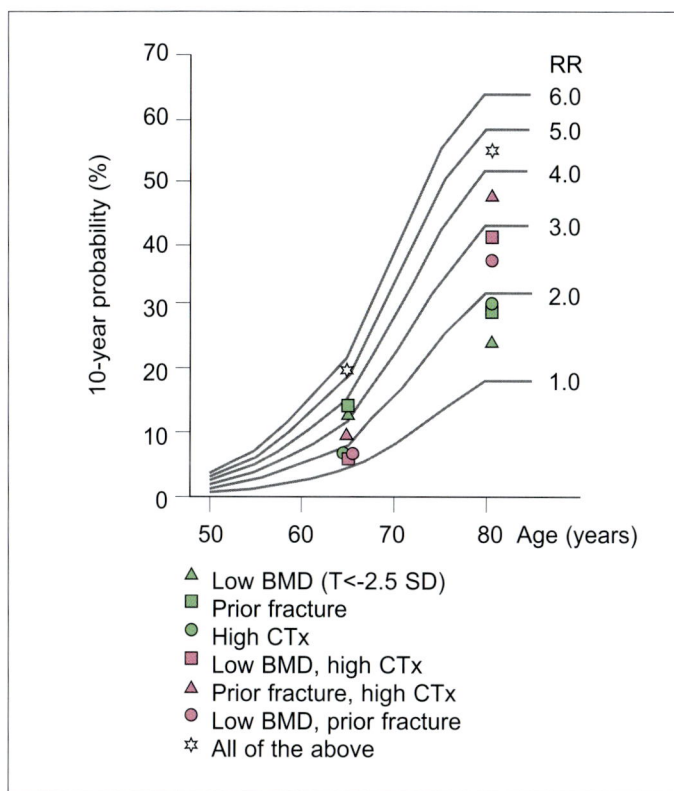

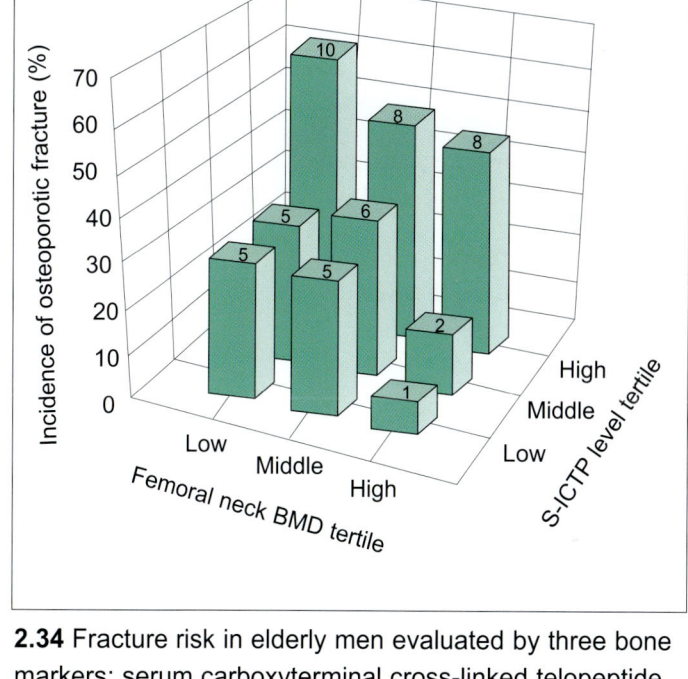

2.33 With any type of risk factor, the question is for how long is it a predictor of outcome. Age is the overall strongest predictor of fracture, whereas bone markers can be added in the estimation of 10-year probability. In this study, the effect of risk factors on 10-year probability of hip fracture is derived from women aged 65 years (OFELY study) or 80 years (EPIDOS study) in Swedish women according to age and relative risk. (Adapted from Johnell O, *et al.* (2002). Biochemical indices of bone turnover and the assessment of fracture probability. *Osteoporos Int* **13**:523–526.)

2.34 Fracture risk in elderly men evaluated by three bone markers: serum carboxyterminal cross-linked telopeptide of type I collagen (ICTP), carboxyterminal type I collagen telopeptide (CTx), and aminoterminal propeptide of type I procollagen (PINP). There was a 10-fold increase in fracture risk in those with high bone resorption and low femoral bone density. (Adapted from Meier C, *et al.* (2005). Bone resorption and osteoporotic fractures in elderly men: the dubbo osteoporosis epidemiology study. *J Bone Mineral Res* 2005;**20**(4):579–587.)

Bone markers are also of value in the elderly. In the population-based Malmö OPRA cohort of elderly women that were followed over almost 5 years, the markers TRAP 5b, serum CTx, and osteocalcin fragments were significantly higher in those women prospectively sustaining a fracture. The resorption markers, TRAP 5b and urine osteocalcin, were also independent predictors of vertebral fractures (OR 2.02–2-25), indicating a doubling of risk and regardless of BMD[39] (**2.30**).

Bone resorption markers, assessed in either urine or serum, are also predictive of hip fracture (**2.32**). Osteocalcin is dependent on post-translational carboxylation for its hydroxyapatite affinity, a process that has been shown to decrease with age. High levels of under-carboxylated osteocalcin are seen in hip fracture patients and associated with an increased fracture risk, particularly in those over 80 years and with a sustained risk increase for 3–5 years[40,41]. Bone markers have also been included in models calculating 10-year fracture probability, with resorption markers significantly contributing to risk[42] (**2.33**). Studies evaluating fracture risk in men based on bone markers are scarce, but in one study of elderly men a pattern similar to that of women was seen, with a steep increase in risk when bone resorption markers were combined with measurements of bone mass. There was also an increased risk independent of bone mass[43] (ICTP RR 1.8 (1.4–2.3)) (**2.34**).

Rapid loss of bone over a defined period of time is also an indicator of disease and markers can be used to demonstrate this. Bone markers have been shown to provide information about fracture risk, independent of and beyond that provided by bone mass measurement alone. Studies have also shown a highly significant correlation between bone

Table 2.8 Secondary causes of osteoporosis

Genetic disorders
Ehlers–Danlos syndrome
Glycogen storage diseases
Gaucher's disease
Haemochromatosis
Homocystinuria
Hypophosphatasia
Marfan syndrome
Osteogenesis imperfecta
Porphyria

Hypogonadal states
Androgen insensitivity
Anorexia nervosa/bulemia
Athletic amenorrhoea
Hyperprolactinaemia
Panhypopituitarism
Premature menopause
Turner and Kleinfelter syndromes

Endocrine disorders
Acromegaly
Adrenal insufficiency
Cushing syndrome
Diabetes mellitus
Hyperparathyroidism
Thyroid disease

Gastrointestinal diseases
Gastrectomy
Inflammatory bowel disease
Malabsorption
Coeliac disease
Primary biliary cirrhosis

Rheumatologic diseases
Ankylosing spondylitis
Rheumatoid arthritis

Haematological disorders
Sickle cell disease
Thalassaemia
Haemophilia
Multiple myeloma
Leukaemias and lymphomas
Systemic mastocytosis

Nutritional deficiencies
Anorexia nervosa
Calcium
Magnesium
Vitamin D

Drugs
Anticoagulants (heparin and warfarin)
Anticonvulsants
Cyclosporines and tacrolimus
Cytotoxic drugs
Glucocorticoids
Gonadotropin-releasing hormone agonists
Thyroxine

Miscellaneous
Alcoholism
Amyloidosis
Chronic metabolic acidosis
Cystic fibrosis
Emphysema
End-stage renal disease
Idiopathic hypercalciuria
Idiopathic scoliosis
Immobilization
Multiple sclerosis
Organ transplantation
Parenteral nutrition
Sarcoidosis

(Adapted from Stein E, Shane E (2003). Secondary osteoporosis. *Endocrinol Metab Clin North Am* **32**(1):115–134.)

turnover markers and subsequent rates of bone loss, with up to 50% of the variance explained by bone turnover in 80-year-old women[44]. In postmenopausal women in their sixties, it has been shown that the differences in bone mass between those with high versus those with low turnover were close to 10% (8±14%), and that bone resorption markers were predictive of bone loss in the hip after 4 years[45].

In summary, bone markers provide information beyond that of a single bone density measurement as they provide information on the cellular process leading to bone loss. Increased levels of bone resorption markers allow for estimation of fracture risk in the elderly for up to 5 years and of bone loss, especially in early menopause. In combination with BMD measurement, the prediction of fracture risk is further enhanced. In a clinical perspective, bone markers should have role in patient evaluation as a complement to other risk factors, particularly as new drugs that are differentially targeting bone formation and bone resorption are becoming available.

Secondary causes of osteoporosis

There are a variety of conditions or interventions that are associated with osteoporosis and increased fracture risk (*Table 2.13*). The risk may relate to the condition itself or to a consequence of the condition, such as immobility, or to its treatment, such as steroid therapy. These conditions should be sought when assessing anyone with osteoporosis. There is more commonly a secondary cause in men and premenopausal women with osteoporosis, but as many as one-third of postmenopausal women have been found to have specific reasons for developing osteoporosis apart from age and postmenapausal bone loss.

The causes include hypogonadism, endocrine disorders, gastrointestinal diseases, transplantation, inflammatory diseases, immobilizing disorders, and certain drugs, most importantly glucocorticosteroids.

Steroid-induced osteoporosis

Cushing, when first describing the features of adrenal cortical hyperactivity in 1932, noted the increases risk of fracture and marked thoracic kyphosis. Cortisone-induced osteoporosis and fractures were reported in 1950, within 1 year of its first use. Glucocorticoids are now very widely used. The prevalence of oral glucocorticoid use in the UK, using a primary care database, is almost 1% of the total adult population at any one time, with one-quarter taking more than 7.5 mg daily[46]. The most frequent reason was respiratory disease but musculoskeletal and skin problems are other common reasons for their use. Most received short-term courses, but over 20% continued for longer than 6 months.

The use of glucocorticoids significantly increases the risk of future fracture, in particular the hip. This effect is greater at higher doses and with greater duration of use but it is not possible to say that there is a safe dose. Fracture risk increases rapidly after initiation of glucocorticoid therapy and declines rapidly after treatment is stopped (*Table 2.14, 2.35, 2.36*)[47].

Table 2.14 Relative risk of fracture in glucocorticosteroids users in General Practice Research Database (GPRD)

	Relative risk (95% CI)
Any fracture	1.33 (1.29–1.38)
Hip	1.61 (1.47–1.76)
Vertebra	2.60 (2.31–2.92)
Forearm	1.09 (1.01–1.17)

(Adapted from van Staa *et al.* (2002). The epidemiology of corticosteroid-induced osteoporosis: a meta-analysis. *Osteoporos Int* **13**(10):777–787.)

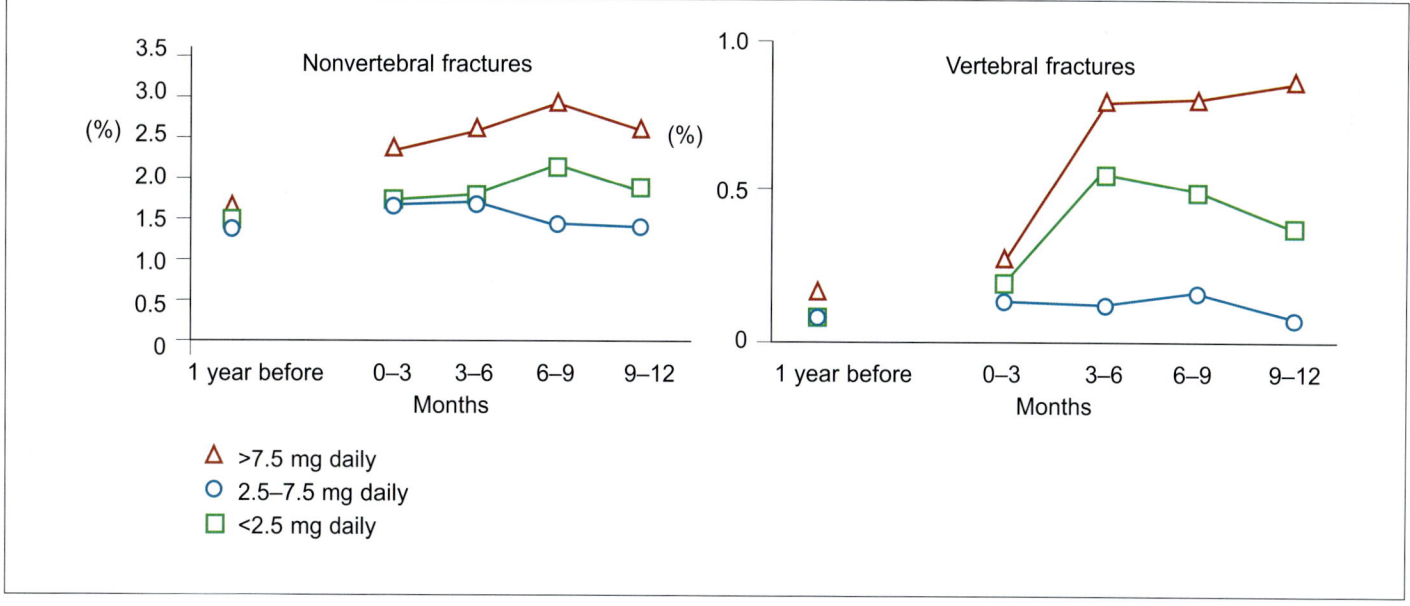

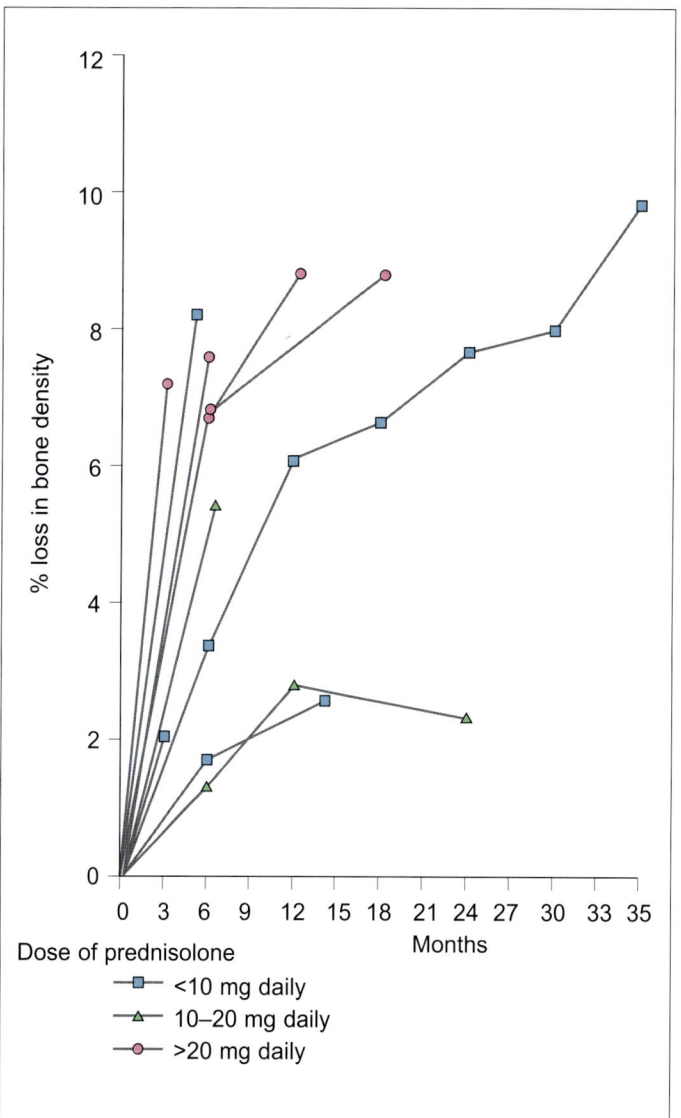

2.35 The rapid dose-related increase in risk of nonvertebral (**A**) and vertebral fracture (**B**) is demonstrated before *vs.* during first year of glucocorticoid therapy. In people using prednisolone (≥7.5 mg), the risk of nonvertebral fractures was increased by 54% in the first year. (Adapted from van Staa TP, *et al.* (2002). The epidemiology of corticosteroid-induced osteoporosis: a meta-analysis. *Osteoporos Int* **13**(10):777–787.)

Glucocorticoid therapy results in a rapid loss of BMD; the rate of loss is may be as high as 30% in the first 6 months, with higher than normal rates of loss persisting for the duration of treatment. These effects are at least partially reversible on cessation of glucocorticoids. Bone loss occurs at both cortical and trabecular sites, although loss is most marked at the latter. However, the increased risk of fracture associated with glucocorticoid therapy is greater than that explained by the effect on bone density[48], which has therapeutic implications when considering who to treat (see Chapter 5).

Glucocorticoids affect the skeleton in other ways (*Table 2.15*), with retardation of growth in children and an

2.36 The rapid loss of spine BMD after start of corticosteroid therapy is demonstrated in ten longitudinal studies. (Adapted from van Staa TP, *et al.* (2002). The epidemiology of corticosteroid-induced osteoporosis: a meta-analysis. *Osteoporos Int* **13**(10):777–787.)

increased risk of avascular necrosis. The drugs also affect the connective tissues, the most apparent manifestation being skin thinning (**2.37**) with fragility of subcutaneous vessels, resulting in 'steroid purpura'. Glucocorticoids affect bone through multiple pathways, influencing both bone formation and bone resorption (*Table 2.16*).

Glucocorticoids have inhibitory effects on the differentiation of osteoblast precursors and osteoblast lifespan, with direct inhibitory effects on bone formation demonstrated in histomorphometric studies. Osteocyte apoptosis is induced. Glucocorticoids also decrease intestinal absorption of calcium and, by direct effects on the kidney, increase urinary phosphate and calcium loss. Together these lead to secondary hyperparathyroidism. This, in combination with gonadal and adrenal hormone changes, results in increased osteoclast maturation and activity with an increase in bone resorption.

It is therefore likely that the net bone loss with glucocorticoid use is the combination of enhanced activation frequency of bone remodelling units due to secondary hyperparathyroidism, together with an inadequate amount of new bone synthesis due to the suppression of osteoblastic function. In addition, low serum testosterone levels have been reported in glucocorticoid-treated men and are believed to be due both to direct effects on the testis and indirect effects on testosterone production mediated via suppression of gonadotropin hormone secretion.

Fracture risk with glucocorticoids is determined by several factors and is not just dependent on bone mass and its loss. Factors include:
- Bone density – its starting value before glucocorticoids therapy and the subsequent loss.
- Glucocorticoid dose – bone loss is dependent on cumulative and daily dosage.
- Duration of exposure – a short course of will cause reversible bone loss, but long-term glucocorticoid use increases reduction in bone density, increasing the likelihood that a fracture will occur eventually.
- Effects of glucocorticoids on the bone tissue independent to bone density.
- Underlying disease for which glucocorticoids have been prescribed – this may be independently associated with increased fracture risk.

Fractures due to glucocorticoids occur at a higher bone density and this is relevant when deciding at what threshold of bone density to initiate bone sparing therapy.

Table 2.15 The effects of glucocorticoids on bone

- Bone mass reduced
- Fracture risk increased
- Growth retardation
- Avascular necrosis

Table 2.16 The effects of glucocorticoids and bone – possible mechanisms

Direct effects
- Decreased number and function of osteoblasts
- Increased apoptosis of osteocytes
- Increased osteoclast activity

Indirect effects
- Reduced intestinal calcium absorption
- Increased renal calcium excretion
- Secondary hyperparathyroidism and bone resorption
- Decreased sex hormones by suppression of gonadotrophic and adrenotrophic hormones

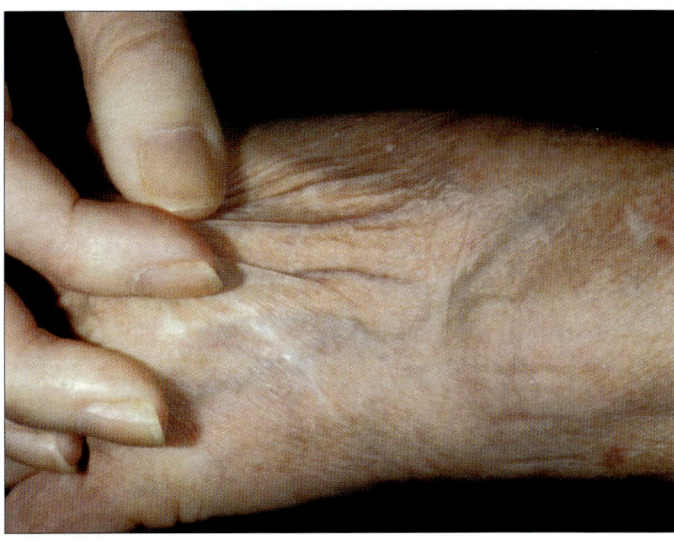

2.37 Thinning of the skin due to steroid-induced changes in connective tissue.

Rheumatoid arthritis

There is both localized bone loss around the inflamed joints and generalized bone loss in rheumatoid arthritis (RA), with a twofold increase in prevalence of osteoporosis in males and females[49] (**2.38**). There is also an increased risk of vertebral fracture as well as appendicular fracture, most clearly demonstrated for the hip. In addition, stress fractures occur in the pelvis or related to biomechanically abnormal joints such as the fibula adjacent to the knee and ankle (**2.39**).

The possible mechanisms for increased bone loss in RA relate to the direct effects of inflammation and tissue damage, the secondary effects of immobility, and iatrogenic effects such as glucocorticoid therapy. Clearest associations have been shown with age, weight, functional status, and long-term glucocorticoid therapy. The increased occurrence of fracture relates to this bone loss but some relate to local abnormal stresses from joint deformity. Risk of falls is also increased with arthritis and the impact is probably greater.

Transplantation

Organ transplantation is an increasingly common and successful treatment of end-stage renal, hepatic, cardiac, and pulmonary disease. As a result, it is clear that osteoporosis is a major long-term complication. The reasons are multiple: the disease that resulted in transplantation and prior therapies, immobilization, and lifestyle factors such as alcohol and smoking but, most importantly, the immunosuppressive therapy with glucocorticosteroids and antirejection agents such as cyclosporine and tacrolimus.

Athletes

Elite athletes are at increased risk of osteoporosis and fracture. This is typically endurance athletes and is also seen amongst ballet dancers. Although increased physical activity is associated with higher bone density, women who exercise excessively may develop hypothalamic amenorrhea. The risk

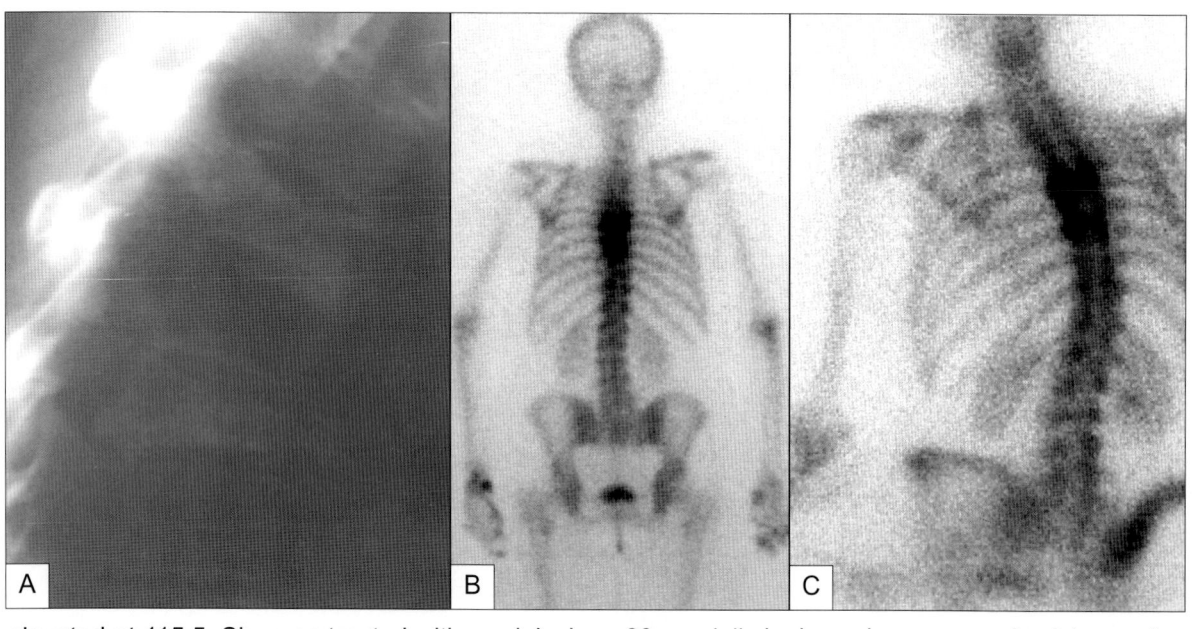

2.38 At the age of 69 the patient developed symptoms of polymyalgia rheumatica with pain and stiffness across her shoulders and in the buttocks and thighs which affected everyday activities in the mornings. Her CRP was elevated at 115.5. She was treated with prednisolone 30 mg daily by her primary care physician and responded dramatically to this. She continued on prednisolone 30 mg daily for 1 month, 27.5 mg daily for 1 month, 20 mg daily for 2 months and then 20 mg alternating with 15 mg daily. After 6 months of having started steroids when on this dose she then sustained severe back pain in the midthoracic spine and X-ray showed wedge fractures of T7 and T9. When seen in the rheumatology clinic a month later, she was still getting severe disabling back pain for which she had commenced slow release morphine. She had been put on prophylactic alendronate when she commenced prednisolone. When seen she had a thoracic kyphosis with protuberant abdomen and skin thinning with steroid purpura. There was marked tenderness in the midthoracic spine. She had a past history of breast cancer and therefore had an isotope bone scan (**B, C**) which showed increased uptake at the sites of vertebral deformity but no other bony lesions.

of developing this is greater if there is a low body weight with low calorie intake and a previous history of amenorrhea. The combination of disordered eating, amenorrhea, and bone loss in athletes is called the 'female athlete triad'.

Anorexia nervosa

Anorexia nervosa is associated with osteoporosis and fracture (**2.40**). If anorexia develops during adolescence, they may be severely osteoporotic as that is the stage of acquiring peak bone mass. Recovery of bone mass may be incomplete even if anorexia is successfully overcome. There are multiple mechanisms but the key ones are malnutrition, low body mass, and oestrogen deficiency. When low body mass is associated with amenorrhea there is a significant risk of developing osteoporosis. It is recommended that women have a body mass index of 18 or over to avoid this.

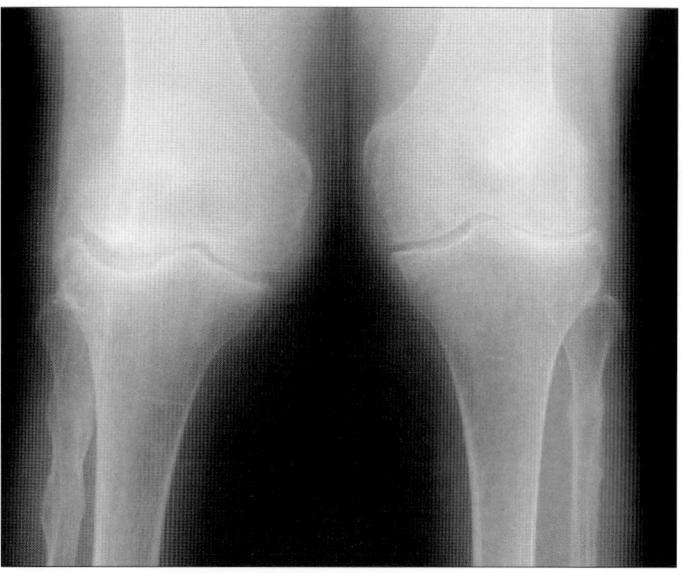

2.39 Stress fractures of both fibula in a 68-year-old woman with long-standing erosive rheumatoid arthritis. There is marked loss of joint space of the lateral compartment of the knee, resulting in valgus deformities of the knees with abnormal loading on the fibula.

2.40 The patient presented at 50 years of age with severe persistent back pain and was found to have suffered multiple lower thoracic vertebral fractures. She had sustained a spontaneous rib fracture 3 years previously. She now was very restricted and had to lie flat on her back most of the time. She had lost about 15 cm in height. She had suffered from anorexia nervosa from her late teens until her early 20s and, in 1999, she had possible inflammatory bowel disease which was treated for 1 year with oral corticosteroids. When seen she was very thin with a BMI of 16.5 and had a marked kyphosis and skin ulceration over the lower thoracic spine. Bone density assessment showed bone mass in the proximal femur of 0.226 g/cm^2 (T-score -5.87) and her bone mineral density in the lumbar spine (L1–L4) of 0.557 g/cm^2 (T-score of -4.45).

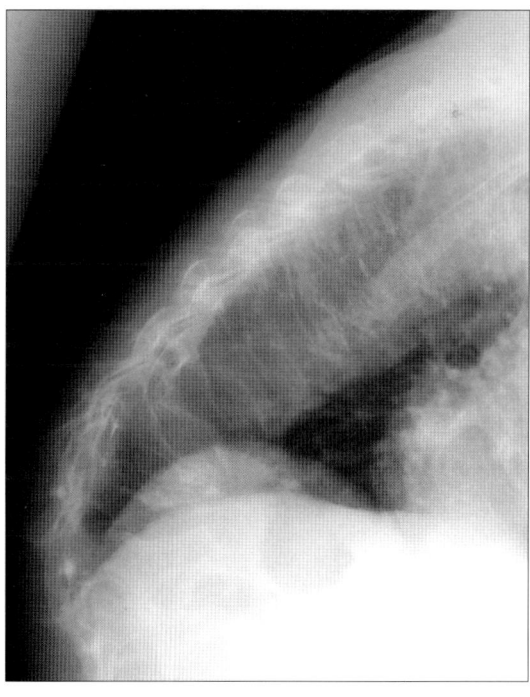

Men, osteoporosis, and fracture

Although osteoporosis is less common in men, they sustain significant bone loss with ageing: lifetime fracture risk at 50 years is 13%, and 20% of symptomatic vertebral fractures and 30% of hip fractures occur in men. The age-related increase occurs later than in women. The major osteoporotic fractures are of the vertebrae and hip. The number of men sustaining osteoporotic fractures is increasing due to demographic changes.

Osteoporosis in men is more frequently associated with a secondary cause than in women (*Table 2.17*). These may relate to hypogonadism, concomitant conditions and diseases and lifestyle factors such as excess alcohol, often taken in combination with excess smoking. Comorbid diseases, such as stroke, Parkinson's disease, dementia, and poor vision are important risk factors for hip fracture in men. Underlying causes are identified in many men with vertebral fractures, of which steroid therapy, hypogonadism, excess alcohol consumption, and smoking are important factors. Hypogonadism is a well established cause of osteoporosis in men, occurring in up to 20% of men with vertebral fractures and 50% of elderly men with hip fractures. Mortality following fracture is greater in men than women. However, because fractures are less common in men and they are usually associated with moderate trauma, osteoporosis is often not considered and the person not investigated.

As secondary causes are common in men, they need to be looked for in the assessment of any male presenting with a low-trauma fracture, or who has been identified as having osteoporosis (see *Case Study*).

References

1 World Health Organization Study Group (1994). Assessment of fracture risk and its application to screening for postmenopausal osteoporosis: *WHO Technical Report Series* No. **843**. World Health Organization, Geneva, Switzerland.

2 World Health Scientific Group (2003). The burden of musculoskeletal diseases at the start of the new millenium. Report of a WHO Scientific Group. *WHO Technical Report Series* No. **919**. World Health Organization, Geneva, Switzerland.

3 Kanis JA, Johnell O, Oden A, Jonsson B, De Laet C, Dawson A (2000). Risk of hip fracture according to the World Health Organization criteria for osteopenia and osteoporosis. *Bone* **27**(5):585–590.

Table 2.17 Causes of male osteoporosis

Secondary causes: very common – 55% of vertebral fractures in selected series
- Steroid therapy – respiratory disease
- Excess alcohol
- Smoking
- Hypogonadism: 20% of cases of secondary osteoporosis:
  - primary or secondary hypogonadotrophic hypogonadism
  - hyperprolactinaemia
  - haemochromatosis
  - primary testicular failure
  - Klinefelters
- Myeloma
- Gastric surgery
- Anticonvulsants

Case Study

A 42-year-old man presented with the sudden onset of severe back pain. He worked in the dockyard and was lifting a heavy crate. The pain persisted for several weeks without much improvement and an X-ray revealed a compression fracture of L3. His bone density was assessed and was 0.475 g/cm^2 (T-score -5.84) in the lumbar spine and 0.643 g/cm^2 (T-score -3.50) in the total hip. He admitted to having been a heavy drinker since 16 years of age and smoked 20–40 cigarettes daily.

4 Gerdhem P, Brandstrom H, Stiger F, *et al.* (2004). Association of the collagen type 1 (COL1A 1) Sp1 binding site polymorphism to femoral neck bone mineral density and wrist fracture in 1044 elderly Swedish women. *Calcif Tissue Int* **74**(3):264–269.

5 Cooper C, Dennison EM, Leufkens HG, Bishop N, van Staa TP (2004). Epidemiology of childhood fractures in Britain: a study using the general practice research database. *J Bone Mineral Res* **19**(12):1976–1981.

6 O'Neill TW, Felsenberg D, Varlow J, Cooper C, Kanis JA, Silman AJ (1996). The prevalence of vertebral deformity in European men and women: the European Vertebral Osteoporosis Study. *J Bone Mineral Res* **11**(7):1010–1018.

7 The European Prospective Osteoporosis Study Group (2002). Incidence of vertebral fractures in Europe: results from the European Prospective Osteoporosis Study (EPOS). *J Bone Mineral Res* **17**:716–724.

8 O'Neill TW, Cooper C, Finn JD, *et al.* (2001). Incidence of distal forearm fracture in British men and women. *Osteoporos Int* **12**(7):555–558.

9 Gullberg B, Johnell O, Kanis JA (1997). Worldwide projections for hip fracture. *Osteoporos Int* **7**(5):407–413.

10 Johnell O, Kanis JA (2004). An estimate of the worldwide prevalence, mortality, and disability associated with hip fracture. *Osteoporos Int* **15**(11):897–902.

11 van Staa TP, Dennison EM, Leufkens HG, Cooper C (2001). Epidemiology of fractures in England and Wales. *Bone* **29**(6):517–522.

12 Rose SH, Melton LJ, III, Morrey BF, Ilstrup DM, Riggs BL (1982). Epidemiologic features of humeral fractures. *Clin Orthop Relat Res* **168**:24–30.

13 Court-Brown CM, Garg A, McQueen MM (2001). The epidemiology of proximal humeral fractures. *Acta Orthop Scand* **72**(4):365–371.

14 Kanis JA, Johnell O, Oden A, De Laet C, Jonsson B, Dawson A (2002). Ten-year risk of osteoporotic fracture and the effect of risk factors on screening strategies. *Bone* **30**(1):251–258.

15 Lau EM, Lee JK, Suriwongpaisal P, *et al.* (2001). The incidence of hip fracture in four Asian countries: the Asian Osteoporosis Study (AOS). *Osteoporos Int* **12**(3):239–243.

16 Sernbo I, Johnell O (1993). Consequences of a hip fracture: a prospective study over 1 year. *Osteoporos Int* **3**(3):148–153.

17 Kanis JA, Oden A, Johnell O, De Laet C, Jonsson B, Oglesby AK (2003). The components of excess mortality after hip fracture. *Bone* **32**(5):468–473.

18 Olsson C, Nordquist A, Petersson CJ (2005). Long-term outcome of a proximal humerus fracture predicted after 1 year: a 13-year prospective population-based follow-up study of 47 patients. *Acta Orthop* **76**(3):397–402.

19 Morris RO, Sonibare A, Green DJ, Masud T (2000). Closed pelvic fractures: characteristics and outcomes in older patients admitted to medical and geriatric wards. *Postgrad Med J* **76**(900):646–650.

20 Taillandier J, Langue F, Alemanni M, Taillandier-Heriche E (2003). Mortality and functional outcomes of pelvic insufficiency fractures in older patients. *Joint Bone Spine* **70**(4):287–289.

21 Johnell O, Kanis JA, Jonsson B, Oden A, Johansson H, De Laet C (2005). The burden of hospitalized fractures in Sweden. *Osteoporos Int* **16**(2):222–228.

22 Wiktorowicz ME, Goeree R, Papaioannou A, Adachi JD, Papadimitropoulos E (2001). Economic implications of hip fracture: health service use, institutional care, and cost in Canada. *Osteoporos Int* **12**(4):271–278.

23 Tosteson AN (1999). Economic impact of fractures. In: *The Effects of Gender on Skeletal Health*. E Orwoll (ed). Academic Press, San Diego, CA, pp. 15–27.

24 Dolan P, Torgerson DJ (1998). The cost of treating osteoporotic fractures in the United Kingdom female population. *Osteoporos Int* **8**(6):611–617.

25 European Communities (1998). Report on Osteoporosis in the European Community: action for prevention. European Communities, Luxembourg.

26 Johnell O (1997). The socioeconomic burden of fractures: today and in the 21st century. *Am J Med* **103**(2A):20S–25S.

27 Kanis JA, Johnell O, Oden A, Dawson A, De Laet C, Jonsson B (2001). Ten-year probabilities of osteoporotic fractures according to BMD and diagnostic thresholds. *Osteoporos Int* **12**(12):989–995.

28 Kanis JA, Johnell O, De Laet C, *et al.* (2004). A meta-analysis of previous fracture and subsequent fracture risk. *Bone* **35**(2):375–382.

29 Lindsay R, Silverman SL, Cooper C, *et al.* (2001). Risk of new vertebral fracture in the year following a fracture. *JAMA* **285**(3):320–323.

30 Ismail AA, Cockerill W, Cooper C, *et al.* (2001). Prevalent vertebral deformity predicts incident hip though not distal forearm fracture: results from the European Prospective Osteoporosis Study. *Osteoporos Int* **12**(2):85–90.

31 Ross PD, Davis JW, Epstein RS, Wasnich RD (1991). Pre-existing fractures and bone mass predict vertebral fracture incidence in women. *Ann Intern Med* **114**(11):919–923.

32 Cumming RG, Cummings SR, Nevitt MC, *et al.* (1997). Calcium intake and fracture risk: results from the study of osteoporotic fractures. *Am J Epidemiol* **145**(10):926–934.

33 Dargent-Molina P, Favier F, Grandjean H, *et al.* (1996). Fall-related factors and risk of hip fracture: the EPIDOS prospective study. *Lancet* **348**(9021):145–149.

34 Åkesson K, Vergnaud P, Gineyts E, Delmas PD, Obrant KJ (1993). Impairment of bone turnover in elderly women with hip fracture. *Calcif Tissue Int* **53**(3):162–169.

35 Åkesson K, Kakonen SM, Josefsson PO, Karlsson MK, Obrant KJ, Pettersson K (2005). Fracture-induced changes in bone turnover: a potential confounder in the use of biochemical markers in osteoporosis. *J Bone Mineral Metab* **23**(1):30–35.

36 Garnero P, Hausherr E, Chapuy MC, Marcelli *et al.* (1996). Markers of bone resorption predict hip fracture in elderly women: the EPIDOS Prospective Study. *J Bone Mineral Res* **11**(10):1531–1538.

37 Garnero P, Sornay-Rendu E, Claustrat B, Delmas PD (2000). Biochemical markers of bone turnover, endogenous hormones and the risk of fractures in postmenopausal women: the OFELY study. *J Bone Mineral Res* **15**(8):1526–1536.

38 Riis BJ, Overgaard K, Christiansen C (1995). Biochemical markers of bone turnover to monitor the bone response to postmenopausal hormone replacement therapy. *Osteoporos Int* **5**(4):276–280.

39 Gerdhem P, Ivaska KK, Alatalo SL, *et al.* (2004). Biochemical markers of bone metabolism and prediction of fracture in elderly women. *J Bone Mineral Res* **19**(3):386–393.

40 Luukinen H, Kakonen SM, Pettersson K, et al. (2000). Strong prediction of fractures among older adults by the ratio of carboxylated to total serum osteocalcin. *J Bone Mineral Res* **15**(12):2473–2478.

41 Vergnaud P, Garnero P, Meunier PJ, Breart G, Kamihagi K, Delmas PD (1997). Undercarboxylated osteocalcin measured with a specific immunoassay predicts hip fracture in elderly women: the EPIDOS Study. *J Clin Endocrinol Metab* **82**(3):719–724.

42 Johnell O, Oden A, De Laet C, Garnero P, Delmas PD, Kanis JA (2002). Biochemical indices of bone turnover and the assessment of fracture probability. *Osteoporos Int* **13**(7):523–526.

43 Meier C, Nguyen TV, Center JR, Seibel MJ, Eisman JA (2005). Bone resorption and osteoporotic fractures in elderly men: the Dubbo Osteoporosis Epidemiology Study. *J Bone Mineral Res* **20**(4):579–587.

44 Garnero P, Sornay-Rendu E, Chapuy MC, Delmas PD (1996). Increased bone turnover in late postmenopausal women is a major determinant of osteoporosis. *J Bone Mineral Res* **11**(3):337–349.

45 Bauer DC, Sklarin PM, Stone KL, *et al.* (1999). Biochemical markers of bone turnover and prediction of hip bone loss in older women: the study of osteoporotic fractures. *J Bone Mineral Res* **14**(8):1404–1410.

46 van Staa TP, Leufkens HG, Abenhaim L, Begaud B, Zhang B, Cooper C (2000). Use of oral corticosteroids in the United Kingdom. *QJM* **93**(2):105–111.

47 van Staa TP, Leufkens HG, Cooper C (2002). The epidemiology of corticosteroid-induced osteoporosis: a meta-analysis. *Osteoporos Int* **13**(10):777–787.

48 Kanis JA, Johansson H, Oden A, et al. (2004). A meta-analysis of prior corticosteroid use and fracture risk. *J Bone Mineral Res* **19**(6):893–899.

49 Haugeberg G, Uhlig T, Falch JA, Halse JI, Kvien TK (2000). Bone mineral density and frequency of osteoporosis in female patients with rheumatoid arthritis: results from 394 patients in the Oslo County Rheumatoid Arthritis register. *Arthritis Rheum* **43**(3):522–530.

How to assess and monitor osteoporosis and risk of fracture

Introduction

The aim in clinical practice is to identify those who are at high risk of fracture who will benefit from treatment. Is this high risk because of osteoporosis, high risk of falling, or a combination of both?

The ideal is to identify and treat before the first fracture, but for many the first suspicion of osteoporosis is raised by a long bone fracture following a fall or a spontaneous vertebral fracture. People sustaining a traumatic or low trauma fractures need to be assessed for the cause, in particular osteoporosis, to decide about the need for treatment to prevent another fracture. If osteoporosis is identified, then any underlying factors that may worsen the patient's condition need to be recognized and managed. Finally, there is a need to monitor treatment to ensure the desired outcome is being achieved.

This chapter will attempt to answer these questions (*Table 3.1*) on a scientific basis, to give practical guidance for clinical management. Each medical unit will have to develop their own strategy from this for managing people with osteoporosis.

Assessing risk of osteoporosis and fracture

Fractures are increasingly common with ageing; one in three women and one in eight men over the age of 50 years will sustain a fracture. People who are osteoporotic are more at risk but not all those with osteoporosis will sustain a fracture during their lifetime and, conversely, not all those who fracture are osteoporotic. For a treatment that will prevent fracture, it must be targeted at those who are at greatest risk

Table 3.1 Key clinical questions

- Are they at high risk of future fracture?
- Do they have osteoporosis?
- If they have osteoporosis, is there a reason?
- Was their fracture due to osteoporosis?
- Was there any other reason why they sustained a fracture?
- Do they need an intervention to reduce their risk of fracture?
- What intervention is most appropriate?
- Have they responded to treatment for osteoporosis?
- Are they at less risk of fracture?

if it is to offer most benefit for that individual and to be cost-effective. The need is to identify those individuals who are at highest risk of fracture.

The risk of fracture can be expressed in terms of the probability of this happening in the following 10 years – the 10-year probability of fracture, given as a percentage or odds ratio. This timeframe is meaningful for the patient, and there is also evidence of the effectiveness of various treatments over this period of time.

The strongest risk factors for fracture are age and female sex. It is therefore appropriate to estimate the 10-year probability of fracture in those over 65 years, in particular in women. With an estimate of future fracture probability it will be possible to have an informed discussion about the potential benefits of any treatment. This is, however, only appropriate if the person is willing and capable to take a treatment long-term. Any decision by the person around this balance of risk and benefit will be influenced by other factors such as the individual's personal experiences and subsequent anxieties about sustaining a fracture or suffering side-effects from treatment. It is not possible to predict for the individual whether they will sustain a fracture or benefit from a treatment, but we can estimate probabilities by the application of knowledge of the risk factors to the individual. Once the level of risk is estimated, it requires careful explanation to have any meaningful value for the patient.

There are various factors that have been identified in epidemiological studies that are associated with an increased risk of fracture, in addition to age and sex (see Chapter 2), which can be used to aid this clinical decision-making process about whom to treat. These risk factors relate to bone strength, risk of falling, and the impact of any fall (**3.1**). Bone density has the strongest association with fracture risk, but no risk factor alone is of sufficient strength to identify those at highest risk in whom treatment to prevent fracture will be cost-effective.

Algorithms have, therefore, been developed to help identify those individuals most at risk (see Chapter 1 and *vide infra*). The algorithms rely on a combination of these clinical risk factors and assessing bone density when indicated. Such individuals will therefore gain most from any intervention, and interventions are also most cost-effective in this situation.

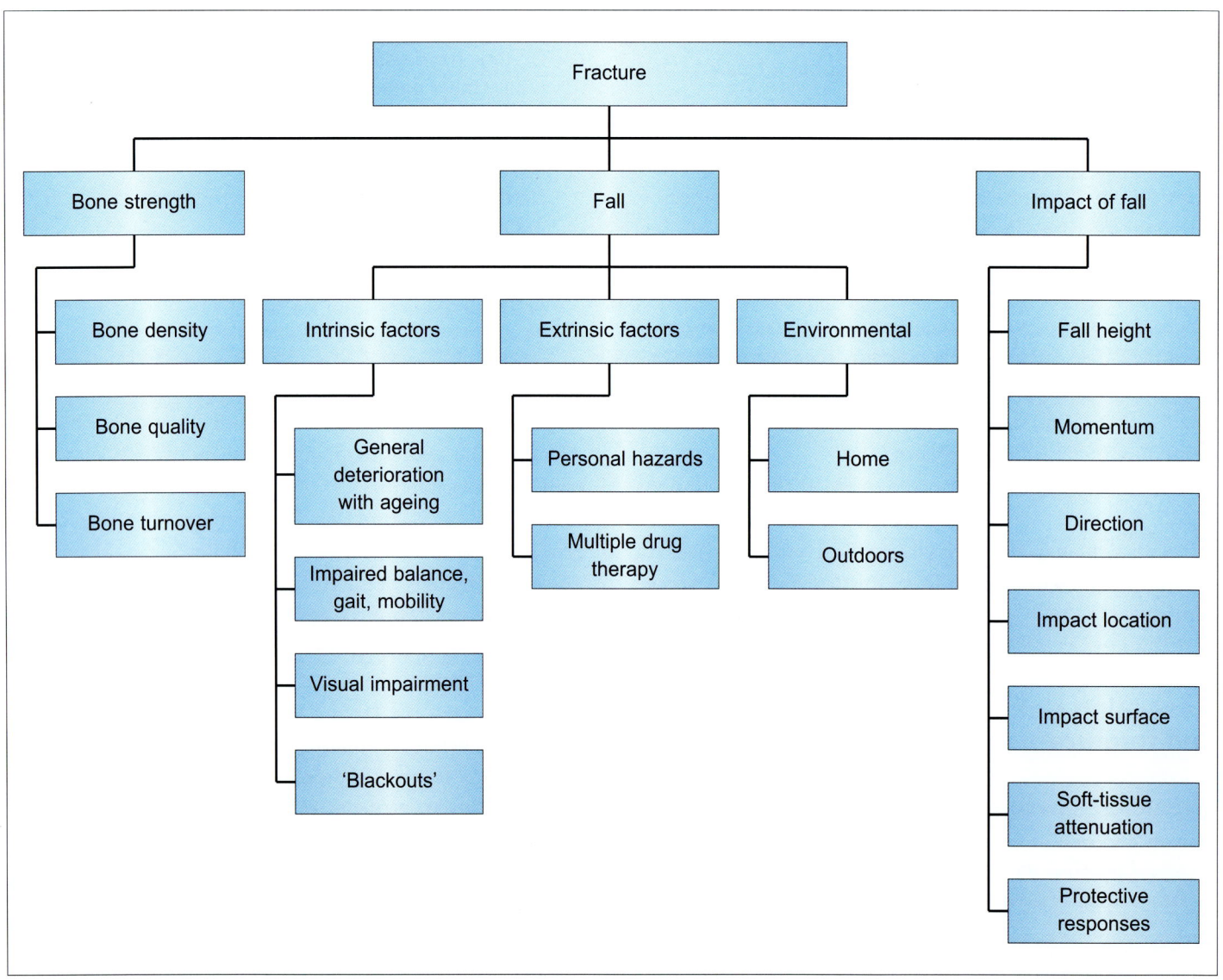

3.1 Factors relating to risk of fracture.

In practice when should risk of future fracture be assessed?

Those at highest risk are more likely to be identified if this is done later in life. The 10-year risk of fracture in a 50-year-old women is 9.8%, whereas it is 21.7% in an 80-year-old[1]. Fracture risk can be reduced within a year by various treatments in such older people. Such a 'high risk' strategy aimed at older people will prevent the greatest number of fractures and give the most personal and economic potential benefit.

Bone density measurement is not appropriate if a woman is premenopausal with no major risk factors as there is no proven specific intervention; general advice should suffice. However, it may be appropriate in a young woman with an eating disorder as this may influence her future behavior, or a person following transplantation or receiving high-dose corticosteroids as this may influence the use of a bisphosphonate. Compliance with treatment is generally increased following such informed decision-making. There is less of a reason to assess risk of fracture in perimenopausal women now that long-term hormone replacement therapy (HRT) is not considered appropriate as a routine way of reducing fracture risk.

Clinical risk factors for osteoporosis and fracture

Age and female gender are the strongest risk factors for fracture. In addition, previous low energy fracture, glucocorticosteroid therapy, reduced lifetime oestrogen exposure, anorexia nervosa, low body mass index, maternal hip fracture, smoking, low levels of physical activity, and certain diseases such as rheumatoid arthritis and diabetes mellitus increase the risk of osteoporosis and fracture (*Table 3.2*). Although these factors are associated with increased personal risk, they cannot singly predict which individual will fracture, and are of limited value alone in deciding who will benefit most from an intervention. As risk of fracture is increased in those with clinical risk factors and low bone density, these clinical risk factors can be used to identify who should be assessed for their future risk of fracture by bone densitometry.

The absolute risk of fracture for any individual during the next 10 years will be a consequence of several of these factors, and the contribution to that absolute risk of each of these factors will vary. In an 80-year-old, age and risk of falling are most important, whereas in a 60-year-old, premature oestrogen deficiency and specific conditions such as steroid treated rheumatoid arthritis may be more relevant. The risk associated with some risk factors, such as smoking, is far less than the risk associated with others, such

---

Table 3.2 Clinical risk factors for osteoporosis and fracture

Lifestyle
- Level of physical activity now and in the past
- Dietary calcium intake
- Smoking
- Alcohol consumption (current and past)

General health (past or present)
- Previous fracture(s)
- Comorbidities and general health status
- Corticosteroids (dose and duration)
- Low BMI
- Anorexia or over-exercise
- Height loss in an older person
- Fall history in an older person
- Primary or secondary (<45 years) amenorrhoea
- Male hypogonadism
- Drugs, e.g. sedatives, diuretics, aromatase inhibitors
- Prolonged immobilization – chair or bedbound

Specific conditions
- Endocrine, e.g. hyperparathyroidism, thyroid disease
- Gastrointestinal, e.g. coeliac disease, inflammatory bowel disease, primary biliary cirrhosis
- Rheumatological, e.g. rheumatoid arthritis, ankylosing spondylitis, Ehlers–Danlos syndrome

Family history
- Osteoporosis and low-trauma fracture (maternal hip fracture)

Examination
- Height (compare to that as young adult)
- Weight (BMI)
- Balance and coordination
- 'Get Up and Go' test (see page 67)
- Hypermobility
- Skin laxity

as associated with a previous low-energy trauma fracture. The goal is to develop algorithms that consider all the different risk factors and can enable a person to be given their 10-year probability of fracture. This work is ongoing.

In an individual over 75 years who has sustained a low-energy trauma fracture, the risk of future fracture is high enough that some guidelines, such as the NICE Guidelines in the UK, recommend treatment as it will be cost-effective to prevent further fracture. In younger people, other risk

factors need to be present, including low bone mass, to identify those with a sufficiently high risk to justify treatment. (See also *Table 2.13*.)

Bone mass measurements

The presence of osteoporosis can be determined by bone mineral density. The WHO definition of osteoporosis is based on measurement by dual energy X-ray absorptiometry (DXA) at the hip and lumbar spine. Bone mass accounts for

3.2 Bone mineral density at the hip is a strong predictor of hip fractures in both men and women. The risk is greater at 50 years than 80 years, as other factors become more important in the elderly. (Adapted from Johnell O, *et al.* (2005). Predictive value of BMD for hip and other fractures. *J Bone Mineral Res* **20**(7):1185–1194.)

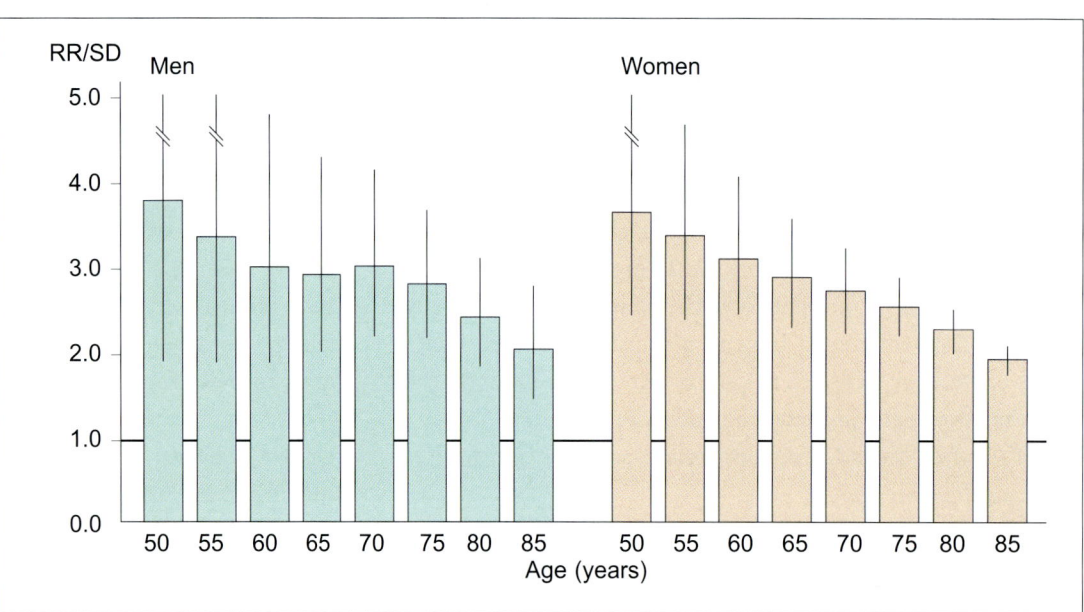

Table 3.3 Bone density measurement: a comparison of methods (including qualitative parameters)

	Osteoporosis (according to WHO definition)	Fracture prediction shown	Defined reference populations	Treatment studies with fracture outcome	Correlation to DXA hip	Estimated cost to acquire (Euro)	Precision	Radiation
DXA hip	+	+	+	+	Reference	70–100,000	0.5–3%	+
DXA spine	+	+	+	+	0.6–0.8	60–90,000	0.5–3%	+
QUS heel	-	+	+	-	0.4–0.7	25–30,0000	1.5–6%	-
DXA heel	-	+	-	-	0.6–0.7	25–30,000	1.2%	+
QUS finger	-	-	-	-	0.2–0.4	9,000	1%	-
QCT	-	-	-	-	0.6–0.7	300,000	2–6%	+++
Radio-grammetry	-	+	-	-	0.4–0.5	NA	1%	+
SPA/SXA	+	+	+	-	0.5–0.6	NA	1–2%	+

DXA of the hip is regarded as the golden standard and it is only DXA of the hip and spine that are thoroughly evaluated in relation to treatment, i.e. pharmacological trials with fracture as end-point

75–90% of the variance of bone strength, and for each decrease of 1 standard deviation in bone density at the proximal femur there is a 2–4-fold increase in fracture risk depending on age (**3.2**).

There are several methods of assessing bone mineral density (*Table 3.3*, **3.3–3.7**). Measurement at any site is the best predictor of fracture at that site, the reason why DXA of the hip and lumbar spine are preferred. Measurement of the lumbar spine is best around 50–65 years, as vertebral factures are most common at an earlier age. The hip is more suitable in older people because the typical age of hip fracture is 80 years and because age-related degenerative changes of the lumbar spine result in overestimates in bone density. Measurement of the total hip by DXA is regarded as most reliable for monitoring bone mass, because of

changes in disc spaces and joints of the lumbar spine with advancing age. The axial skeleton can also be assessed by quantitative computed tomography (QCT).

Other measures of bone density and quality can be made of the peripheral skeleton to predict risk such as peripheral single (SXA) or dual energy (DXA) X-ray absorptiometry, digital X-ray radiogrammetry (DXR), peripheral QCT (pQCT), or quantitative ultrasound (QUS). The specificity of these other methods however, is less than DXA of the lumbar spine or proximal femur for predicting fractures at these sites. They will misclassify people if used alone to diagnose osteoporosis and level of fracture risk. A low bone mass combined with other clinical risk factors identifies those with a significant risk of future fracture in whom treatment is likely to be cost-effective.

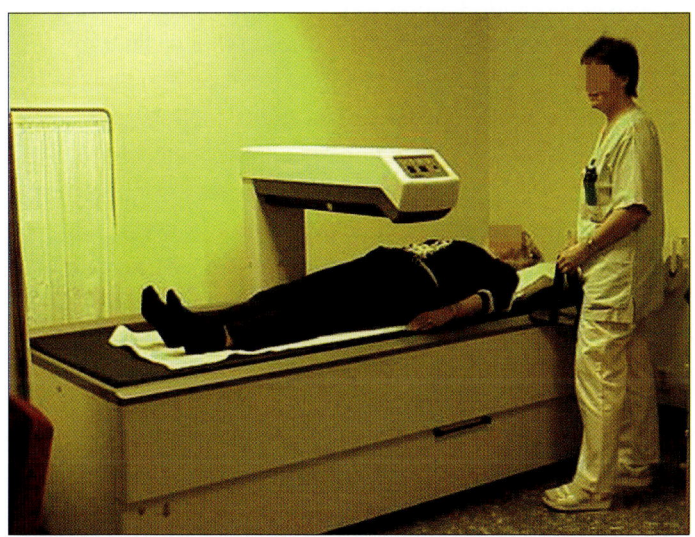

3.3 Dual energy X-ray absorptiometry (DXA) depends on the differential attenuation of low-energy and high-energy X-rays by bone mineral and soft tissues. Either a fan or pencil beam of X-rays is used, with detectors the other side of the object to be measured. The dual energies overcome the problem of differential soft tissue attenuation by allowing for variable thickness of the soft tissues around the bone object being measured, as well as for varying amounts of fat. DXA technology can measure virtually any skeletal site, but the hip and lumbar spine are the preferred sites for diagnosing osteoporosis and predicting risk of the important fractures at those sites. Some machines can also give vertebral morphometry measurements. Whole-body composition can also be measured with some machines. Radiation dosage is low, precision is high.

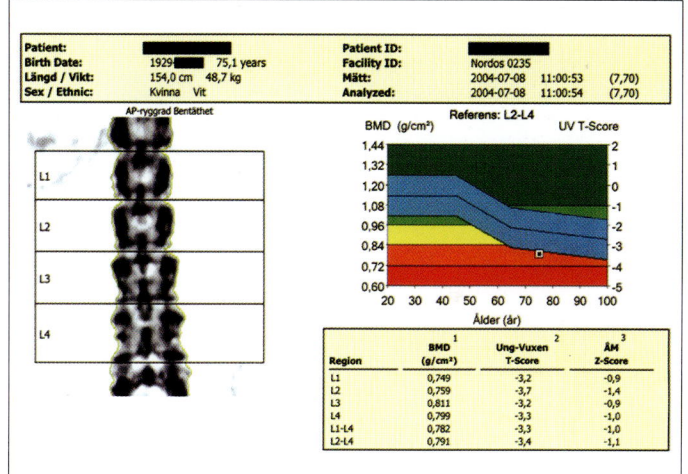

3.4 The usual scans are a postero-anterior view of the lumbar spine and the proximal femur. Various parts of the proximal femur can be analysed separately. These parts vary in the cortical to trabecular bone ratio. Lateral spine DXA is possible with some machines. This enables just the vertebral body to be measured so that the results are not influenced by changes in the posterior elements such as osteophytes, facet joint hypertrophy, and aortic calcification. The bone density measurement, expressed in g/cm^2 (areal density) can be compared to the normal population from large databases. This 'normal' population should relate to the local population. The comparison is expressed as a T-score when comparing it to peak bone mass (the mean bone density of a 35-year-old of the same sex and ethnicity), and as a Z-score when compared to the mean bone density of others of similar age and same sex and ethnicity.

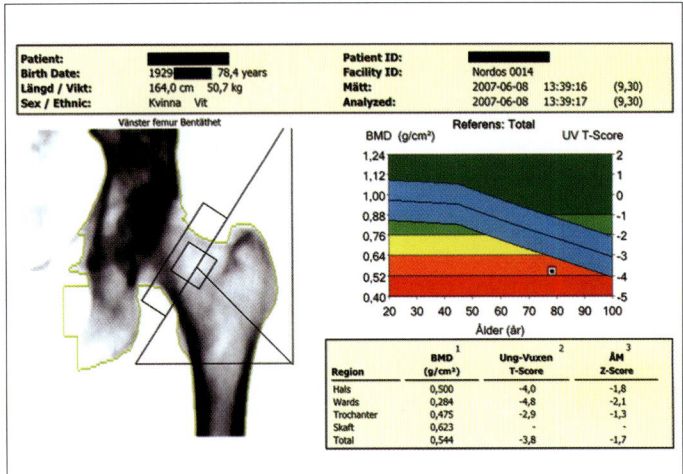

3.5 Hip DXA – print-out from the DXA machine. Measurement of the hip is reported for the total hip and for three standard regions: femoral neck, trochanter and Wards triangle. Total hip and femoral neck are most commonly used for clinical purposes.

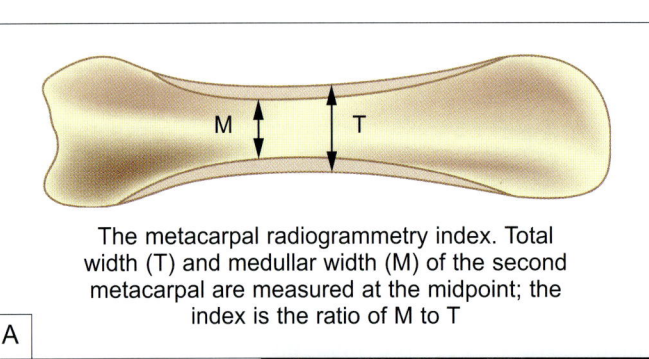

The metacarpal radiogrammetry index. Total width (T) and medullar width (M) of the second metacarpal are measured at the midpoint; the index is the ratio of M to T

A

3.7 X-ray radiogrammetry is one of the oldest methods to estimate bone density. Bone volume is calculated from measurements of cortical thickness of the metacarpals (**A**). A computerized automated analysis has been developed for this method (**B**). It therefore gives a measurement of peripheral bone density.

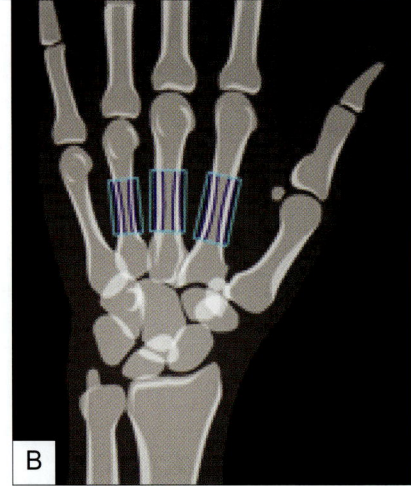

B

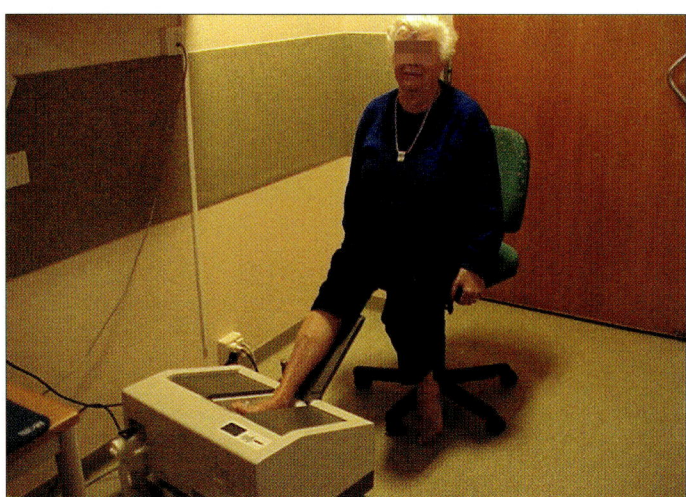

3.6 Ultrasound has been used for many years to study the mechanical properties of various materials in engineering, and it has been developed to study the properties of bone. Clinical ultrasound measures the transmission of high frequency sound through bone. In this clinical application, quantitative ultrasound devices mainly measure the heel as there needs to be minimal and consistent soft tissue covering. The transmission of ultrasound is affected by bone mass, bone structure, and bone material features, and this is used to give a measurement of bone mass and quality. Measurements made are of broadband ultrasound attenuation (BUA) and or speed of sound (SOS). Only peripheral sites can be assessed. Advantages are that the equipment is mobile and does not involve radiation, but there is a lack of standardization between different machines available, and variation limits its use for repeated measurements. QUS measurements correlate with bone density at the same site, but not so well with bone density at other sites and it cannot therefore be used to diagnose osteoporosis which is defined in terms of bone density at the hip or lumbar spine. QUS gives an estimate of hip fracture risk that is, in part, independent of bone density. It may be measuring other aspects of bone quality.

There are several methods of assessing bone strength by measuring various aspects of its structure. Bone densitometry by DXA measures an arial bone density, and the usual sites are the lumbar spine and proximal femur. The WHO definition of osteoporosis is based on this technique. Bone density can also be measured peripherally in the forearm or heel by X-ray absorptiometry, and this correlates with measurements in the spine and hip and predicts fracture risk. QCT, usually of the forearm or lumbar spine, can be used, but exposes the person to more radiation. QUS can be used to measure the quality of bone at several peripheral sites and this predicts fracture; however, QUS does not correlate closely enough with bone density measurements by DXA to be used to diagnose osteoporosis. Radiogrammetry measures the cortical bone in the metacarpals, and this correlates with bone density measured by DXA.

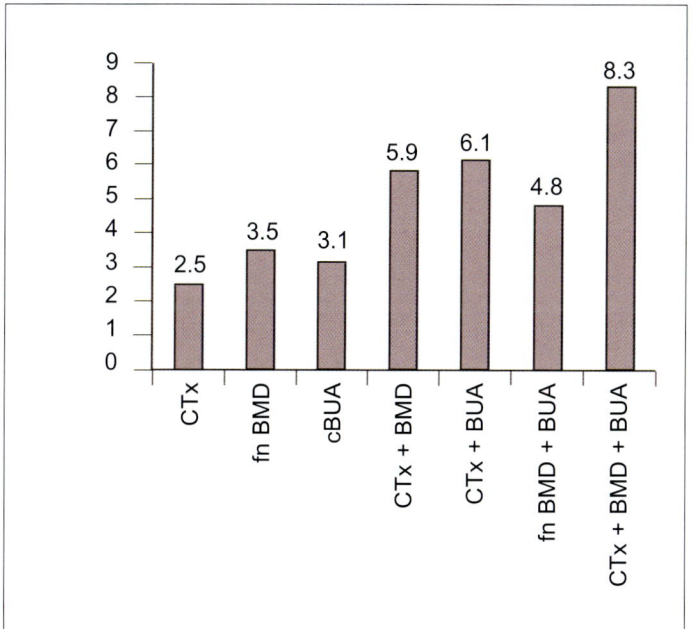

3.8 Prediction of hip fracture – combination of bone resorption marker, bone density and ultrasound. Seventy-five women with hip fracture *vs.* 3 age match controls. (Adapted from Garnero P, *et al.* (1996). Markers of bone resorption predict hip fracture in elderly women: the EPIDOS Prospective Study. *J Bone Mineral Res* **11**(10):1531–1538.)

Bone markers of turnover

Bone loss may be predicted by biochemical markers of high bone turnover (**3.8**). They may be independent measures of future fracture risk, but their predictive power for the individual is poor. Used in combination with bone density, biochemical bone markers are more predictive of fracture and may strengthen the indication for treatment.

Fall risk assessment

Fracture is a result of bone fragility and a force, usually due to a fall. Falls cause other problems in the elderly (see page 14). There are variety of intrinsic and extrinsic risk factors for falls (see *Table 1.4*) and these should be looked for so that those most at risk of falling can be identified (*Table 3.4*, **3.9**, **3.10**). Intrinsic risk factors should be sought by a general examination including checks on pulse, postural blood pressure, vision, and neuromuscular function. A careful description of any fall from the patient or an eyewitness is essential. The drug history is important. A formal home assessment for extrinsic risk factors may be needed, for example by an occupational therapist, if someone is at risk of falling.

   The best predictors of falls are having already experienced a fall in the previous year and decreased neuromuscular function, measured as an inability to rise unaided from a chair without using the arms – the 'Get Up and Go' test. If the person is at high risk of falling, then measures must be taken to reduce that risk (see page 67), by targeting intrinsic and extrinsic risk factors as well as by a general approach to improve muscle strength, balance, and coordination.

Table 3.4 Identifying older people at high risk of falling

- Fallen within 1 year
- Lower limb weakness
- Poor gait
- Impaired balance
- Impaired coordination
- Poor vision
- The 'Get Up and Go Test' (see **3.10**)

Case/risk identification in general services
Ask if fallen in the past year and about frequency, context, and characteristics of the fall

Observe for balance and gait deficit and potential to benefit from interventions to improve balance and mobility

Falls service
All healthcare professionals dealing with patients known to be at risk of falling should develop and maintain basic professional competence in falls assessment and prevention

Primary and community care

Case/risk identified at health screen

Case/risk identified opportunistically at presentation with fall/other problem

Case/risk identified opportunistically at presentation with fall/other problem

Secondary care

Presentation at A&E with fall injury

Multifactorial falls risk assessment
Offer multifactorial falls assessment. This may include:
• Falls history
• Gait, balance, mobility, muscle weakness
• Osteoporosis risk*
• Perceived functional ability
• Fear of falling
• Visual impairment
• Cognitive impairment
• Neurological examination
• Continence
• Home hazard
• Cardiovascular examination
• Medication review

*Refer as necessary

Multifactorial interventions
Offer individualized multifactorial intervention to older people at risk including:
• Strength and balance training
• Home hazard assessment and intervention
• Vision assessment and referral
• Medication review/withdrawal

After medical treatment for injurious fall, patients should be offered multidisciplinary assessment and intervention

Strength and balance training

Home hazard intervention and follow-up

Medication review/withdrawal

Cardiac pacing

Education and information
To promote participation of older people, falls prevention programmes should:
• Discuss changes a person is willing to make to prevent falls
• Information should be relevant and available in languages in addition to English
• Address potential barriers such as low self-efficacy and fear of falling

Programmes should be flexible to accommodate different needs

Information on the following should be provided orally and in writing:
• Measures to prevent falls
• Motivation
• Preventable nature of some falls
• Physical/psychological benefits of modifying risk
• Further advice and assistance
• How to cope with a fall

3.9 Identifying those who have fallen or at high risk is important to preventing falls and consequent injuries. This care pathway has been proposed in the UK NICE Clinical Guideline on the assessment and prevention of falls in older people (November 2004), giving the strength of evidence for the recommendations made (Grade A recommendation based on a meta-analysis of RCT's or at least one RCT down to Grade D based on expert opinions or extrapolated from studies) (*Table 3.5*, page 66). (Adapted 3 NICE (2004). Falls: the Assessment and Prevention of Falls in Older People. NICE Clinical Guideline **21**.)

The specialist services for falls and for osteoporosis should be operationally linked or dovetailed

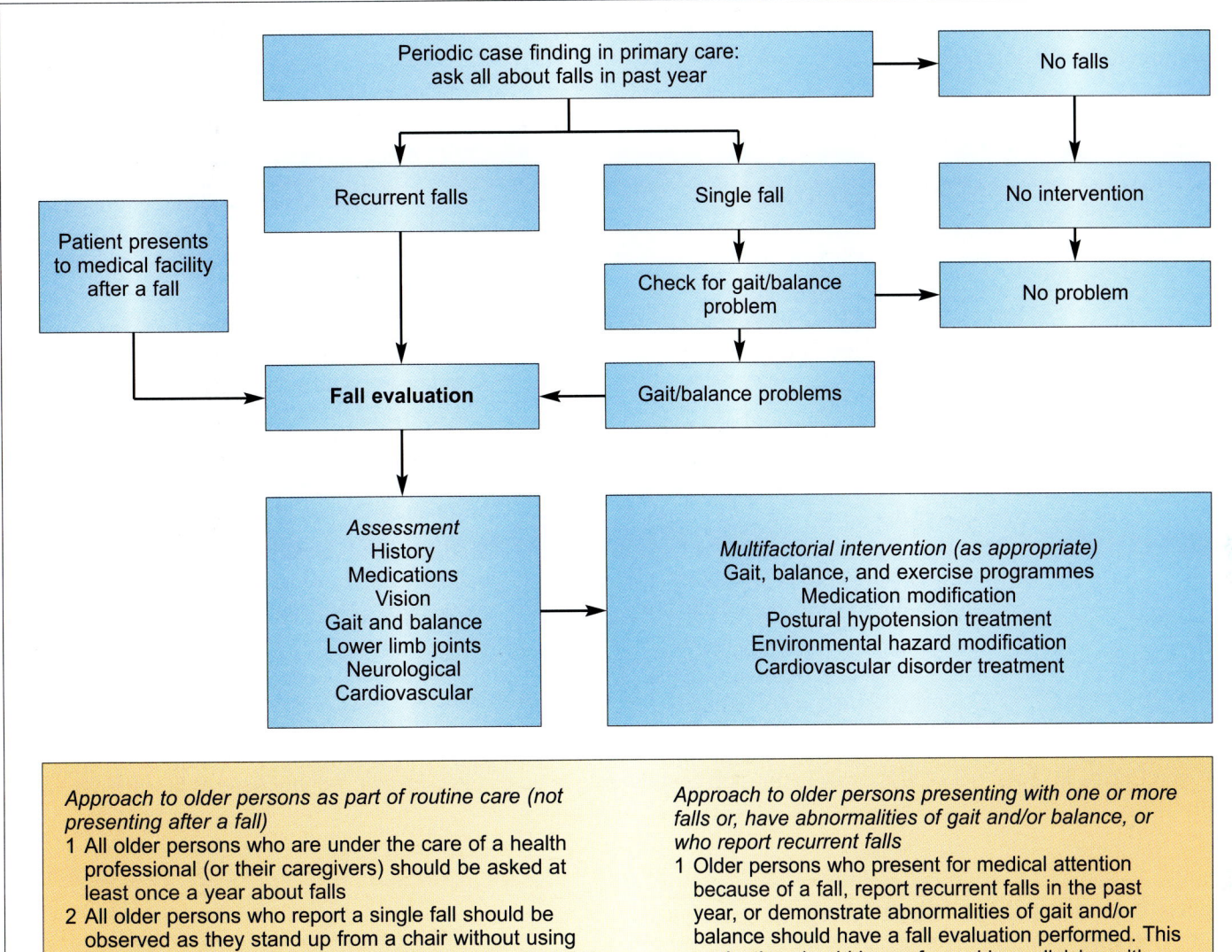

Periodic case finding in primary care:
ask all about falls in past year

No falls

Recurrent falls

Single fall

No intervention

Patient presents
to medical facility
after a fall

Check for gait/balance
problem

No problem

Fall evaluation

Gait/balance problems

Assessment
History
Medications
Vision
Gait and balance
Lower limb joints
Neurological
Cardiovascular

Multifactorial intervention (as appropriate)
Gait, balance, and exercise programmes
Medication modification
Postural hypotension treatment
Environmental hazard modification
Cardiovascular disorder treatment

Approach to older persons as part of routine care (not presenting after a fall)
1 All older persons who are under the care of a health professional (or their caregivers) should be asked at least once a year about falls
2 All older persons who report a single fall should be observed as they stand up from a chair without using their arms, walk several paces, and return (i.e. the 'Get Up and Go Test'). Those demonstrating no difficulty or unsteadiness need no further assessment
3 Persons who have difficulty or demonstrate unsteadiness performing this test require further assessment

Approach to older persons presenting with one or more falls or, have abnormalities of gait and/or balance, or who report recurrent falls
1 Older persons who present for medical attention because of a fall, report recurrent falls in the past year, or demonstrate abnormalities of gait and/or balance should have a fall evaluation performed. This evaluation should be performed by a clinician with appropriate skills and experience, which may necessitate referral to a specialist (e.g. geriatrician)
2 A fall evaluation is defined as an assessment that includes the following: a history of fall circumstances, medications, acute or chronic medical problems, and mobility levels; an examination of vision, gait and balance, and lower extremity joint function; an examination of basic neurological function, including mental status, muscle strength, lower extremity peripheral nerves, proprioception, reflexes, tests of cortical, extrapyramidal, and cerebellar function; and assessment of basic cardiovascular status including heart rate and rhythm, postural pulse and blood pressure and, if appropriate, heart rate and blood pressure responses to carotid sinus stimulation

3.10 The guideline for the prevention of falls in older persons of the American Geriatrics Society, British Geriatrics Society, and American Academy of Orthopaedic Surgeons Panel on Falls Prevention recommends a simple regular assessment to identify those at risk of falling and a full assessment for those who have already sustained a fall. (Adapted from AGS, BGS, AAOS Panel on Falls Prevention (2001).Guideline for the Prevention of Falls in Older Persons. *J Am Geriatr Soc* **49**(5):664–672.)

Table 3.5 The grading of evidence: a scheme for the hierarchy of evidence for developing recommendations in guidelines

Recommendation grade	Evidence	Evidence category	
A	Directly based on category I evidence	I	Evidence from: • Meta-analysis of randomized controlled trials, or • At least one randomized controlled trial
B	Directly based on: • Category II evidence, or • Extrapolated recommendation from category I evidence	II	Evidence from: • At least one controlled study without randomization, or • At least one other type of quasi-experimental study
C	Directly based on: • Category III evidence, or • Extrapolated recommendation from category I or II evidence	III	Evidence from nonexperimental descriptive studies, such as comparative studies, correlation studies and case–control studies
D	Directly based on: • Category IV evidence, or • Extrapolated recommendation from category I, II, or III evidence	IV	Evidence from expert committee reports or opinions and/or clinical experience of respected authorities
GPP	Recommended good practice based on clinical experience of the Guideline Development Group		

(Adapted from NICE (2004). Falls: the Assessment and Prevention of Falls in Older People. NICE Clinical Guideline 21; and Eccles M, Mason J (2001). How to develop cost-conscious guidelines. *Health Technol Assess* 5(16):1–69.)

Fracture probability: identifying who to treat

The methods described above can be used to estimate patients at highest risk of osteoporosis and fracture and whether they will benefit from treatment. The higher the risk, the more cost-effective is the treatment and there is therefore potentially more to be gained from intervention (see Chapter 4). However, no method of assessing risk has both good sensitivity and specificity and many fractures will occur in people who it is not possible to identify from these known risk factors. Because of this and because osteoporosis and fracture are so common, people at all ages should maximize their bone strength and try to reduce their risk of future fracture. It is essential that all of us take at least some measures to avoid future fracture.

The practicality of finding those at highest risk needs to be considered. Screening the whole population has been shown to be inefficient; large resources will be needed to find a few people, many of whom may not want to undertake long-term treatment. A sequential approach can be used, first identifying clinical risk factors in those who are willing and able to undertake treatment, and then confirming the size of the risk by bone density assessment if there is uncertainty (**3.11, 3.12**). For example, the risk may be sufficient to justify treatment in an elderly person starting high-dose glucocorticoid treatment or an elderly person with several vertebral fractures, but may not be sufficient without confirmation of underlying osteoporosis in a 60-year-old woman who has sustained a Colles' fracture.

A WHO fracture risk assessment tool has been recently developed based on population-based cohorts from different countries that estimates the 10-year probability of major osteoporotic fracture[2]. It is based on clinical risk factors and bone density at the femoral neck. It is available as a computer-driven tool and can be accessed at http://www.shef.ac.uk/FRAX/.

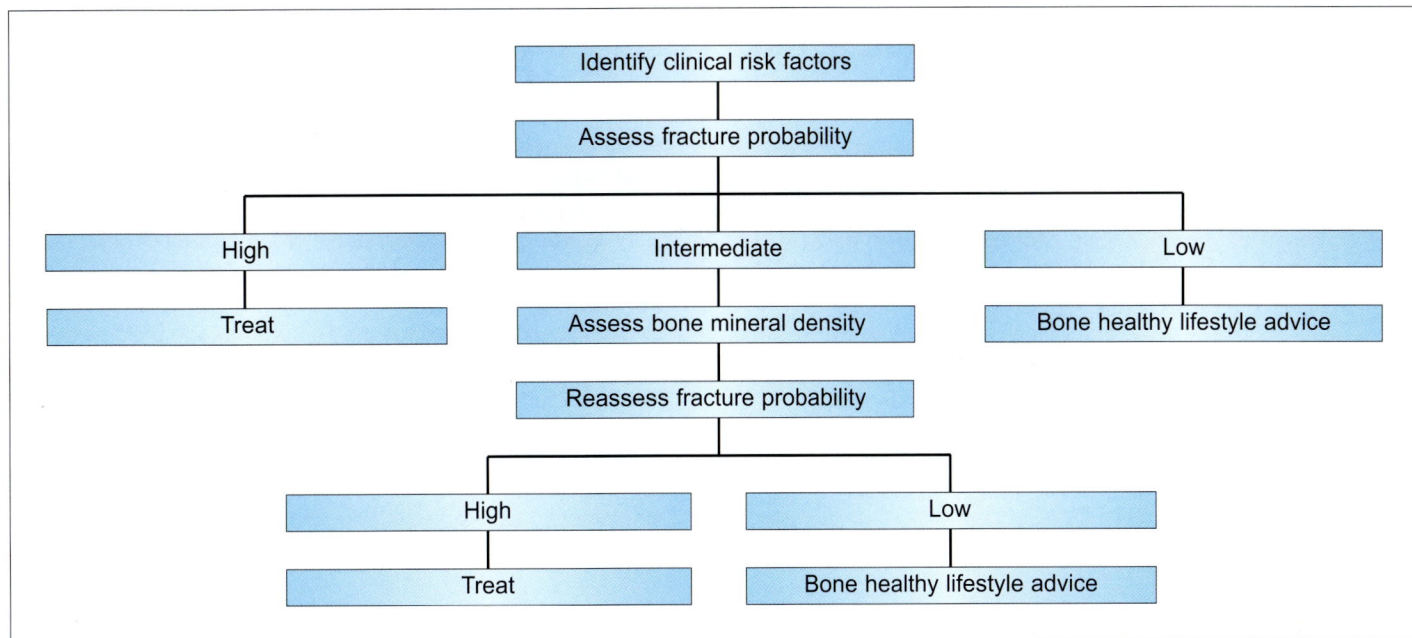

3.11 A sequential approach can be used to identify those at the highest risk of fracture. If there is concern about the risk of future fracture, then clinical risk factors can be used to separate those with a sufficiently high risk to justify treatment and those with a low risk who should follow a bone healthy lifestyle (see Chapter 4). There will be many where a bone density assessment will contribute to the risk assessment.

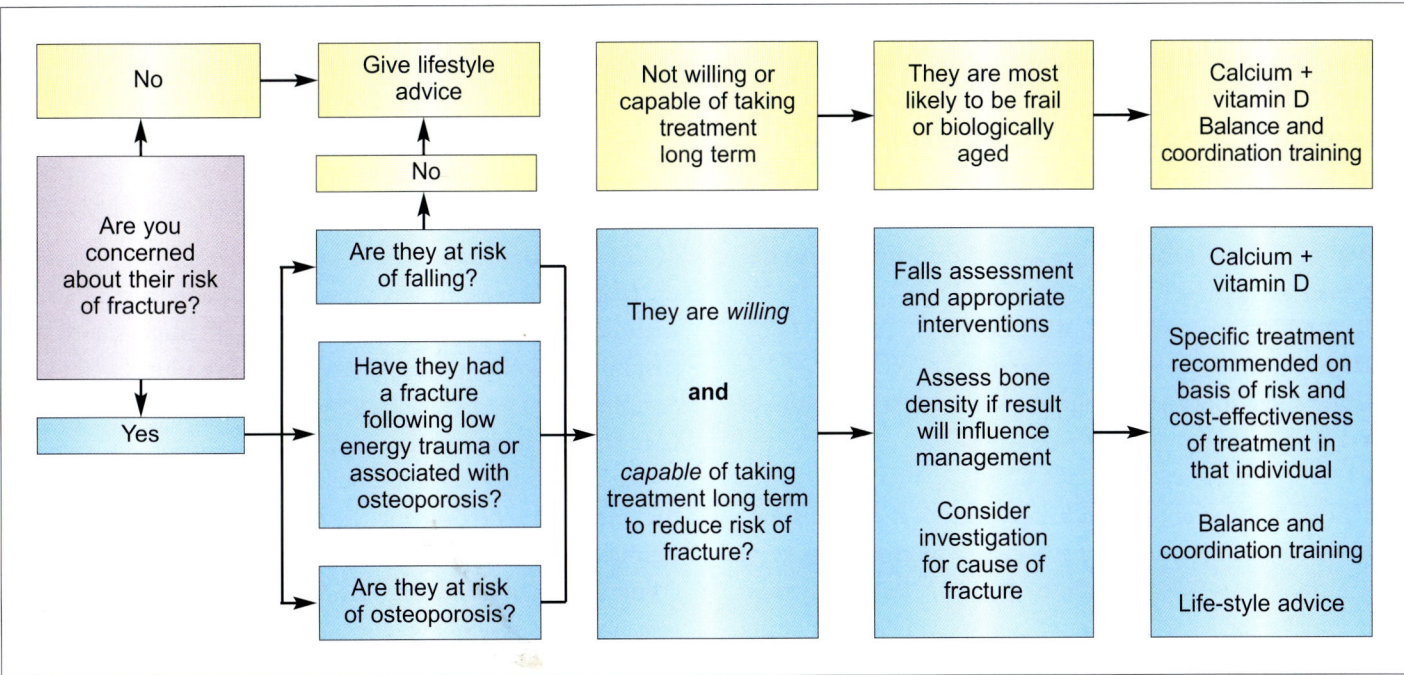

3.12 This flow chart can be used to aid clinical decision making. Those who are not willing or capable of taking a treatment are likely to be the frail elderly and measures should be taken to improve balance and coordination; and correct any dietary lack of calcium or vitamin D deficiency. If the person is considered to be at sufficient risk from clinical risk factors alone, then a bone density measurement is not needed as it will not affect any clinical decision about treatment. The IOF One-Minute Test (**3.13**) can be used to help identify those with clinical risk factors who need further assessment. (Adapted from Woolf AD, Akesson K (2003). Preventing fractures in elderly people. *BMJ* **327**(7406):89–95.)

Are you at risk of osteoporosis?
Take the One-Minute Osteoporosis Risk Test

1 Have either of your parents broken a hip after a minor bump or fall?
  ❑ Yes   ❑ No

2 Have you broken a bone after a minor bump or fall?
  ❑ Yes   ❑ No

3 Have you taken corticosteroid tablets (cortisone, prednisone, etc) for more than 3 months?
  ❑ Yes   ❑ No

4 Have you lost more than 3 cm (just over an inch) in height?
  ❑ Yes   ❑ No

5 Do you regularly drink heavily (in excess of safe drinking limits)?
  ❑ Yes   ❑ No

6 Do you smoke than 20 cigarettes a day?
  ❑ Yes   ❑ No

7 Do you suffer frequently from diarrhoea (caused by problems such coeliac disease or Crohn's disease)?
  ❑ Yes   ❑ No

For women:
8 Did you undergo menopause before the age of 45?
  ❑ Yes   ❑ No

9 Have your periods stopped for 12 months or more (other than because of pregnancy)?
  ❑ Yes   ❑ No

For men:
10 Have you ever suffered from impotence, lack of libido or other symptoms related to low testosterone level?
  ❑ Yes   ❑ No

If you answered 'yes' to any of these questions, it does not mean that you have osteoporosis. Diagnosis of osteoporosis can only be made by a physician through a bone density test.

We recommend that you show this test to your doctor, who will advise whether further tests are necessary. The good news is that osteoporosis can be diagnosed easily and treated.

Talk to your local osteoporosis society about what changes you might make in your lifestyle to reduce osteoporosis risk. You can contact your national osteoporosis society via: www.osteofound.org

3.13 The One-Minute Osteoporosis Risk test, developed by the International Osteoporosis Foundation, can be used to identify those who may have osteoporosis and be at risk of fracture. It can be used to identify those who need a bone density assessment as part of their risk assessment. (http://www.osteofound.org/osteoporosis/risk_test.html)

Assessing a person with osteoporosis and fracture

There are three reasons to assess someone who has sustained a fracture.
- To establish the impact on the person.
- To establish the cause of the fracture.
- To estimate the risk of recurrence and whether treatment is indicated to reduce that risk.

For this a medical and social history, physical examination, and some investigations are necessary. A person presenting with a fracture is in pain with the sudden loss of function. This may be the sudden onset of back pain following lifting something heavy and awkwardly or may be the sudden onset of groin pain with inability to walk following a fall, such as tripping over a rug. The severity of pain needs to be recognized to ensure it is effectively controlled. The impact on the quality of life in the short-, medium- and long-term must also be monitored, and rehabilitation techniques as well as good fracture management be used to minimize this. A strong focus on the individual and their pain and quality

of life is needed, rather than just on the healing process of the fracture or treating any underlying osteoporosis. Patients want to be independent and mobile, although many who sustain an osteoporotic fracture may have already lost this. Simple pain charts and quality of life instruments can be used to help with assessing the impact.

The cause of fracture should be considered. What were the circumstances of the fracture? Was it related to a significant degree of force that you would expect to result in a fracture, such as a down the stairs, or was it a low-energy trauma, such as tripping over a rug, that suggests underlying bone fragility? Was it spontaneous without any force apart from normal loading? Fractures following significant trauma do not suggest any underlying skeletal cause and prevention of recurrent fractures would relate to reducing the risk of accidents, not by increasing skeletal strength. Fractures occurring spontaneously are indicative of an underlying skeletal problem. This is most typical of pathological fractures in the appendicular skeleton or vertebral fractures in an osteoporotic skeleton. Fractures occurring following low-energy trauma, typically affecting the appendicular skeleton, may indicate reduced skeletal strength.

However, such low-energy fractures may also relate to the characteristics of the forces applied upon the bone at the time of trauma, and further evaluation of bone strength by densitometry is needed to ascertain the likely predominant cause. If due to underlying bone weakness, then treatment is indicated to improve bone strength to prevent further fracture. The occurrence of a low-energy fracture in the presence of reduced bone density is a strong predictor of further fracture. Other causes of spontaneous or low-energy fractures must also be considered such as osteomalacia and infiltrative lesions such as primary and secondary bone cancer and bone cysts (*Table 3.6*). This may require investigation (*Table 3.7, 3.8*). If the fracture relates to underlying osteoporosis, then causes of this need to be considered and looked for (*Table 2.13*). It is more frequent

to identify a secondary cause in men with osteoporosis. It must not be forgotten that the person presenting with a low-energy fracture is likely to have fallen, and correctable causes need to be looked for and dealt with, if possible.

If someone over the age of 75 years sustains a low-trauma fracture, the likelihood of this being related to underlying osteoporosis is high; this may be sufficient to be an indication for long-term pharmacological treatment to reduce the risk of another fracture. Vertebral fractures at this older age are, in particular, usually associated with underlying osteoporosis. These fractures, however, need to be confirmed on X-ray as loss of height at this age is frequently due to degenerative disc disease and not loss of vertebral body height due to fracture.

The need for treatment to prevent a further fracture may be guided by establishing the reasons for fracture. If bone strength is reduced, then the target for therapy is to improve that, whereas if bone strength is good but the person has

---

Table 3.6 Differential diagnosis of low-trauma fracture and vertebral deformity

Low-trauma fracture
- Osteoporosis
- Metastatic malignancy
- Myeloma
- Osteomalacia
- Paget's disease
- Osteomyelitis
- Bone cyst

Vertebral deformity
- Osteoporosis
- Metastatic malignancy
- Myeloma
- Osteomalacia
- Paget's disease
- Osteomyelitis
- Traumatic vertebral fracture earlier in life
- Scheuermann's osteochondritis of the spine

Table 3.7 Investigation of osteoporosis

Baseline
- Examination:
  - Look for features of secondary causes of osteoporosis
- Haematology:
  - Full blood count
  - ESR
- Biochemistry:
  - Serum calcium, phosphate
  - Serum alkaline phosphatase
  - Serum creatinine
  - Serum albumin
  - Testosterone and SHBG in men (not very elderly)

Further assessment in selected patients
- Liver function tests
- Serum protein electrophoresis
- Gonadotrophins
- Vitamin D metabolites
- Thyroid function tests
- Urine Bence–Jones protein

Investigation of fracture or bone pain
- Full examination, in particular breasts or prostate
- X-ray of affected site
- Further imaging:
  - Isotope bone scan if any concern of metastases
  - CT scan or MRI to characterize lesion
- Biochemistry:
- Serum protein electrophoresis
  - Urine Bence–Jones protein
  - PSA in men with vertebral fractures

Table 3.8 Typical biochemical changes in bone conditions

Disease	Plasma calcium	Plasma phosphate	Plasma alkaline phosphatase	Viscosity or ESR	Other investigations
Osteoporosis	N	N	N	N	DXA
Osteomalacia	N or ↓	N or ↓	N or ↑	N	Serum vitamin D; bone biopsy
Paget's disease	N or ↑	N	↑	N	
Primary hyperthyroidism	↑	N or ↓	N or ↑	N	PTH↑
Myeloma	N or ↑	N or ↑	N or ↑	N or ↑	Serum protein electrophoresis; urine Bence–Jones protein
Malignancy	N or ↑	N	N or ↑	N or ↑	Breast examination; PSA; chest x-ray; bone scintigraphy; MRI

frequent falls, then a fall prevention programme is needed. These approaches are not usually mutually exclusive. Anyone who is a frequent faller needs as strong a skeleton as possible and someone with osteoporosis needs to take care to avoid any significant trauma.

Methods of monitoring treatment

The aim of treatment is to reduce the occurrence of fractures, but the end-point of fracture is too late for the individual. Reducing risk is measurable in a population but is not as meaningful for the individual, because it is not easy to appreciate an event which has not happened.

When evaluating the efficacy of any new treatment for osteoporosis, the key outcome measure that is required is evidence of fracture prevention. In clinical trials, therefore, fracture rates are the primary outcome. A surrogate end-point of bone mineral density (BMD) is often used for shorter and small studies as changes in a treatment group can be seen in months, BMD correlates with bone strength, and the absolute value of BMD reflects fracture risk. However, changes in BMD with treatment such as bisphosphonates only explains a minority of the observed reduction in fracture risk. In addition, the correlation of BMD with bone strength and fracture rate are not perfect. This limits the role of BMD in assessing the effectiveness of any treatment both in clinical trials and in the management of the individual patient. Changes in BMD do reflect a treatment response and can be used to assess if the patient is responding in any way. The interpretation is, however, difficult as a lack of increase in

BMD will not necessarily mean that there is no reduction in fracture risk. In addition, for the individual, the rate of change in bone mass and the precision of the measurement, although very good, means that it is not meaningful to monitor their response by bone densitometry except in the long-term, at intervals of at least 2 years, but preferably 4–6 years.

Falls should be monitored and reasons of any falls need to be looked for and modified if possible. Bone markers are, as yet, of limited value in the routine monitoring of individuals. Of particular interest is their use to look at the patient's early response to therapy and check upon concordance with treatment.

The general fitness and wellbeing of the person with osteoporosis needs to be monitored as they are often frail individuals with other pathologies. Comorbidity is an indicator of poor outcome following a fall or fracture. It is also important to monitor their quality of life. A key goal of treating osteoporosis and preventing fracture is to enable the person to have a good quality of life, avoiding dependency and maintaining mobility.

References

1 van Staa TP, Dennison EM, Leufkens HG, Cooper C (2001). Epidemiology of fractures in England and Wales. *Bone* **29**(6):517–522.
2 Kanis JA, Oden A, Johnell O, *et al.* (2007). The use of clinical risk factors enhances the performance of BMD in the prediction of hip and osteoporotic fractures in men and women. *Osteoporos Int* **18**:1033–46.

Chapter 4

Management of osteoporosis

Introduction

Bone loss with ageing is universal and many will become osteoporotic in later life with increased risk of fracture. Measures therefore need to be taken by all to maximize bone mass and strength at all ages and to reduce risk of injuries when older. This needs to be at all stages of life. In this chapter we review the lifestyle interventions that all should follow to reduce risk at the population level. Some people are at greater risk and have most to lose if they do sustain a fracture and most to gain by preventative measures. For them, a more effective intervention may be appropriate. We have considered how to identify such individuals at most risk and in the next chapter chapter we review the evidence of what specific interventions will increase bone density and reduce fracture risk.

When assessing the evidence for the effectiveness of any intervention, there are several issues that need to be considered: (1) the characteristics of the study population compared with the target population; (2) the level of risk of the study population for sustaining a fracture; and (3) were the outcome measures used meaningful and standard? Bone density changes are a surrogate for the clinically relevant goal of fracture prevention. Studies to demonstrate fracture prevention have to be very large and over long periods of time and, as a consequence, data are deficient for some interventions. There are few comparative studies of the different treatments. For lifestyle risk factors, evidence of increased risk of osteoporosis or fracture does not mean that correcting the risk factor will necessarily reduce that risk – direct evidence of efficacy is needed although often the appropriate studies have not been done. A difficulty of epidemiological studies is that the various lifestyle factors are confounders of each other as, for example, many

smokers also consume alcohol, are thin, and are less physically active. Concordance is very important when considering if an intervention will be effective in clinical practice in contrast to a clinical trial. This is very important when treatment has to be long term and there is no easily recognized clinical response to encourage the person to continue with treatment.

It is important to remember that treatment of osteoporosis is not just about prevention of another fracture. Many patients will have already sustained a fracture and they require optimal fracture management and rehabilitation to minimize the impact in the short and long term.

LIFESTYLE INTERVENTIONS

Increase in life expectancy is the result of increased economic wealth and improved health care from birth onwards. However, increased wealth has also brought lifestyle changes such as urbanization, a more sedentary way of living, poor diet, smoking, and alcohol abuse, which counteract bone health. Undernutrition in developing countries and the fashion for excessive thinness in westernized countries also increase the risks of osteoporosis and future fracture. Maintaining a bone healthy lifestyle at all ages (*Table 4.1*) is an important part of mitigating the expected increase in osteoporosis and fracture in all countries, but is most important where change is likely to be greatest.

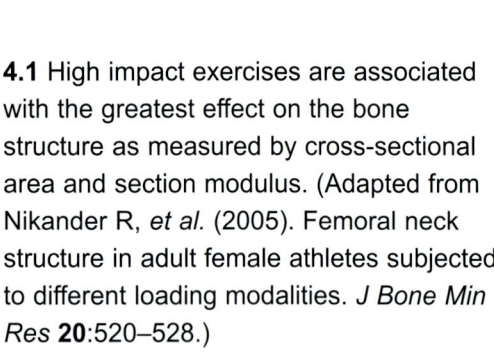

Table 4.1 Bone healthy lifestyle

- Adequate dietary calcium
- Adequate vitamin D through diet `and sunlight exposure
- Regular weight bearing exercise
- Avoid smoking
- Avoid excess alcohol

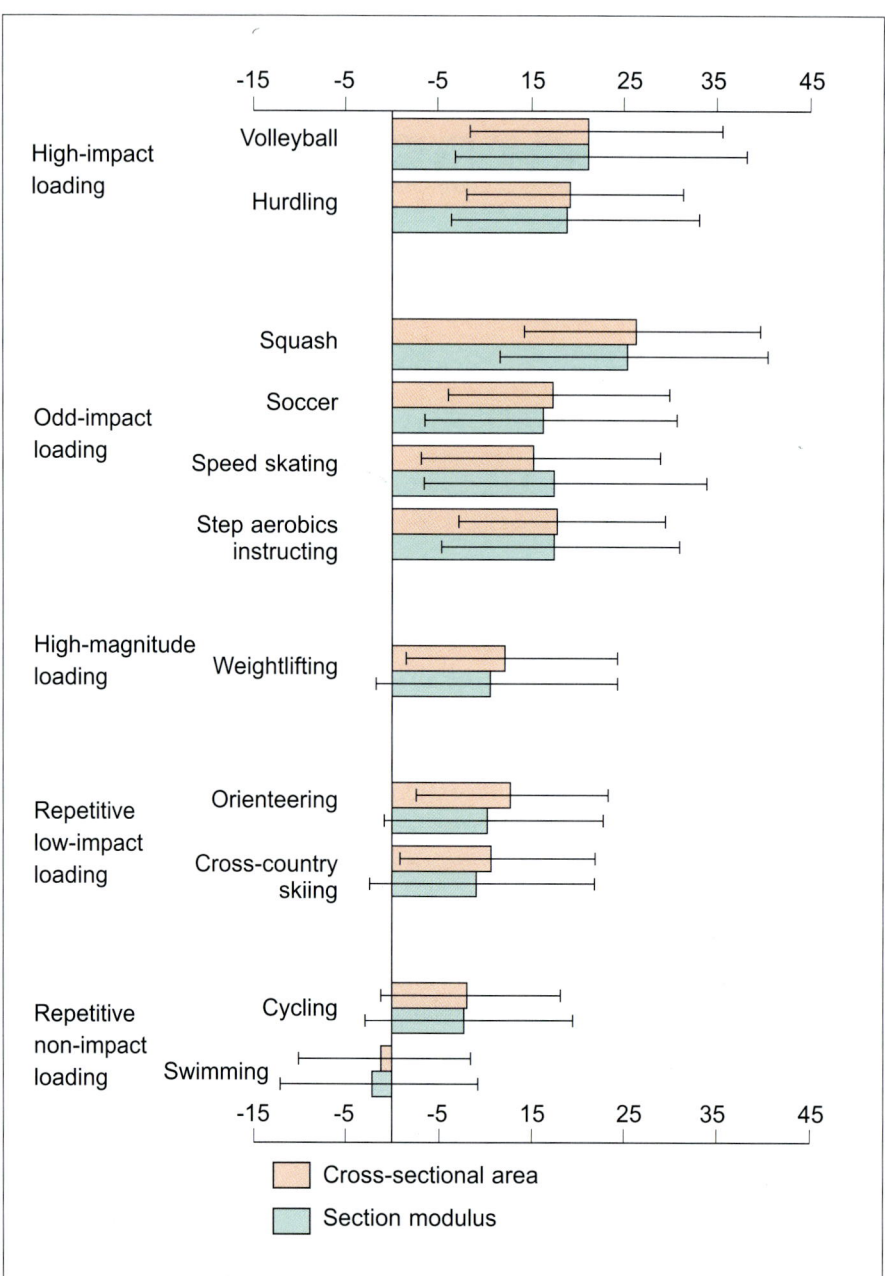

4.1 High impact exercises are associated with the greatest effect on the bone structure as measured by cross-sectional area and section modulus. (Adapted from Nikander R, *et al.* (2005). Femoral neck structure in adult female athletes subjected to different loading modalities. *J Bone Min Res* **20**:520–528.)

Physical activity and exercise

Maintaining a strong skeleton at all ages relies on mechanical stimuli from weight bearing and physical activity. The risk of falling is reduced by maintaining physical fitness. Risk of fracture is increased in those physically inactive; walking for 4 hours a week was found to be associated with a 41% lower risk of hip fracture in postmenopausal women aged 40–77 years[1]. Immobility, such as bed rest, rapidly causes bone loss that can only be slowly regained. People are, however, becoming less physically active and fit in all countries and cultures. It is estimated that 17% of adults in the world are physically inactive and only an average of 41% of adults are doing some, but insufficient physical activity (<2.5 hours per week of moderate activity)[2]. Physical activity declines with ageing.

Physical activity increases bone mass, density, quality, and strength. The benefit of physical activity is greatest at or before puberty[3]. The response of the skeleton in adulthood to physical activity is less but maintenance of, or increases in, bone density has been demonstrated with impact and nonimpact exercise regimes in pre- and postmenopausal women[4-6]. A greater benefit is seen in those with high calcium intake[7]. The effect of exercise is site specific, benefiting most the loaded site, but the characteristics of the exercise that is most effective is not clear. Impact type sports are probably best at improving bone strength, such as tennis, aerobics, basketball, gymnastics, or weight training (4.1), and for older people brisk walking and using stairs are probably of benefit. The frequency and duration required are unclear. The long-term benefits are uncertain; in some studies stopping exercise has shown that the bone density returns to baseline levels[8]. Whether the improvements in bone density translate into a reduction in fracture risk is not yet established.

Although physical exercise programs may only increase bone mass by a marginal percent, the additional benefits from improved gait, balance, coordination, and muscle strength contribute to a potential antifracture effect. Poor balance and quadriceps weakness are predictors of falls and fracture. Programmes of muscle strengthening and balance retraining, individually prescribed by a trained health professional and Tai Chi exercises are likely to prevent falls in elderly people[9], but there is little evidence for other forms of exercise. Although these measures may prevent falls, there is little evidence that this results in prevention of fractures. Epidemiological studies do, however, show that past and present physical activity does relate dose dependently to risk of hip fracture.

From these studies it is recommended to be physically active at all stages of life, with vigorous activities in early years and moderate activity in older life such as regular brisk walking of at least 30 minutes daily (4.2). Greatest benefits are during growth and development, and establishing lifelong exercise habits will have long-term benefit. Those who are less active, especially the sedentary elderly, will also benefit from increasing their level of physical activity. To be effective, physical activity should be weight bearing, easy, enjoyable, sociable, and fit into everyday routines so that it is sustainable throughout life. There are also other health benefits of increasing physical fitness such as reducing the risk of heart disease. The utility of a formal exercise intervention beyond this in maintaining or increasing bone mass and reducing fractures in later life in the general population is problematic, as long-term sustainability is necessary for real benefits and the best way to influence such behaviour is not clear[10].

Diet, nutrition, and body weight

Body weight and nutrition are important determinant of bone mineral density (BMD) and risk of fracture and their outcome. They are important at all stages of life. Bone density is closely related to body weight[11] in men and women across all ages and throughout the skeleton. Changes in bone density also relate to body weight: the risk of hip fracture is greater with low body weight and with weight loss[12,13]. Women who were relatively thin when 50–64 years and had lost at least 10% of their body weight had the highest risk of hip fracture[12]. The fracture risk is in part related to osteoporosis and bone strength, but also to less protective soft tissue. Anorexia nervosa can be associated with severe osteoporosis and premature occurrence of fractures (see 2.41), which is a consequence of poor nutrition, low body weight, and sex hormone deficiency.

Normal nutrition is important for the development and maintenance of the skeleton (*Table 4.2*). Undernutrition is associated with a reduced peak bone mass and acceleration of age-related bone loss[14,15]. People with hip fracture are often under- or malnourished. Undernutrition may increase the propensity to falls, possibly a consequence of impaired

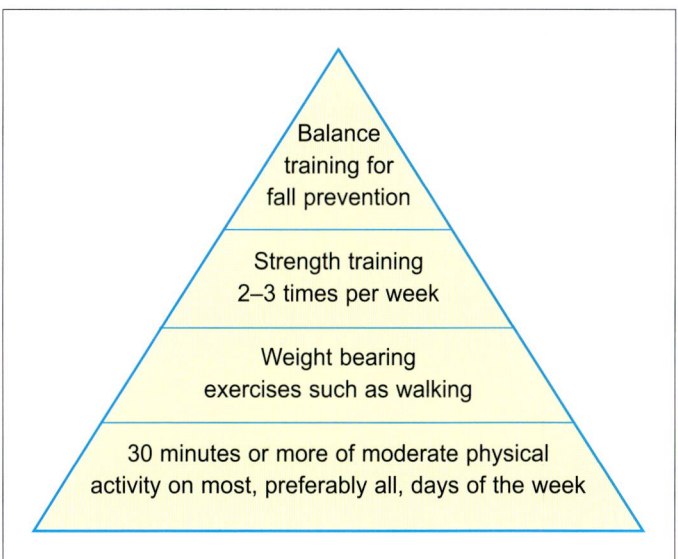

4.2 General recommendations for physical activity in adults. (Adapted from U.S. Department of Health and Human Services (2004). *Bone Health and Osteoporosis: A Report of the Surgeon General*. Rockville MD: Department of Health and Human Services, Office of the Surgeon General.)

coordination and reduced muscle strength. The consequences of falls are worse due to less protective soft tissue, and the outcome following fracture is worse with prolonged hospital stays, more complications, and increased mortality. Undernutrition increases with advancing age and may relate to the spontaneous reduction of food intake, to malabsorption, or to intercurrent illnesses. Protein–calorie malnutrition is the most common problem in the elderly but there are also deficiencies in micronutrients such as calcium and vitamin D (see below). Low intakes of vitamin K may also increase the risk of hip fracture in women. Low body weight and undernutrition are also associated with comorbidity and general frailty in an ageing population, all of which will increase the risk of fracture and worsen the outcome.

Ensuring adequate nutrition with a balanced diet to provide the needed macro- and micronutrients and that will maintain an ideal body weight is therefore recommended[16] (*Table 4.3*). Although energy requirements decrease with advancing age, the recommended dietary allowance of protein increases from 0.8 g/kg of body weight in young adults to 1 g/kg in the healthy elderly. Protein supplementation in patients with recent hip fracture has been shown to improve the clinical outcome with reduction in complications, shorter hospital stays, and reduced subsequent bone loss[14,15]. Dietary protein intake has also been shown to be associated with a reduced risk of hip fracture in men and women aged 50–69 years[17]. The role of other nutritional supplements is not clear. Phytoestrogens are plant products with some oestrogen-like structures and actions including the potential to act on bone. They may have a role in preventing osteoporosis and fracture but there is presently a lack of data on efficacy.

Smoking

Smoking carries a moderate and dose-dependent risk for osteoporosis and fracture[18–20]. In a longitudinal population-based cohort study of men first enrolled at 50 years and followed for 27 years, the risk of any fracture increased linearly with smoking up to about 25 pack-years. At higher rates of consumption there was no further substantial increase in fracture risk per pack-year (**4.3**)[21]. Reduced bone mass has been shown in different populations around the globe[22] at all sites, most marked at the hip[23]. This will increase the risk of fracture; it is estimated that smoking

---

Table 4.2 Nutrition and bone

Undernutrition in older persons:
- Spontaneous reduction in food intake
- Malabsorption
- Intercurrent illness
- Protein–calorie malnutrition most common problem

Effects of undernutrition:
- Reduced peak bone mass
- Accelerated age-dependent bone loss
- Hip fracture cases are often under- or malnourished
- Increased risk of falling
- Impaired coordination
- Reduced muscle strength
- Consequences of falls worse due to less protective soft tissues
- Outcome of fracture worse with increased morbidity and mortality

---

Table 4.3 Nutrients of importance for bone health

Convincing evidence of association with decreased risk of osteoporotic fracture:
- Calcium
- Vitamin D

Possible association with decreased risk of osteoporotic fracture:
- Protein
- Phytoestrogens
- Fruits and vegetables

Plausible association with decreased risk of osteoporotic fracture:
- Zinc
- Copper
- Manganese
- Boron
- Vitamin A
- Vitamin C
- Vitamin K
- B vitamins
- Potassium
- Sodium

(Adapted from: WHO (2003). Diet, nutrition and the prevention of chronic diseases. *WHO Technical Report Series* No. **916**. World Health Organization, Geneva.)

increases the lifetime risk of hip fracture by 31% in women and 40% in men[23]. The increased risk of fracture has been demonstrated at all sites in both men and women, and is greatest for hip fracture, with estimates of a relative risk of 1.84 (95% CI 1.52–2.22). This increased risk is not only explained by effects on bone density and body mass index (BMI)[20]. Past smokers are at intermediate risk[19] and it would, therefore, appear that stopping smoking will reduce the risk of osteoporosis and fracture. However, the benefit may not be seen for 10 years in women[24] but could be up to 30 years in men[21] (**4.4**).

Alcohol

Alcohol affects bone metabolism, whether acute or chronic consumption, moderate or excessive. Chronic alcohol abuse is associated with osteoporosis and fracture, and is a common cause of secondary osteoporosis in men. An increase in osteoporotic (RR 1.38, 95% CI 1.16–1.65) and hip fractures (RR 1.68, 95% CI 1.19–2.336) was found in an analysis of several large population studies[25]. The risk of fracture increases with alcohol intake above a threshold of 2 units daily in both men and women in a study of three

4.3 Risk of fracture associated with smoking in a longitudinal population-based cohort study of men. (Adapted from Olofsson H, *et al.* (2005). Smoking and the risk of fracture in older men. *J Bone Min Res* **20**:1208–1215.)

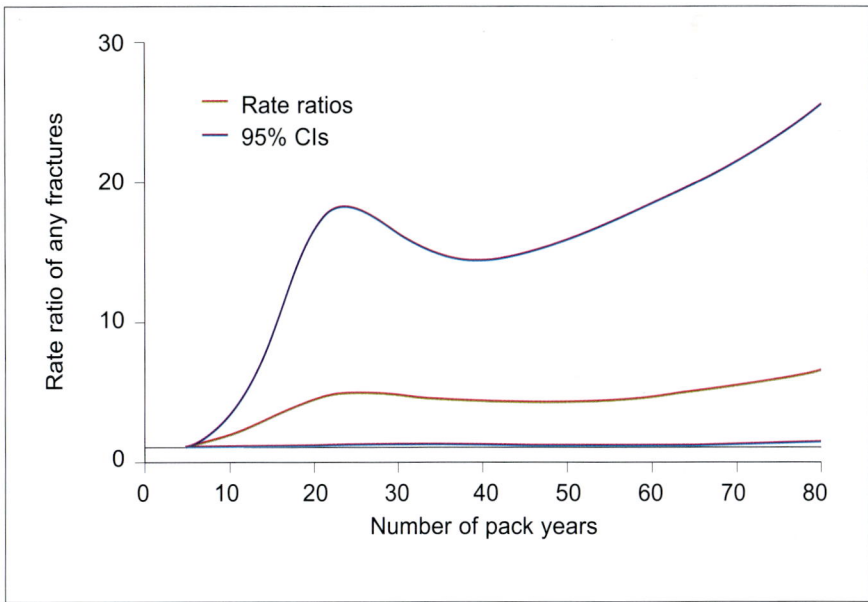

4.4 Risk of fracture following smoking cessation in a longitudinal population-based cohort study of men. (Adapted from Olofsson H, *et al.* (2005). Smoking and the risk of fracture in older men *J Bone Min Res* **20**:1208–1215.)

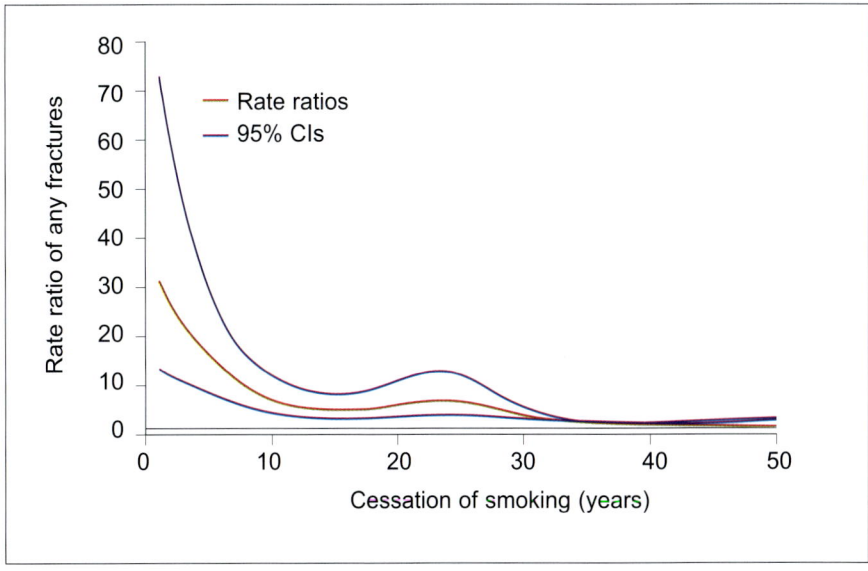

prospective cohorts of 5,939 men and 11,032 women in total, followed for a total of over 75,000 person-years[25] (**4.5**). The effect was nonlinear and seen above an intake of 3 units daily in both men and women.

The effect of chronic heavy drinking on the skeleton during adolescence and young adulthood is particularly harmful leading to future osteoporosis (see **2.42**). The effect is increased because of other frequently coexistent lifestyle risk factors such as smoking, poor diet, and lack of physical activity. People who drink alcohol are more likely to smoke than nondrinkers, and smokers are much more likely to drink than nonsmokers. Eating disorders are common in women who abuse alcohol. The risk of fracture may relate to an increased risk of falls with greater physical impact, in addition to reduced BMD. Moderate alcohol consumption, in contrast, may not be harmful[25,26] and may even be beneficial with increased bone density, but it does not seem to reduce fracture risk. There is little evidence as to the effect of reducing alcohol intake; in the Framingham Study[27] there was no effect on fracture risk of changing from a past heavy to a present light alcohol intake, but avoidance of excess is recommended (which has additional health benefits).

Calcium and vitamin D

Many studies have examined the role of adequate dietary calcium and vitamin D in maximizing bone density and preventing fracture. These have looked at the role of calcium and vitamin D in bone health from an epidemiological perspective, using dietary changes or by the use of supplements in people unselected for their calcium and vitamin D status, or in people known or likely to be deficient. The interest in these dietary constituents is because calcium is the basic requirement for bone mineralization and is needed for the normal development and maintenance of the skeleton, and because of the known role of vitamin D in bone metabolism (see Chapter 1 and see below).

Serum calcium levels are tightly regulated as calcium is essential for transmembrane transportation and cell communication for all cell types throughout the body. Bone tissue is the main calcium reservoir, and the bone mineral content is regulated through feedback systems that involve parathyroid hormone (PTH), calcium, and vitamin D. PTH initiates bone resorption in response to low levels of calcium. Consequently, insufficient calcium intake or absorption to offset the obligatory losses in the urine, digestive juices, and sweat may provoke a continuous upregulation of PTH release, causing increased bone loss. This low-grade secondary hyperparathyroidism is not uncommon in the elderly. This mechanism provides the rationale for calcium and vitamin D treatment as part of a strategy to prevent bone loss, particularly in the elderly.

Adequate calcium intake is important in achieving optimal peak bone mass and an increased calcium intake is

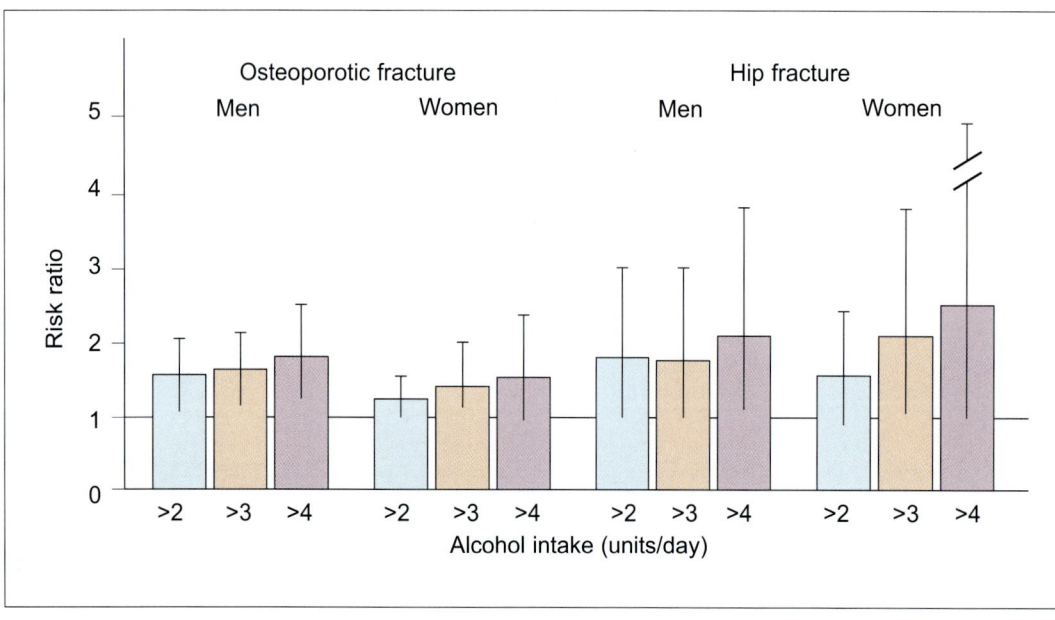

4.5 Risk of fracture with alcohol intake. (Kanis JA, et al. (2005). Alcohol intake as a risk factor for fracture. *Osteopor Int* **16**:737–742).

of benefit if the baseline dietary calcium intake is low. In later life, low calcium intake is associated with an increased risk of fracture[28], including in Asian men and women[29]. Dietary calcium intake declines with ageing and many people consume less than the recommended daily allowance. In addition, there is a decline in efficiency of calcium absorption with ageing.

Vitamin D plays a central role in calcium regulation. It is either provided through the food intake or by exposure of the skin to sunlight. Vitamin D, in the ingested form or from dermal conversion of 7-dehydrocholesterol by ultraviolet light, is biologically inactive until metabolized through several steps in the liver and kidneys (**4.6**). Vitamin D insufficiency is common in the elderly, particularly in northern latitude countries with few hours of sunlight. Skin synthesis is less efficient due to an age-related decline in the amount of 7-dehydrocholesterol (a precursor of vitamin D) in the epidermal layer of the skin, along with older people spending less time outdoors in sunlight. Many older people who are osteoporotic or sustain fractures have low levels of vitamin D. This may not only be relevant to reduced bone strength but there may also be muscle weakness as a consequence, with increased risk of fracture. It is therefore apparent that inadequate calcium and vitamin D are deleterious to bone health but the evidence for the benefit of supplementation to correct this is less clear.

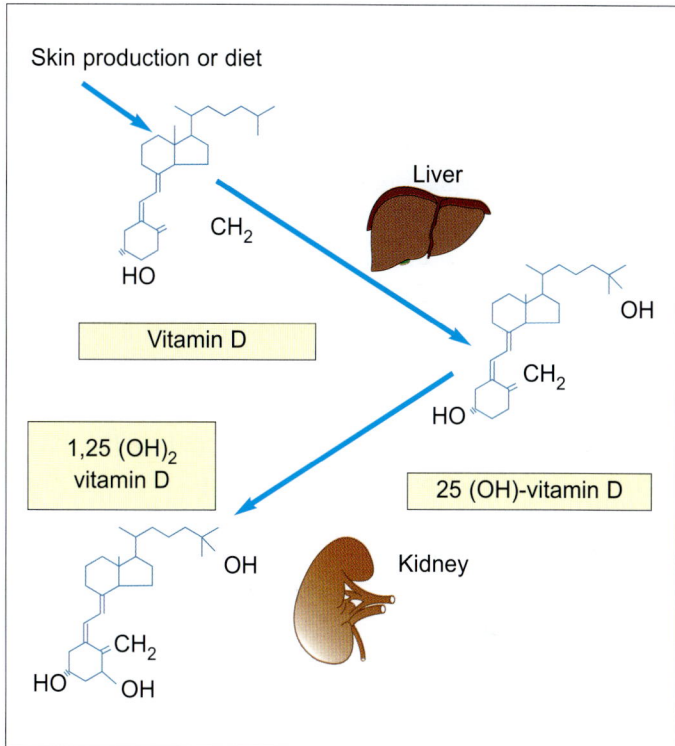

4.6 Metabolic pathway of vitamin D.

Calcium

The effectiveness of calcium supplementation in the prevention and treatment of osteoporosis remains under debate, particularly concerning fracture as outcome. Studies using calcium supplement alone have shown conflicting results. In a recent meta-analysis that included 15 studies and a total of 1806 postmenopausal women, a small but significant effect on bone density was seen at all measured sites[30]. The antifracture effect was estimated at a relative risk of 0.77 (95% CI 0.54–1.09) for vertebral fractures and 0.86 (95% CI 0.43–1.72) for nonvertebral fractures, and was not significant because of a too small sample size. Benefits are greatest in those with a low calcium intake[31]. In almost all randomized controlled trials (RCTs) for bone specific antiresorptive agents, calcium supplementation (400–800 mg) is included in the placebo group that show a 0.5–2 % gain in bone mass.

Vitamin D

Vitamin D_3 supplements alone, usually 400 IU/day with the assumption of an adequate dietary calcium intake, have not been shown to reduce the incidence of fractures in studies of elderly men and women living in the community[32] or in nursing homes[33]. A recent Cochrane review[34] showed no significant effect on hip fracture (seven trials, 18,668 participants), vertebral fracture (four trials, 5698 participants), or any new fracture (eight trials, 18,935 participants).

Vitamin D has, nevertheless, been shown to reduce the risk of fracture in community living men and women given as 100,000 IU oral cholecalciferol every 4 months over 5 years[35]. Vitamin D has also been shown to increase femoral neck bone density (0.2–2.6%) or reduce the rate of loss in elderly women after 2 years of treatment, while other skeletal sites remain similar compared to the placebo groups[36,37]. The dose required to obtain a measurable bone effect over this period was between 400–800 IU/day.

Vitamin D has also been shown to reduce the risk of falls among ambulatory or institutionalized older people by over 20% in a meta-analysis of 5 RCTs including 1237 participants[38]. This effect of vitamin D may explain some of the benefit in studies of calcium combined with vitamin D.

Calcium combined with vitamin D

Calcium and vitamin D in combination is the accepted baseline treatment for osteoporosis and also as a preventive measure, in particular in the frail elderly. Calcium and vitamin D supplementation (1200 mg calcium and 800 IU vitamin D) over 12 weeks in elderly women reduced the risk of falling[39] (**4.7**). This has been confirmed in a meta-analysis[38]. Recent studies have, however, made it less clear as to whether groups other than the frail elderly will benefit.

In a large RCT of elderly French nursing home patients with calcium (1200 mg) and vitamin D (20 µg [800 IU]) there was significant reduction in new hip (RR 0.70 [95% CI 0.62–0.78]) and for all nonvertebral fractures (RR 0.70 [95% CI 0.51–0.91]) after 3 years of treatment, with significant benefit at 18 months[40,41] (*Table 4.4*).

Several recent studies have examined further the effectiveness of calcium and vitamin D in combination. In a large pragmatic RCT in the secondary prevention of osteoporotic fractures[42], 4,481 women and 811 men aged 70 years and over who had sustained a low trauma fracture were randomized to receive (1) 1000 mg calcium daily, (2) vitamin D 800 IU daily, (3) calcium (1000 mg) in combination with vitamin D (800 IU), (4) placebo. The participants were ambulatory and mostly community dwelling. During between 24 months and 62 months follow-up, 13% sustained a new low-trauma fracture, one-quarter of which were of the hip; there was no difference in the incidence of fractures in the three treatment groups (**4.8**). The vitamin D status was only measured in a small sample and compliance with treatment was two-thirds or less at 2 years.

Another large pragmatic open RCT of women aged 70 years and over with risk factors for hip fracture failed to find evidence that supplementation with 1000 mg calcium and 800 IU vitamin D daily over a median follow-up of 25 months reduces the risk of fracture or falls[43]. A total of 3314 patients were included in the study and 1321 were randomized to treatment; the 1993 controls were just given advice on prevention of falls and osteoporosis. At 12 months follow-up, only 63% of the intervention group was adhering to treatment. Vitamin D status of participants was not established either before or during the study.

The recent Cochrane review[34] of seven trials and 10,376 participants, including those studies detailed above, found a small reduction in hip fractures (RR 0.81, 95% CI 0.68–0.96) and nonvertebral fractures (RR 0.87, 95% CI 0.78–0.97). Most recently, the Women's Health Initiative study of more than 36,000 postmenopausal women aged 50–79 years randomly assigned to 1000 mg calcium and 400 IU vitamin D daily or placebo for an average of 7 years has failed to show any reduction in fractures unless just those adhering to treatment were included[44].

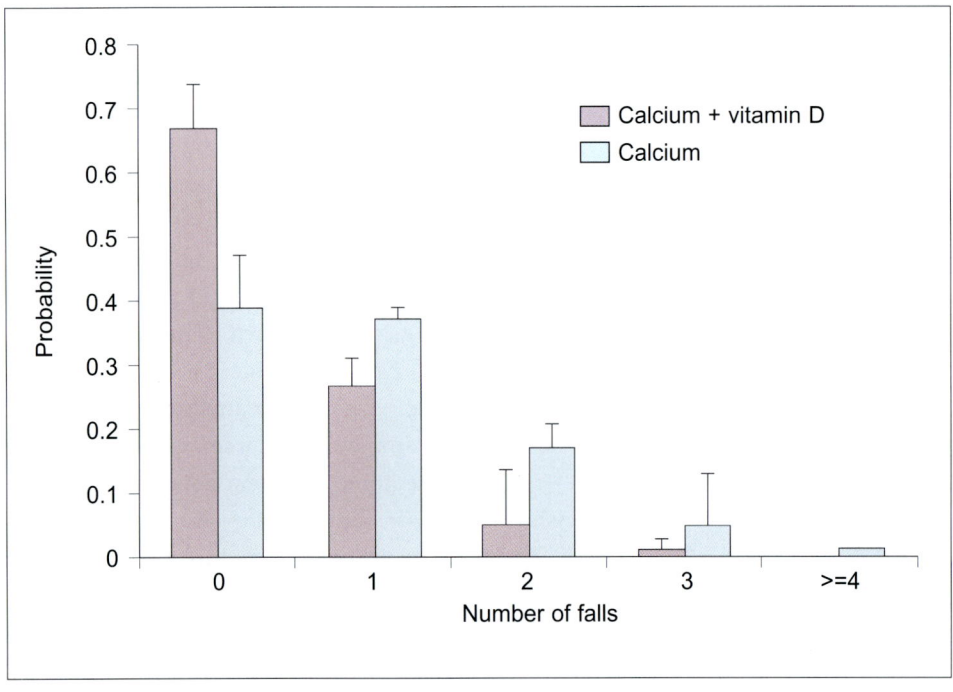

4.7 Effects of calcium and vitamin D supplementation on the risk of falling. (Adapted from Bischoff HA, *et al.* (2003). Effects of vitamin D and calcium supplementation on falls: a randomized controlled trial. *J Bone Min Res* **18**:1342–1343.).

It appears that the vitamin D status of the person and their level of independence makes a difference in response to calcium and vitamin D. It is, however, unfortunate that vitamin D levels were not measured comprehensively in recent studies to help clarify who will benefit most. Effectiveness in clinical practice is also reduced by lack of long-term adherence to treatment. The role of calcium and vitamin D supplements therefore remains unresolved, but it is reasonable to ensure that deficiency is avoided at all stages of life, in particular in the growing skeleton and in the frail elderly. It is easier to achieve sufficiency through dietary intake and sunlight exposure when exercising in younger people but supplements may be needed in the frail elderly. The role of supplementation in those who are mobile with reasonable diets and sunlight exposure, even if elderly, is not proven.

Table 4.4 Calcium and vitamin supplementation in a very elderly population in care

	Vitamin D + calcium	Placebo	P value
Active treatment analysis			
Number of women	872	893	
Hip fracture ≥1	109	153	<0.01
Nonvertebral fractures ≥1	205	270	<0.01
Intention to treat analysis			
Number of women	1176	1127	
Hip fractures ≥1	137	178	<0.02
Nonvertebral fractures ≥1	255	308	<0.02

(Adapted from Chapuy MC, *et al.* (1994). Effect of calcium and cholecalciferol treatment for three years on hip fractures in elderly women. *BMJ* **308**:1081–1082.)

4.8 Effects of calcium, vitamin D, or combination treatment on the incidence of new low-trauma fracture. (Adapted from Grant AM, *et al.* (2005). Oral vitamin D3 and calcium for secondary prevention of low-trauma fractures in elderly people (Randomized Evaluation of Calcium Or vitamin D, RECORD): a randomized placebo-controlled trial. *Lancet* **365**(9471):1621–1628.)

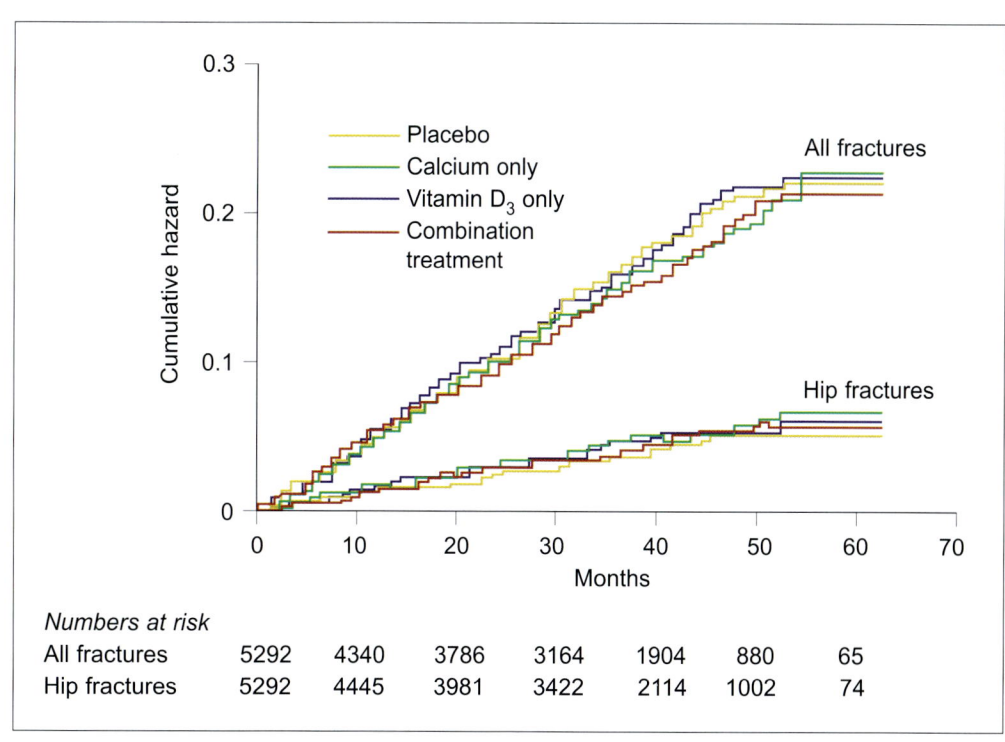

Numbers at risk							
All fractures	5292	4340	3786	3164	1904	880	65
Hip fractures	5292	4445	3981	3422	2114	1002	74

Recommended supplementation if being used is:

- Calcium 500–1000 mg depending on dietary intake to reach above a total of 1000 mg/day.
- Vitamin D 400–800 IU daily – the higher dose may be indicated for institutionalized persons or those receiving equivalent care, or during the winter in northern latitude countries.

A bone healthy lifestyle

There are several potentially modifiable risk lifestyle factors associated with reduced bone density and increased risk of fracture (see above). It has been estimated that if the whole population undertook and achieved a high level of physical activity and calcium consumption that the population risk of hip fractures could be reduced by about 17% in older women[45], and avoiding undernutrition, smoking, and excess alcohol would have greater benefits (**4.9**); the challenge is achieving such changes in peoples behaviour.

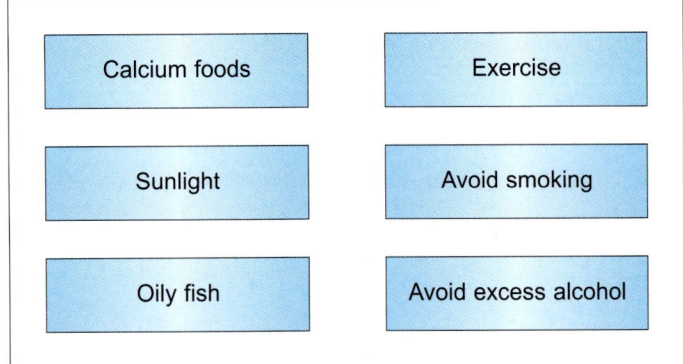

Calcium foods	Exercise
Sunlight	Avoid smoking
Oily fish	Avoid excess alcohol

4.9 A bone healthy lifestyle.

PHARMACOLOGICAL INTERVENTIONS

Pharmacological interventions in osteoporosis rely on targeting osteoclasts, osteoblasts, or both. The rationale for inhibition of osteoclasts stems from a number of observations; most important was the observation that oestrogen withdrawal led to increased osteoclast activation and hence blocking osteoclast differentiation and actions seemed essential. Inhibition of osteoclast action leads to a secondary gain in bone mass. In addition, it has clearly been more difficult to stimulate osteoblasts selectively to obtain a true bone anabolic effect. An ideal bone agent should have a dual effect and preferably increase not only bone mass but also improve bone quality and strength.

Bone turnover is a slow process and, as a consequence, evaluation of treatment effect in terms of bone gain and fracture reduction is extended over time, i.e. 1–3 years. This has an impact on design of trials and outcome evaluation. From an evidence-based perspective, fracture efficacy should be the primary end-point of all studies; however, if fracture efficacy is proven (*Table 4.5*), change in BMD and change in bone markers may serve as surrogate end-points, albeit recognizing the limitations of this approach.

Evidence of effect on fracture is the required end-point for any osteoporosis treatment to be considered of clinical value. The strength of evidence depends on the source. The best evidence is considered to be from the meta-analysis of several RCTs, whereas the weakest evidence is considered to be unsupported expert opinion. Recommendation of treatment should be based on evaluation using these established criteria for evidence of efficacy. This approach is used in guideline development[46].

Table 4.5 Categories of evidence

Ia Evidence from meta-analysis of randomized controlled trials

Ib Evidence from at least one randomized controlled trial

IIa Evidence from at least one controlled study without randomization

IIb Evidence from at least one other type of quasi-experimental study

III Evidence from descriptive studies, such as comparative studies, correlation studies and case-control studies

IV Evidence from expert committee reports or opinions or clinical experience of respected authorities, or both

(Adapted from Eccles M, *et al.* (1998). North of England evidence based guidelines development project: methods of developing guidelines for efficient drug use in primary care. *BMJ*, **316**(7139):1232–1235.)

Bisphosphonates

Bisphosphonates are chemically developed from pyrophosphates, compounds that inhibit precipitation of calcium carbonate and have industrial applications. Bisphosphonates act by binding to the mineral phase of bone, binding to hydroxyapatite. Osteoclast activity is reduced with decreased ruffle border, decreased acid production, and decreased production of lysosomal enzymes and prostaglandins (4.10). Osteoclast numbers are reduced by increased apoptosis and inhibition of osteoclast recruitment. They have little effect on other organ systems. Bisphosphonates are known to markedly suppress bone turnover. It has been estimated that bone resorption must be suppressed by 40–80% in order to obtain a significant effect on BMD. Since bisphosphonates primarily affect the activity of osteoclasts, the effects on bone resorption markers have gained most interest.

Bisphosphonates are, in general, poorly absorbed from the gastrointestinal tract. Only about 0.5–5% of a given dose is absorbed from the stomach, further decreased by food intake (particularly calcium-containing foods) or even drinks such as coffee or juice. Oral bisphosphonates must, therefore, be taken after a food-free interval of an overnight fast and a fast of 30–60 minutes after taking them. The possibilities of less frequent dosing with highly potent oral compounds, as well as the development of intravenous administration are therefore much more convenient from the persons' viewpoint and potentially more effective due to better adherence to therapy. About half of the absorbed drug is excreted unmetabolized in the urine. Bisphosphonates are deposited in bone for a prolonged time, probably up to 10 years or more[47].

A core P-O-P bond, which in bisphosphonates is exchanged with a P-C-P bond, characterizes the basic pyrophosphate structure. This allows for two side chains (R1 and R2), with R1 binding to hydroxyapatite and R2 giving the specific biological and chemical properties (4.11, 4.12). The potency of each bisphosphonate compound depends on side chain substitution. Nitrogen-containing bisphosphonates are most potent and exert their inhibitory effect through the mevalonate pathway. This allows for lower doses and less frequent dosing.

Alendronate

Alendronate, a second generation bisphosphonate, was the first bisphosphonate for which a clear antifracture effect was seen in RCTs.

Effect on bone turnover

Alendronate suppresses bone turnover within 6–12 weeks[48] (4.13). The effect is most pronounced for bone resorption markers, decreasing 40–60% and results in a sustained increase in bone density in the axial and appendicular skeleton[49] (4.14).

Effect on BMD

The first study, which included postmenopausal women with low bone density (T-score < -2.5) with or without prevalent vertebral deformity, showed BMD increases of 8.8% and 5.9% in the spine and hip, respectively. The effect, including reduction in new vertebral fractures was most pronounced in women above age 65 and with at least one vertebral fracture at entry.

* Bisphosphonates

Active osteoclast	Inactive osteoclast	Apoptotic osteoclast
Bisphosphonate taken up by osteoclasts	Osteoclasts lose resorptive function upon bisphosphonate uptake	Osteoclastic apoptosis

4.10 Bisphosphonate mechanism of action.

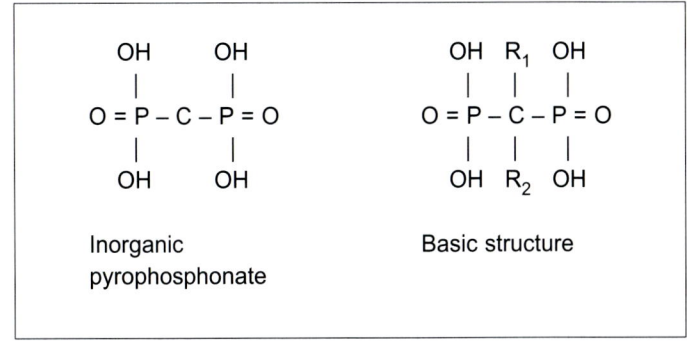

4.11 Basic structure of bisphosphonate.

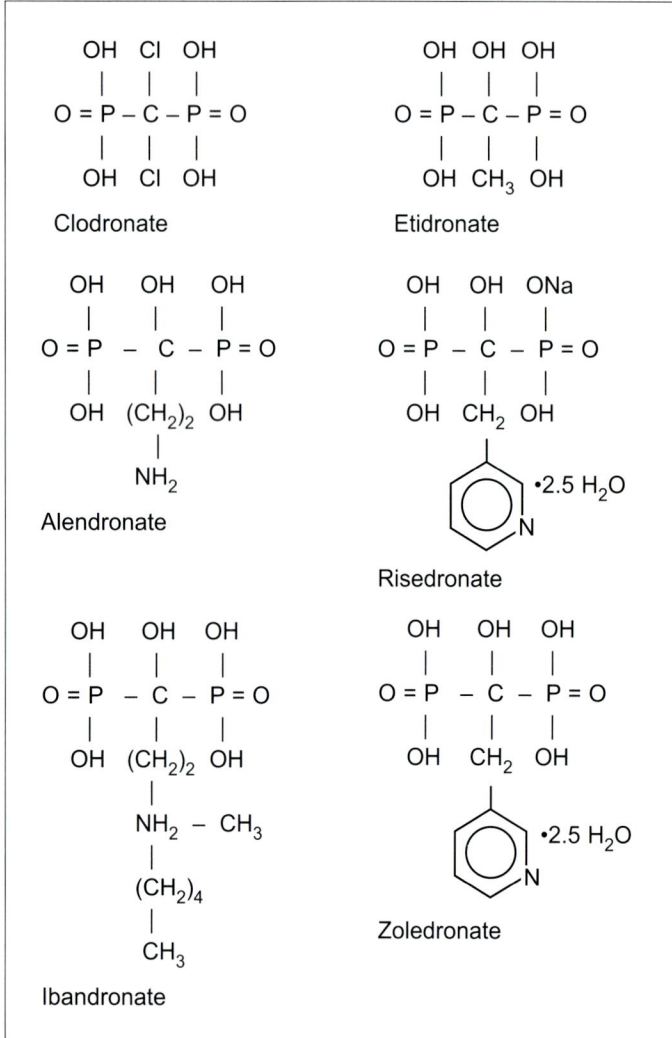

4.12 Structure of clodronate, etidronate, alendronate, risedronate, ibandronate and zoledronate.

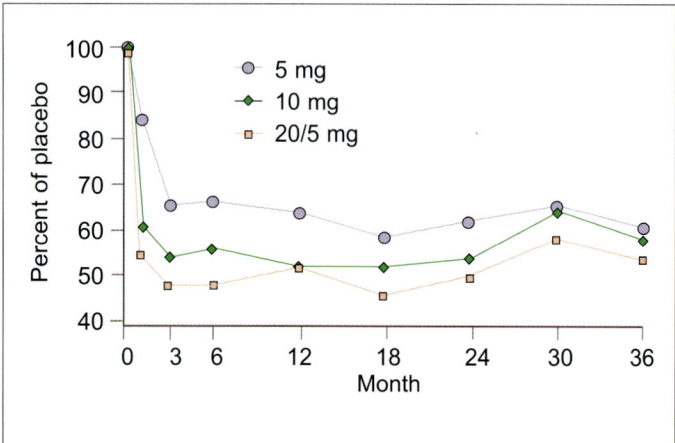

4.13 The effect of alendronate on bone markers. (Adapted from Devogelaer JP, *et al.* (1996). Oral alendronate induces progressive increases in bone mass of the spine, hip, and total body over 3 years in postmenopausal women with osteoporosis. *Bone*, **18**(2):141–150.)

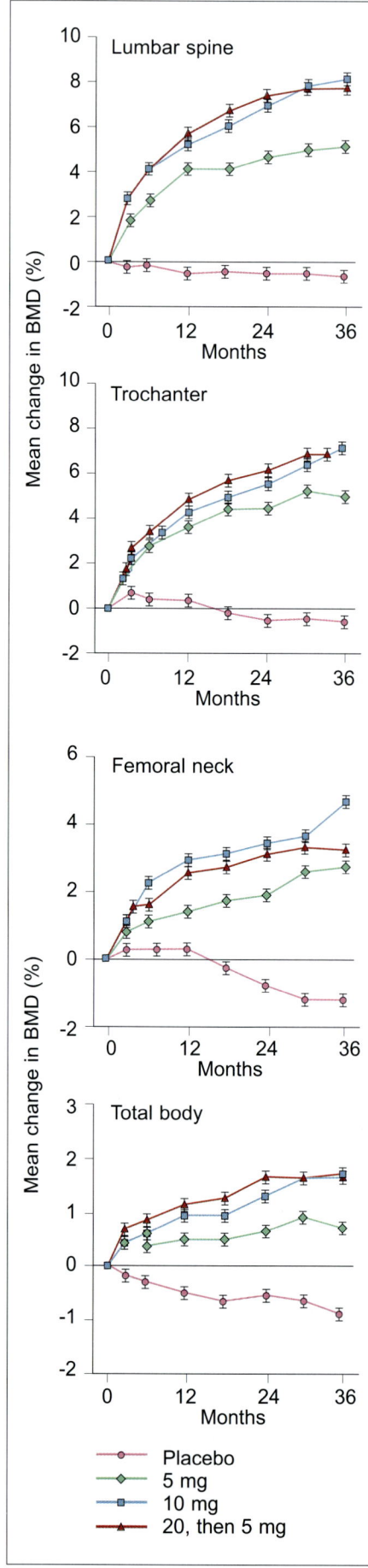

4.14 The effect of alendronate on BMD. (Adapted from Liberman UA, *et al.* (1995). Effect of oral alendronate on bone mineral density and the incidence of fractures in postmenopausal osteoporosis. The Alendronate Phase III Osteoporosis Treatment Study Group. *N Engl J Med,* **333**(22):1437–1443.)

Effect on fracture

Two major trials[49, 50] have shown a reduction in vertebral deformities of about 50%, and prevention of nonvertebral fractures has been demonstrated (**4.15**). In the Fracture Intervention Trial 1 (FIT 1), 2027 women with at least one prevalent vertebral fracture were included. Alendronate treatment over 3 years gave a clear reduction in the number of new radiographic and clinical vertebral fractures (p=0.001) and also a reduction of hip (p=0.047) and wrist fractures (p=0.013), albeit the number of fractures was small. In a meta-analysis of 11 RCTs with alendronate, pooled data favours an antifracture effect from alendronate treatment with 5 mg or greater, with a risk reduction of 47%. Reduction of nonvertebral fractures is also evident in postemenopausal women fulfilling the criteria for osteoporosis[51] (**4.16**).

The effect of alendronate has been shown to be sustained long term[52] (**4.17**). It has been possible to monitor long-term effects of alendronate treatment in a subset of women from some of the early studies. Thus, 10-year treatment effects are reported in 247 women (**4.18**)[53]. The increase in BMD is maintained with an even further increase in spinal BMD (13.7%). Similarly, bone markers stayed depressed. In those discontinuing treatment, the BMD gain remained in the spine, whereas a decrease was obvious in the hip. The BMD effect of 10 mg daily, 35 mg twice weekly, and 70 mg once weekly of alendronate is similar over 2 years in women with postmenopausal osteoporosis (**4.19**). The preferred dosing regimen is now 70 mg once weekly[54, 55].

Risedronate

Risedronate is a third generation, highly potent bisphosphonate that has also been shown to prevent vertebral and nonvertebral fractures. Risedronate is a nitrogen-containing bisphosphonate that, like other nitrogen-containing bisphosphonates, is likely to induce apoptosis through inhibition of farnesyl or geranylgeranyl isoprenoid groups through the mevalonate pathway[56].

Effect on bone turnover

A major 3-year RCT evaluating the antifracture efficacy of risedronate included 2458 postmenopausal women in North America with prevalent vertebral deformities[57]. In this study of risedronate, deoxypyridinoline was dose-dependently suppressed by about 40%, an effect that was evident within 1 month of risedronate treatment (**4.20**, left). The secondary effect on bone formation, as measured by bone-specific alkaline phosphatase was delayed, reaching a

maximum depression at 3–6 months (**4.20**, right). The effect is less pronounced than that of alendronate, which can be interpreted either as a positive or negative outcome; negatively as it indicates a lower efficacy or positively as adverse effects on mineralization from marked long-terms suppression is less likely.

Effect on BMD

The effect of risedronate on bone density is similar to that of alendronate, producing about 4–6% increase in spinal and femoral bone mass after 3 years of treatment. The dose-dependent effect of risedronate evident from bone marker

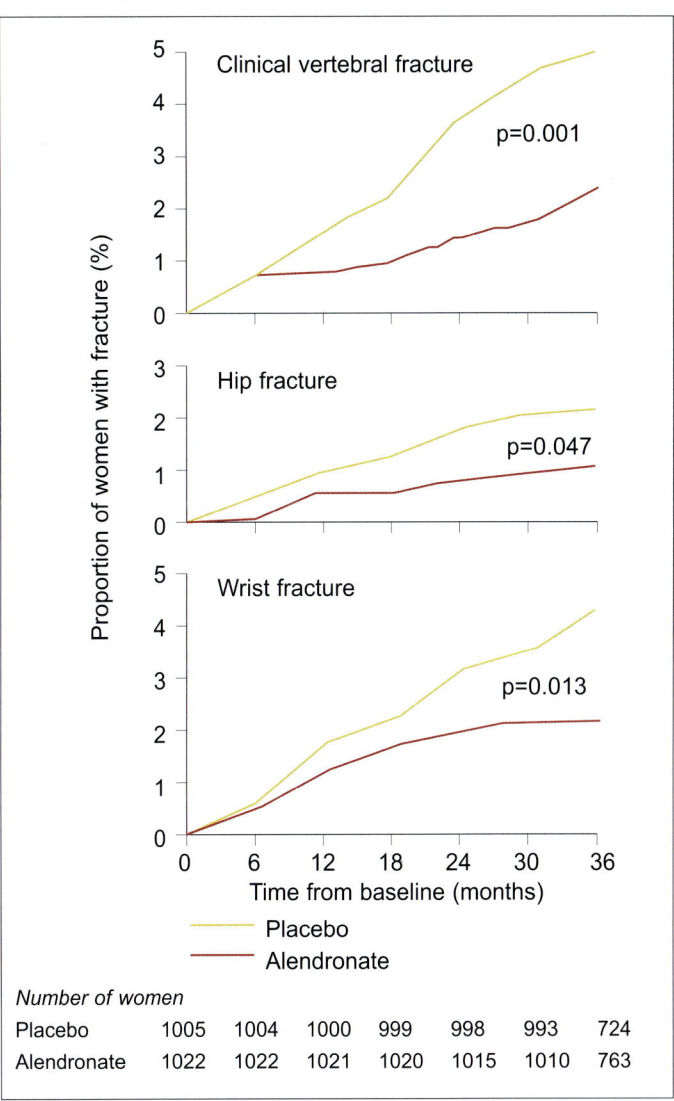

4.15 The effect of alendronate on fracture. (Adapted from Black DM, *et al.* (1996). Randomised trial of effect of alendronate on risk of fracture in women with existing vertebral fractures. Fracture Intervention Trial Research Group. *Lancet*, **348**(9041):1535–1541.)

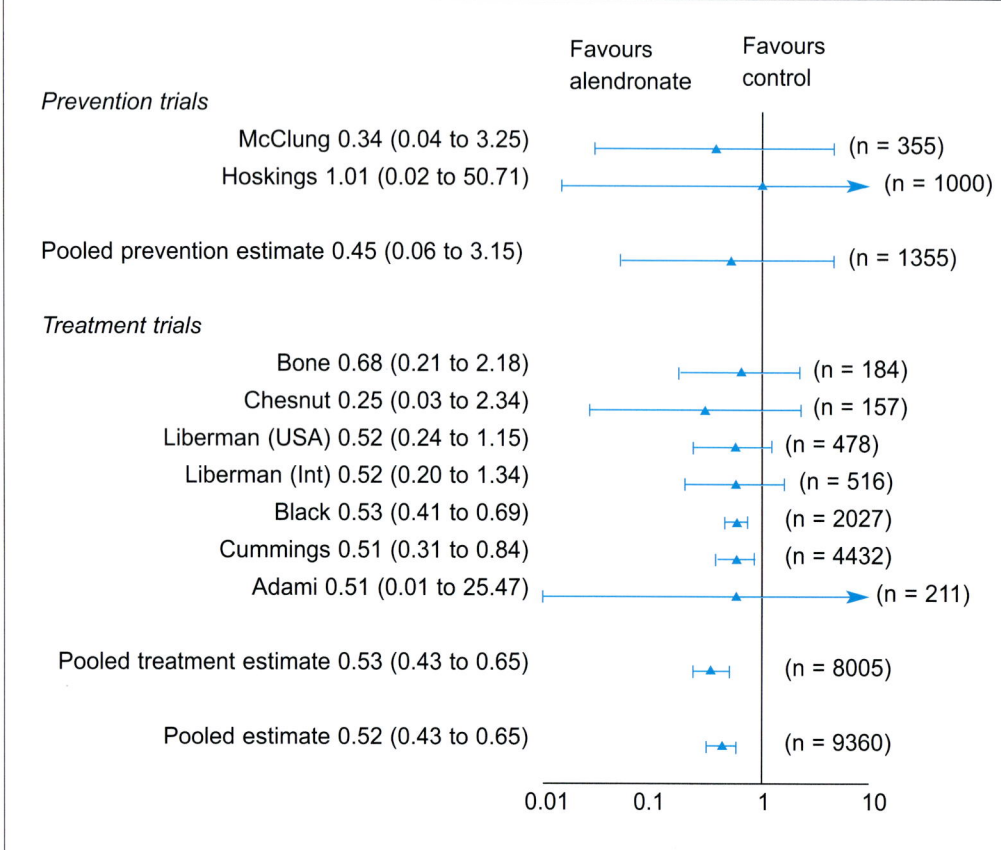

4.16 Alendronate meta-analysis. (Adapted from Cranney A, *et al.* (2002). Meta-analyses of therapies for postmenopausal osteoporosis. II. Meta-analysis of alendronate for the treatment of postmenopausal women. *Endocr Rev*, **23**(4):508-516.)

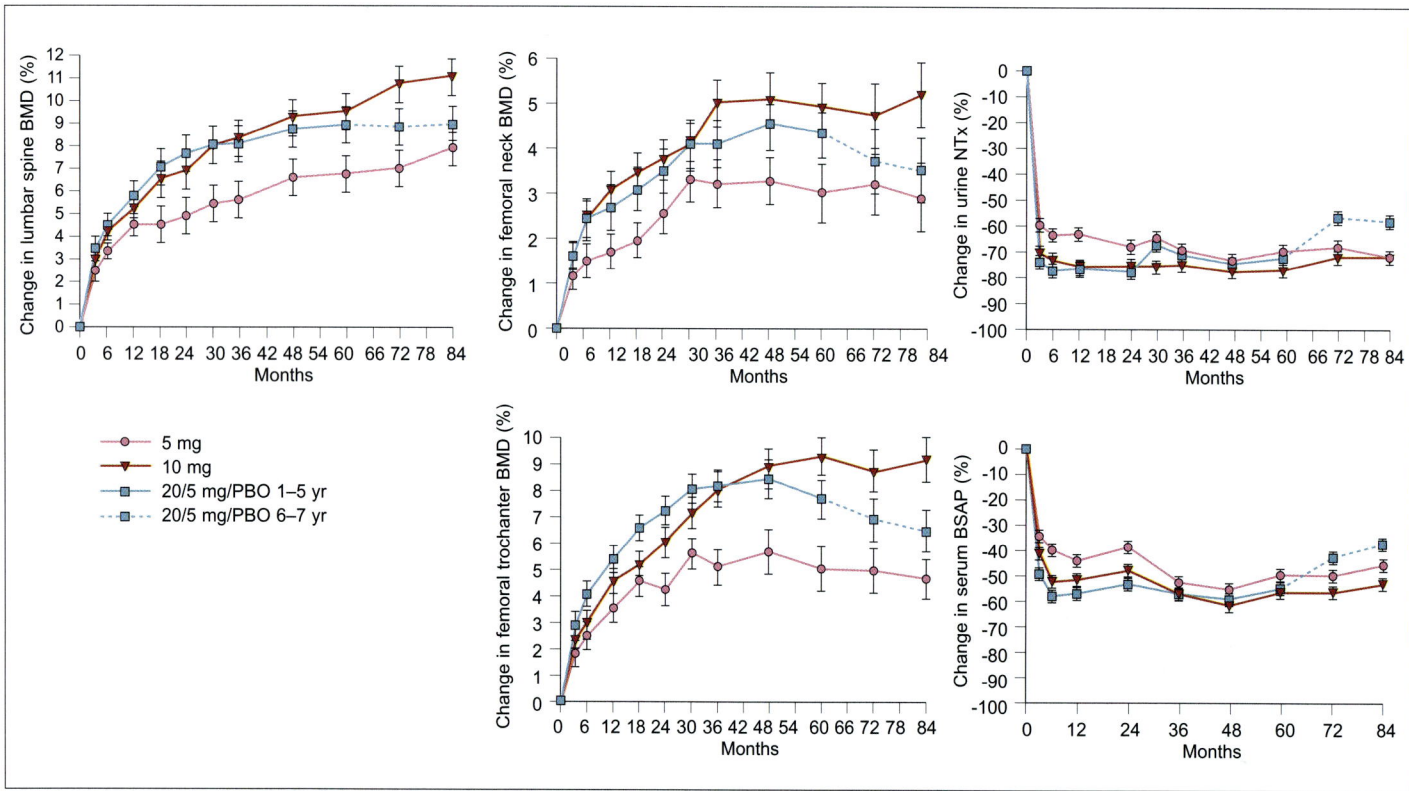

4.17 Alendronate 7-year data. (Adapted from Tonino RP, *et al.* (2000). Skeletal benefits of alendronate: 7-year treatment of postmenopausal osteoporotic women. Phase III Osteoporosis Treatment Study Group. *J Clin Endocrinol Metab*, **85**(9):3109–3115.)

assessment is associated with a similar effect on BMD (**4.21**). Hence, the 2.5 mg/day dose was discontinued within the study, whereas a significant increase in BMD was found for the 5 mg dose. BMD increase was most pronounced in the lumbar spine (5.4%), with a 1.6% increase in the femoral neck and 3.3% in the trochanteric region compared to placebo.

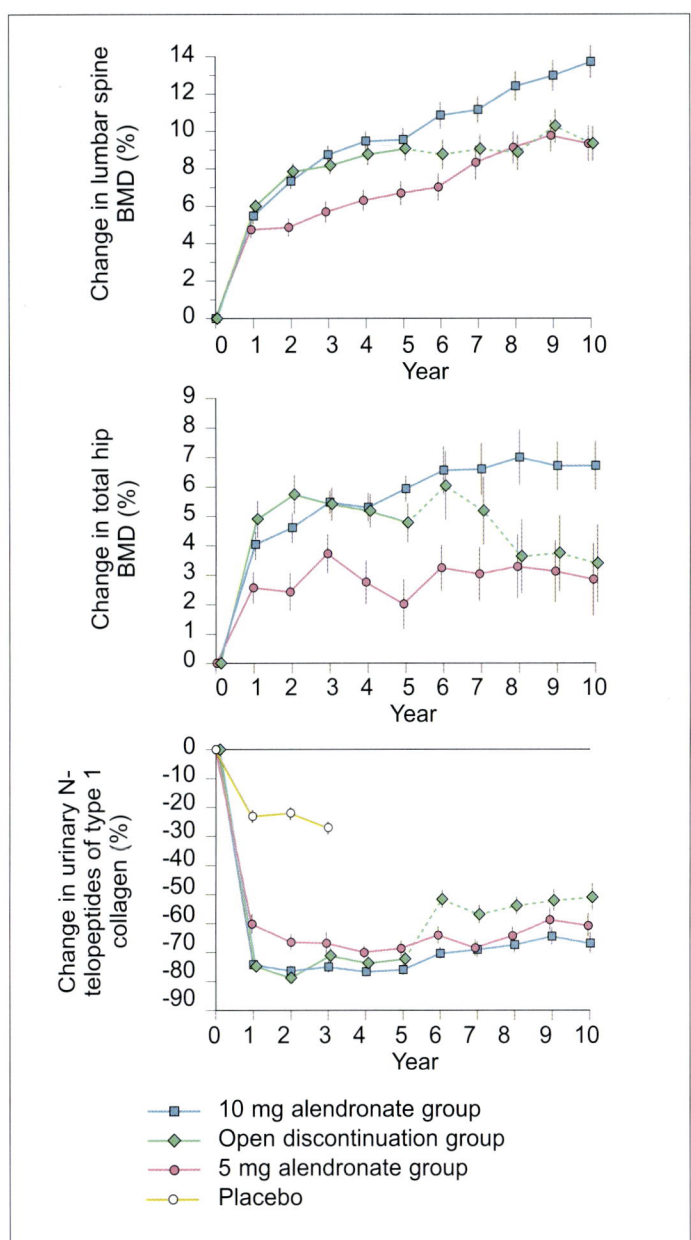

4.18 Alendronate 10-year data. (Adapted from Bone HG, *et al.* (2004). Ten years' experience with alendronate for osteoporosis in postmenopausal women. *N Engl J Med,* **350**(12):1189–1199.)

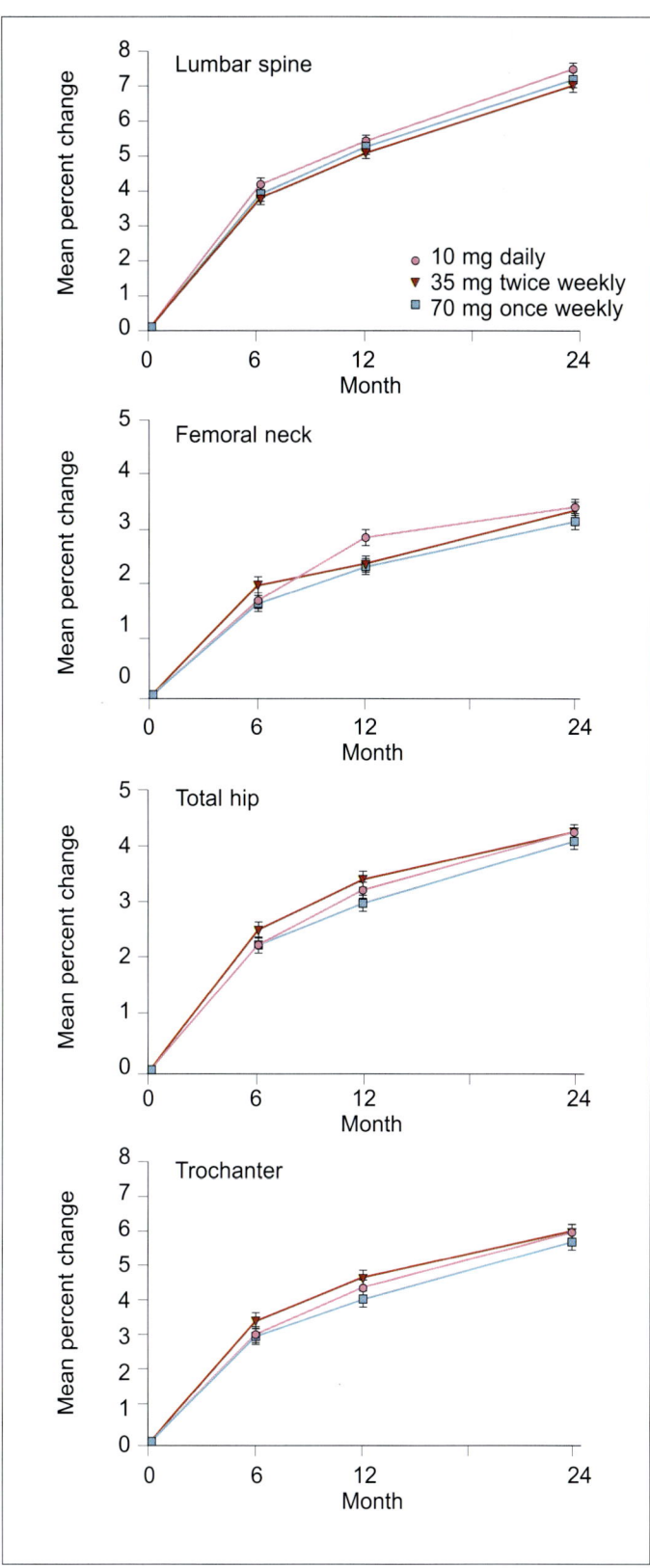

4.19 Alendronate and dosing. (Adapted from Rizzoli R, *et al.* (2002). Two-year results of once-weekly administration of alendronate 70 mg for the treatment of postmenopausal osteoporosis. *J Bone Miner Res* **17**(11):1988–1996.)

Effect on fracture

The antifracture effect on vertebral fracture was evident after 1 year of treatment and sustained at 3 years, with a 41% cumulative decrease in radiographic vertebral fracture incidence (defined as more than 15% loss of vertebral height). Nonvertebral fractures were significantly lower (39%) at 3 years compared to placebo (**4.22**).

The results of the study was to some extent hampered by a rather high discontinuation rate (up to 45%) for various reasons. However, the results of the European and Australian arms of the trial (n=1226) indicates similar effects: vertebral fractures were reduced by 49% in those treated with 5 mg per day. The effect was evident after the first year. Nonvertebral fractures were reduced by 33%; however, this was not significant (p=0.06) (**4.23**)[58].

Hip fracture is the most devastating fracture for the individual with substantial subsequent morbidity and mortality. The effect of risedronate on hip fracture risk was specifically

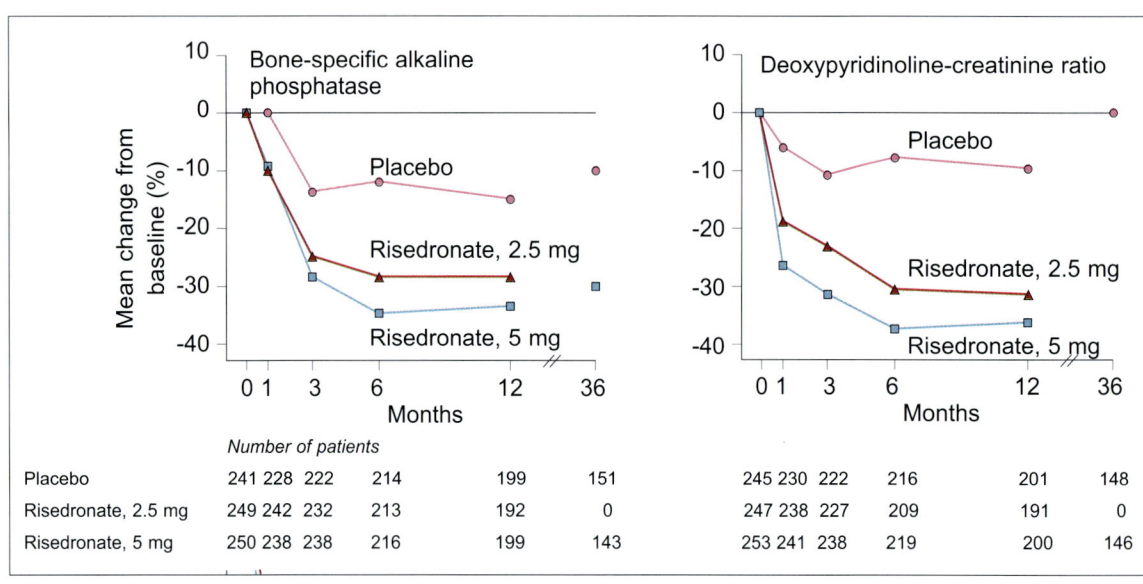

4.20 Risedronate and effect on bone markers. (Adapted from Harris ST, *et al.* (1999). Effects of risedronate treatment on vertebral and nonvertebral fractures in women with postmenopausal osteoporosis: a randomized controlled trial. Vertebral Efficacy With Risedronate Therapy (VERT) Study Group. *JAMA,* **282**(14):1344–1352.)

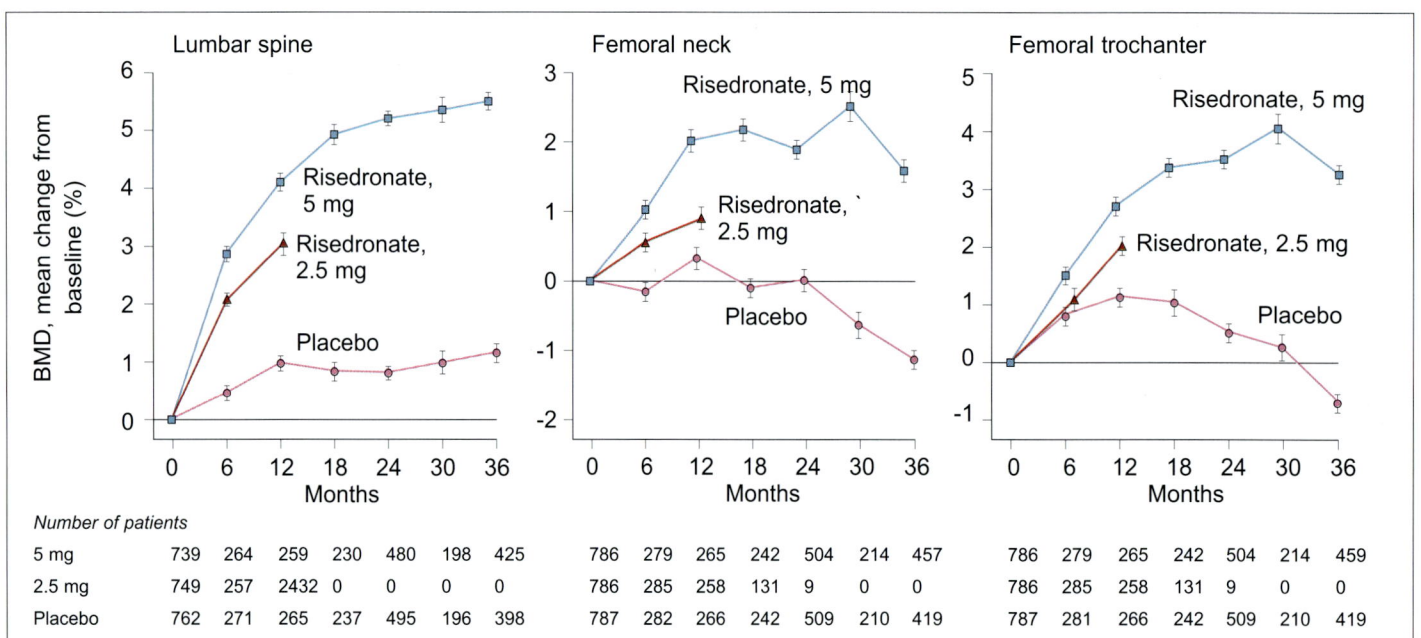

4.21 Risedronate effect on BMD. (Adapted from Harris ST, *et al.* (1999). Effects of risedronate treatment on vertebral and nonvertebral fractures in women with postmenopausal osteoporosis: a randomized controlled trial. Vertebral Efficacy With Risedronate Therapy (VERT) Study Group. *JAMA,* **282**(14):1344–1352.)

evaluated in a high-risk population of 5445 women aged 70–79 years and in 3886 women aged 80 and above (**4.24**). Women were included based on BMD measurement and/or on risk factors. In women aged 70–79 years with osteoporosis, the incidence of hip fracture was reduced by 40% (RR 0.6, 95% CI 0.4–0.9). In women aged 80 and above, included primarily based on risk factors, there was no fracture-sparing effect[59]. Again this study points out that low bone density is a major determinant for the clinical effect of antiresorptive agents.

In a meta-analysis, including eight RCTs fulfilling the inclusion criteria of the analysis, fracture risk for vertebral fractures was reduced by 36% in doses of risedronate above 2.5 mg per day (RR 0.64, 95% CI 0.54–0.77) (**4.25**). The comparable risk reduction for nonvertebral fractures were 27% (RR 0.73, 95% CI 0.61–0.87)[62]. Meta-analyses is the highest level of evidence for a treatment effect, thus it can be concluded that risedronate substantially reduces the risk of both vertebral and nonvertebral fractures.

4.22 Risedronate effect on fracture. (Adapted from Harris ST, *et al.* (1999). Effects of risedronate treatment on vertebral and nonvertebral fractures in women with postmenopausal osteoporosis: a randomized controlled trial. Vertebral Efficacy With Risedronate Therapy (VERT) Study Group. *JAMA,* **282**(14):1344–1352.)

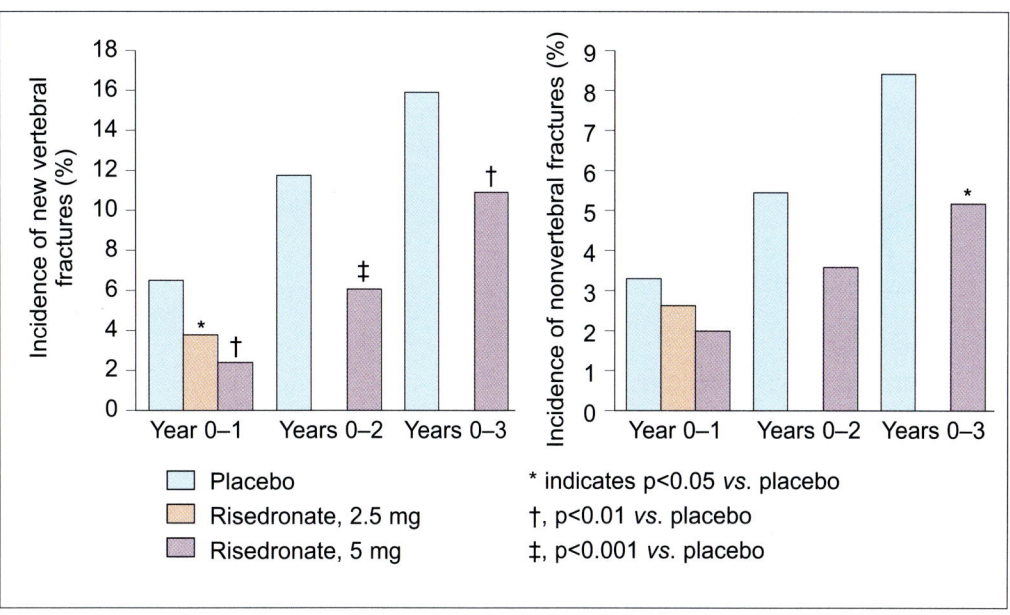

4.23 Risedronate effect on fracture. (Adapted from Reginster JY, *et al.* (2000), Randomised trial of the effects of risedronate on vertebral fractures in women with established postmenopausal osteoporosis. *Osteoporos Int*, **11**:83–91.)

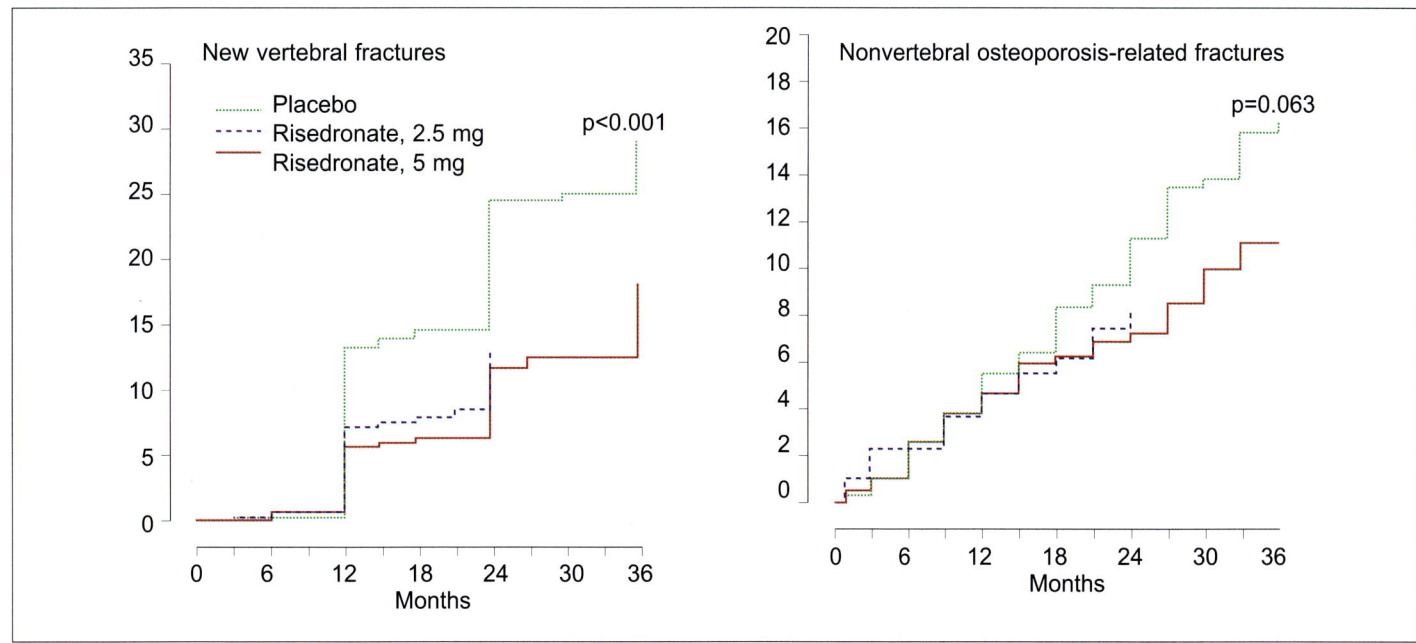

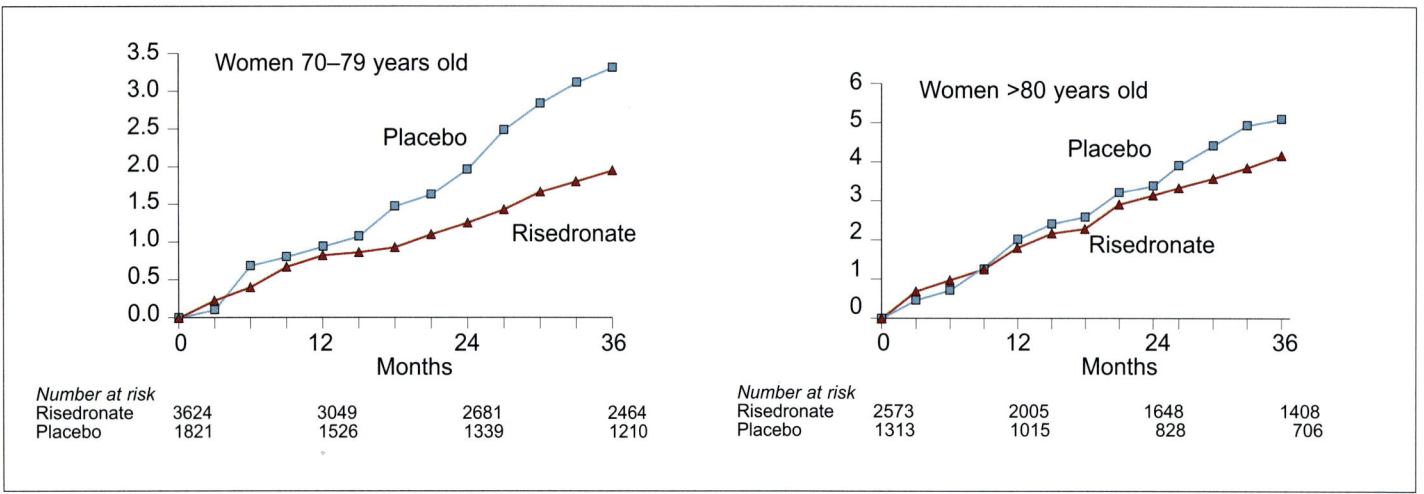

4.24 Risedronate effect on hip fracture. (Adapted from McClung MR, *et al.* (2001). Effect of risedronate on the risk of hip fracture in elderly women. Hip Intervention Program Study Group. *N Engl J Med*, **344**(5):333–340.)

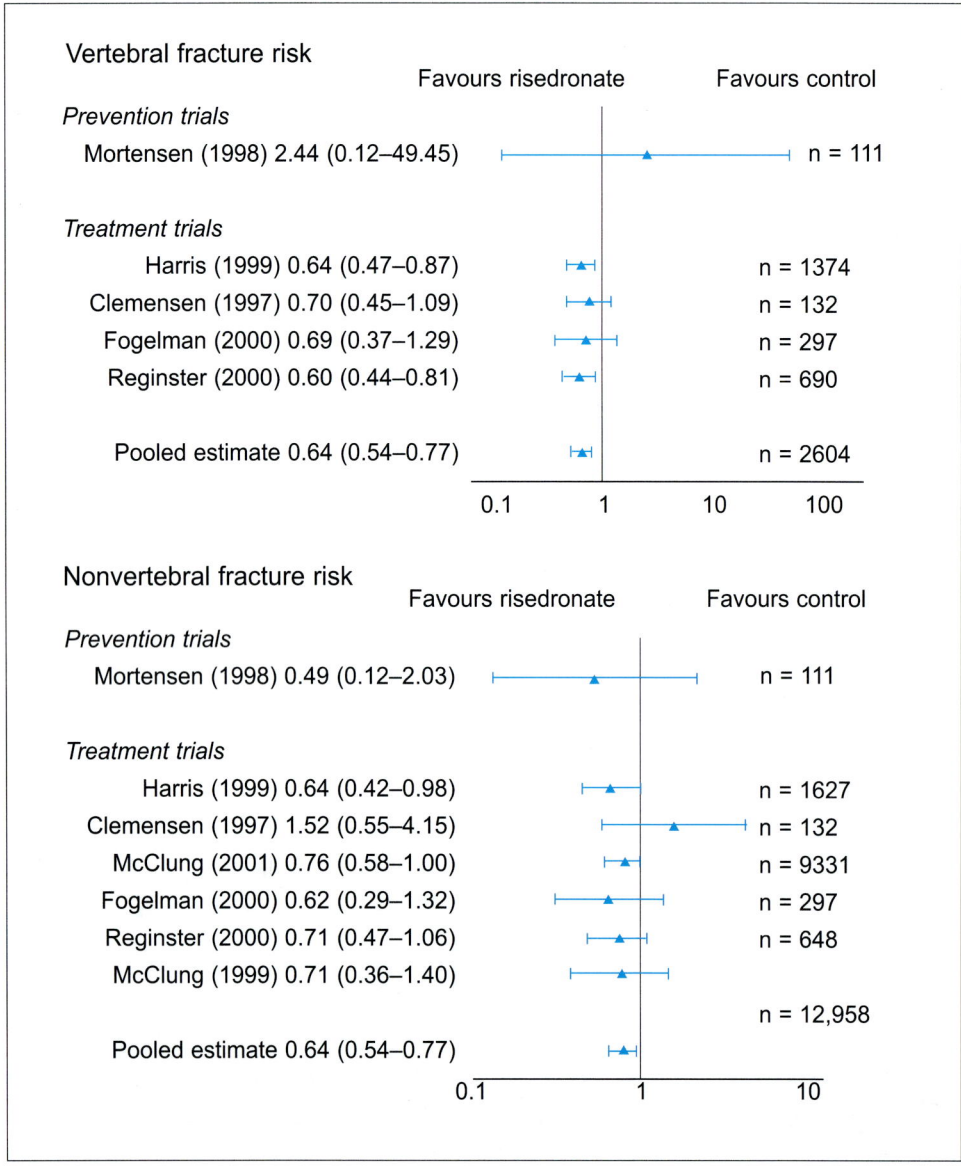

4.25 Risedronate meta-analysis – vertebral fracture risk and nonvertebral fracture risk. (Adapted from Cranney A, *et al.* (2002). Meta-analyses of therapies for postmenopausal osteoporosis. III. Meta-analysis of risedronate for the treatment of postmenopausal osteoporosis. *Endocr Rev*, **23**(4):517–523.)

Safety

Since bisphosphonates are incorporated into the mineralized matrix very long term (up to 10 years), adverse effects from long-term suppression of bone turnover have been a concern. In one study, pretreatment transiliac bone biopsies were compared with biopsies taken after 3 years of risedronate treatment (**4.26**)[60]. Histomorphometric evaluation indicated, as expected, a moderate effect on bone turnover with a 47% decrease in activation frequency. The study did not observe any structural alteration in treated women compared to nontreated women. In an additional study, it has been estimated that changes in lumbar spine BMD only explains 18% of the vertebral fracture efficacy, which may be interpreted as that other qualitative traits may also contribute to fracture risk[61]. In order to further evaluate qualitative traits three-dimensional microcomputed tomography was performed in bone biopsies from treated and nontreated women. In those on placebo, microstructural architecture deteriorated, with for example a 13% increase in trabecular separation, in contrast to those treated with risedronate (**4.27**).

The effect of risedronate treatment has been evaluated up to 7 years in the multinational arm of the Fracture Study[58]. Of the initial study cohort, 164 women were available for the extension study and, after additional randomization, were treated with placebo or risedronate. In those treated with risedronate for 7 years, bone turnover was consistently decreased and BMD remained significantly increased with about 4% increase in the hip and 8–11% in the spine[63]. Weekly dosing of risedronate gives similar changes in bone

markers and a similar BMD response and is the preferred regimen for the purpose of adherence[64]. Risedronate has also been used in men, with similar effects on bone mass and with a significant reduction of vertebral fractures[65].

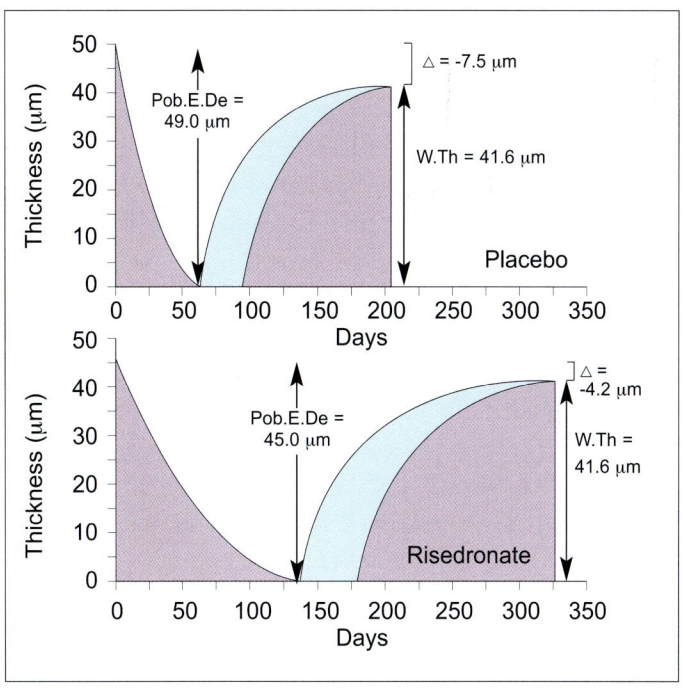

4.26 Effects of long-term risedronate on bone quality and bone turnover in women with postmenopausal osteoporosis. (Adapted from Eriksen EF, *et al.* (2002). Effects of long-term risedronate on bone quality and bone turnover in women with postmenopausal osteoporosis. *Bone*, **31**(5):620–625.)

4.27 Risendronate and effect on bone quality. (From Dufresne TE, *et al.* (2003). Risedronate preserves bone architecture in early postmenopausal women in 1 year as measured by three-dimensional microcomputed tomography. *Calcif Tissue Int* **73**(5):423–432 with permission.)

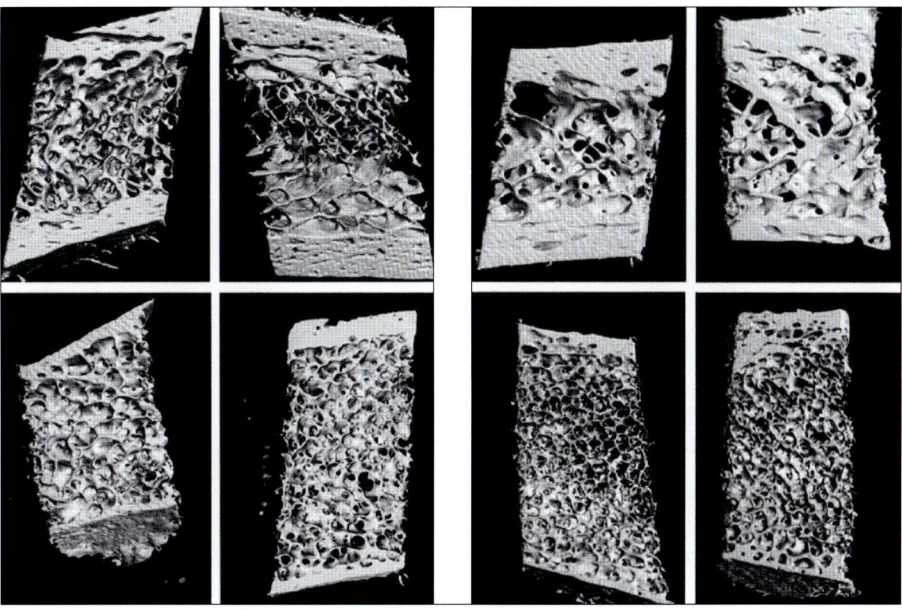

Side-effects

Risedronate, as other bisphosphonates, must be taken according to instructions. It appears to be well tolerated both in the studies and clinically, with no serious side-effects reported. Since negative gastrointestinal effects have been a concern, the gastroduodenal effects have been specifically evaluated in comparison to alendronate and found to be significantly lower[66]. From an observational cohort study conducted using the UK GP database of over 13,000 patients, ophthamological side-effects were specifically evaluated and occurred in a small proportion of the patients (n=313)[67]. This indicates that a number of different side-effects may occur but these are usually mild.

Ibandronate

Ibandronate is a new addition to the nitrogen-containing bisphosphonates for the treatment of osteoporosis. In general, ibandronate has similar properties to other nitrogen-containing bisphosphonates, but is 2-, 10-, and 50-fold more potent than risedronate, alendronate and pamidronate, respectively[68]. Bisphosphonates are poorly absorbed after oral administration, with 0.5–1% absorption when taken according to instructions after an overnight fast and at least 30 minutes before breakfast. For ibandronate this means that efficacy drops and is 100-fold less with oral administration. Hence, ibandronate is suitable for intravenous administration, but based on the high potency, the dosing interval after oral administration can also be increased. Weekly dosing of other bisphosphonates has been available for some time, but from studies it is evident that women would prefer even longer dosing interval as it would fit better with their lifestyle[69]. Similarly, in a comparative study once-monthly ibandronate was preferred over once-weekly alendronate in a cross-over trail[70]. The availability of high-potency bisphosphonates such as ibandronate has promoted development of dosing regimens with extended drug free periods using both intravenous and oral administration. It needs to be borne in mind, however, that the potency in experimental models does not necessarily transfer to a similar difference in potency in clinical effect in patients.

Ibandronate is described as a third generation bisphosphonates with a hydroxyl group at R1 chain and a tertiary nitrogen at the R2 chain. Irrespective of mode of administration, it blocks the osteoclast activity by inhibition of the mevalonate pathway after binding to the mineral phase of bone. Studies using animal models have shown a decrease in bone turnover and an increase in bone mass and bone strength, and that intermittent dosing provides the same benefits as continuous dosing regimens[71]. The potential for increasing the interval between doses has been studied in number of human phase II and III studies in an effort to find the optimal dosing interval with maintained effect on fracture and bone mass. The reports subsequently include different designs with regard to frequency and dose.

Effect on bone turnover

Bone markers serve as early indicator of effect in treatment studies of osteoporosis. In addition, they provide information on the pattern of metabolic response, which is even more interesting to describe when the dosing interval is increased. What occurs in the drug free interval? In a placebo-controlled study evaluating fracture efficacy and safety of daily oral and intermittent ibandronate, the effect on bone markers was also studied. The participants, postmenopausal women (n=2946, aged 55–80 years) were allocated into three groups: 2.5 mg ibandronate daily, 20 mg every other day for 12 days every third month, or placebo[72]. Blood samples were taken prior to dosing in those receiving intermittent dosing and therefore represents the residual effect. Bone resorption is markedly decreased during the entire 3 year treatment period[73] (**4.28**). Both treatments led to a constant suppression of bone resorption, approximately 10% greater in those on daily compared to intermittent dosing. The response is less distinct when evaluated by urinary NTx for all treatments, suggesting a greater assay variability and not necessarily a drug effect, since the pattern is also similar for placebo. Bone formation is suppressed by about 40% but the plateau is delayed until 6 months.

For both bone resorption and bone formation markers, the response pattern is similar to that observed for other nitrogen-containing bisphosphonates. The response to intravenous intermittent dosing measured by bone markers shows a similar pattern. The suppression is dose-related and greater in those receiving 1 mg and 2 mg (**4.29**)[74]. Percentage-wise the suppression is somewhat less when ibandronate is administered intravenously, a finding possibly related to the fact that sampling is done just prior to the next dose and thus after 2–3 months without drug. However, with the 2 mg iv dose, bone resorption is decreased to 60% of baseline, a degree of suppression that is commonly aimed for when using oral bisphosphonates[75]. With monthly dosing, the suppression of bone turnover is significant and the higher concurrent dose (100 mg or 150 mg) induced a consistent >60% suppression[76].

Effect on BMD

Oral daily and intermittent ibandronate produce significant increases in BMD at the spine and the hip as is shown in a 3-year RCT (**4.30**)[72]. Spinal BMD increase by 6.5% and 5.7%, respectively for 2.5 mg given daily and 20 mg given intermittently (see above), an increase that is of similar magnitude to that of other bisphosphonates. The increase is less pronounced in the hip (3.4% and 2.9%, respectively).

In the study by Chesnut *et al.*[72], the intermittent dosing followed a regimen of 20 mg given for 12 consecutive days every 3 months, a dosing regimen that is suboptimal from a patient's perspective despite a drug-free interval extending over 2 months. Modified dosing regimens have subsequently been developed and tested.

In a study of 1609 postmenopausal women, oral ibandronate was used: 2.5 mg daily, 50/50 mg (single dose on two consecutive days), 100 mg or 150 mg once monthly. The primary end-point was a BMD not significantly worse than baseline after 1 year of treatment[76]. Lumbar spine

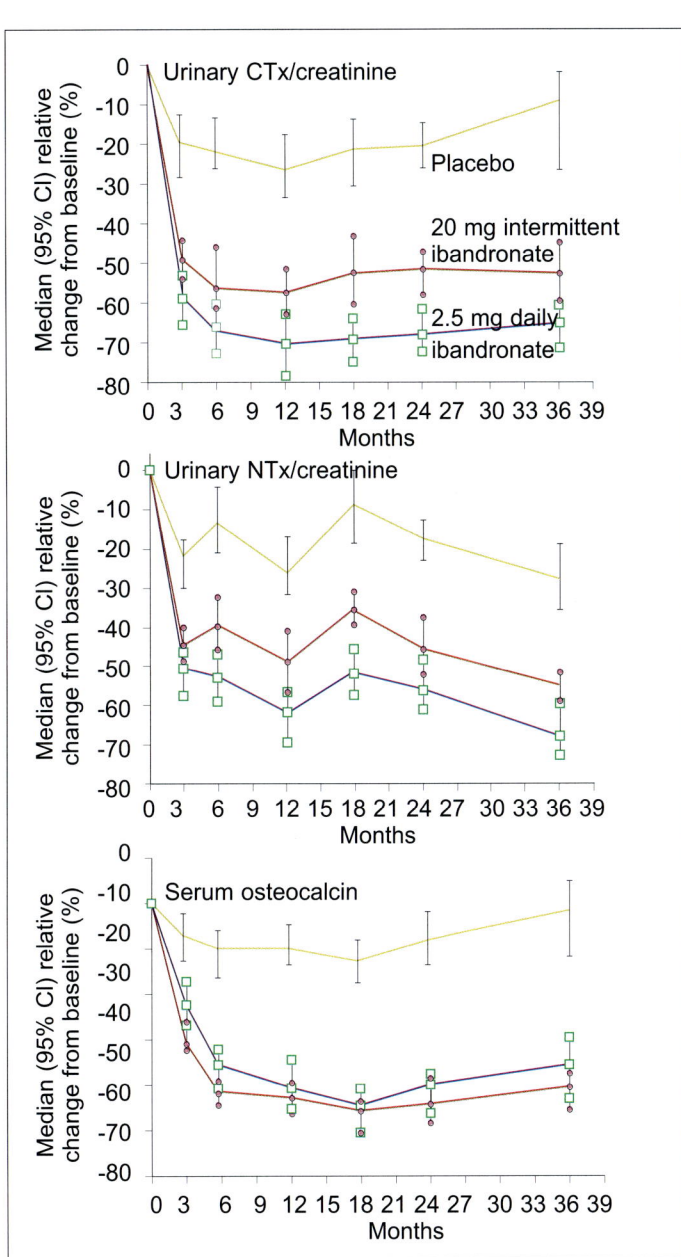

4.28 Ibandronate effect on bone markers. (Adapted from Delmas PD, *et al.* (2004). Daily and intermittent oral ibandronate normalize bone turnover and provide significant reduction in vertebral fracture risk: results from the BONE study. *Osteoporos Int*, **15**(10):792–798.)

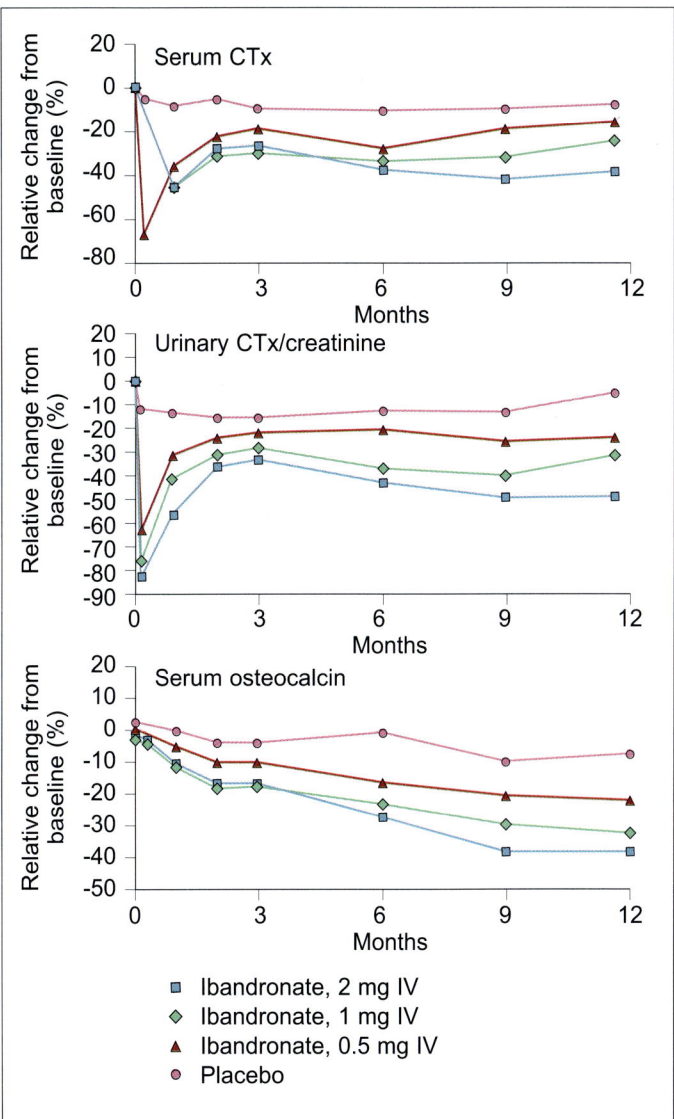

4.29 Ibandronate effect on bone markers. (Adapted from Stakkestad JA, *et al.* (2003). Intravenous ibandronate injections given every three months: a new treatment option to prevent bone loss in postmenopausal women. *Ann Rheum Dis*, **62**(10):969–975.)

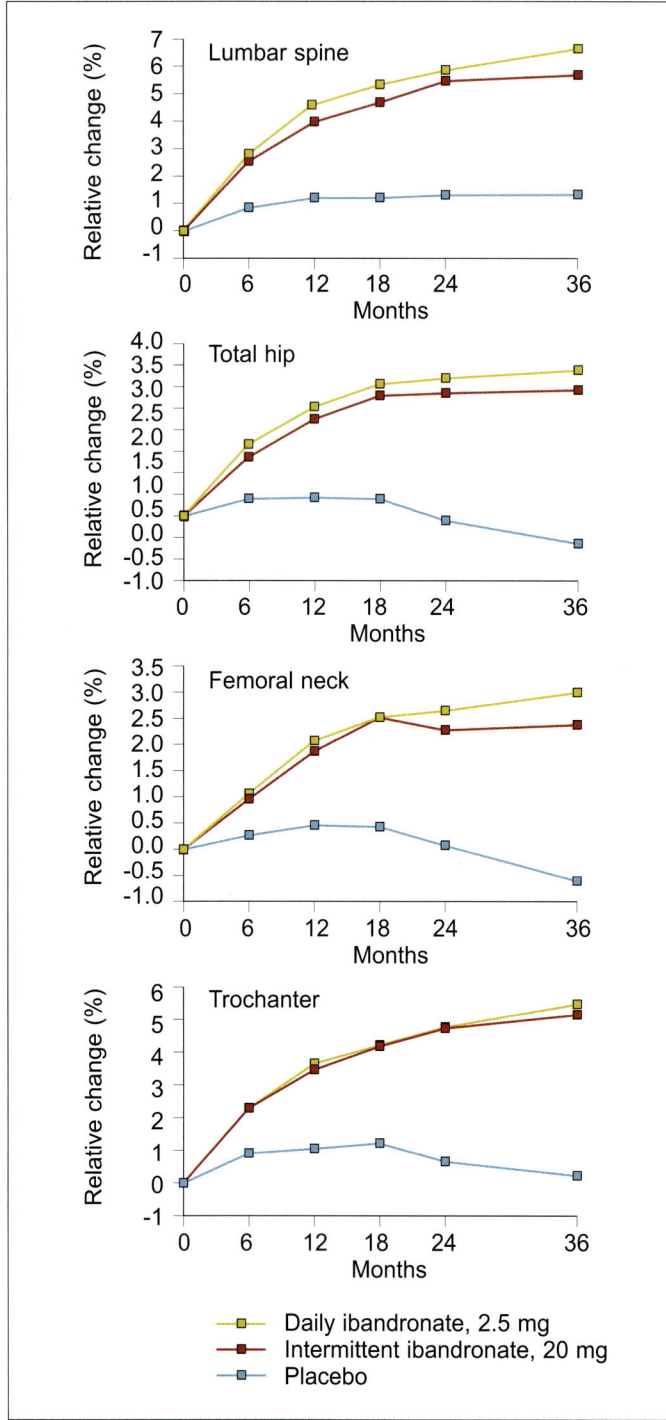

4.30 Ibanronate effect on BMD. (Adapted from Chesnut III CH, *et al.* (2004). Effects of oral ibandronate administered daily or intermittently on fracture risk in postmenopausal osteoporosis. *J Bone Miner Res*, **19**(8):1241–1249.)

BMD increased by 4.1–4.9 % with the monthly regimens, and significantly more patients responded in the 150 mg group. The percentage change in hip BMD was similar, with a larger proportion in the 100 and 150 mg groups achieving a substantial increase (**4.31**, top). This study indicates that

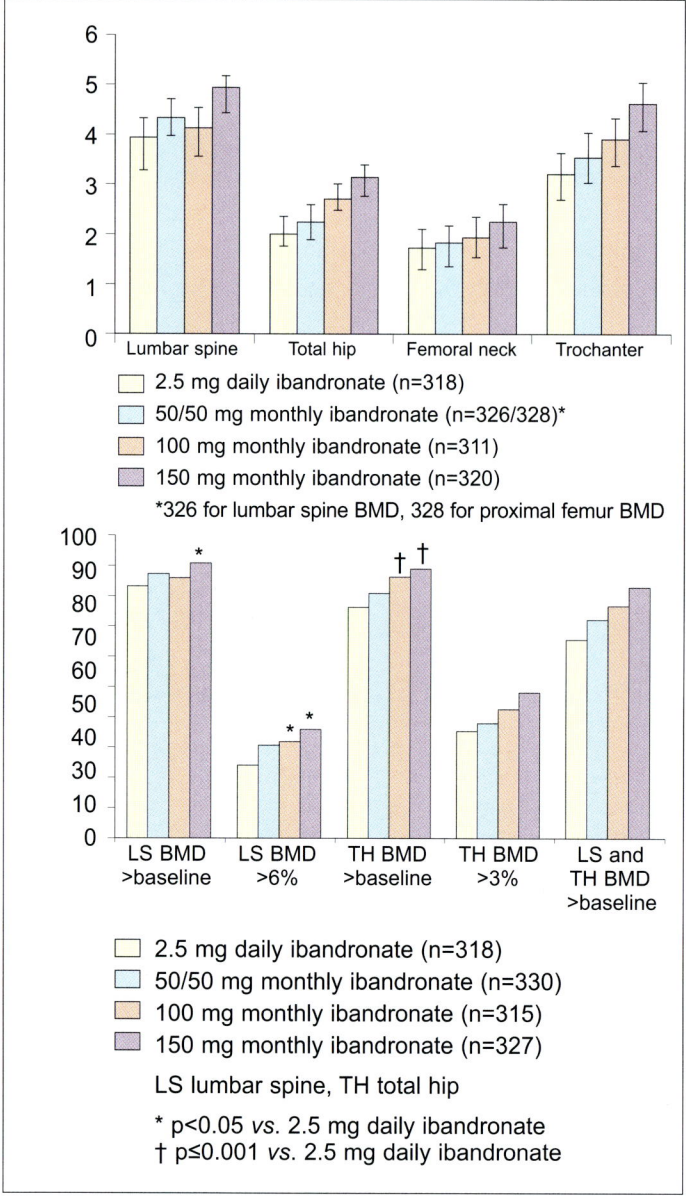

4.31 Ibandronate effect on BMD. (Adapted from Miller PD, *et al.* (2005). Monthly oral ibandronate therapy in postmenopausal osteoporosis: 1-year results from the MOBILE study. *J Bone Miner Res*, 20(8):1315–1322.)

once-monthly oral ibandronate increases BMD over 1 year and is in this respect as effective as daily dosing. The proportion of patients responding is high, up to 90%, with the highest dose slightly superior (**4.31**, bottom).

Effect on fracture

The only study to date sufficiently powered to evaluate the effect of ibandronate on fracture is the study by Chesnut *et al.*[72], which included over 2900 women followed over 3 years, taking oral 2.5mg daily or 20 mg intermittent doses

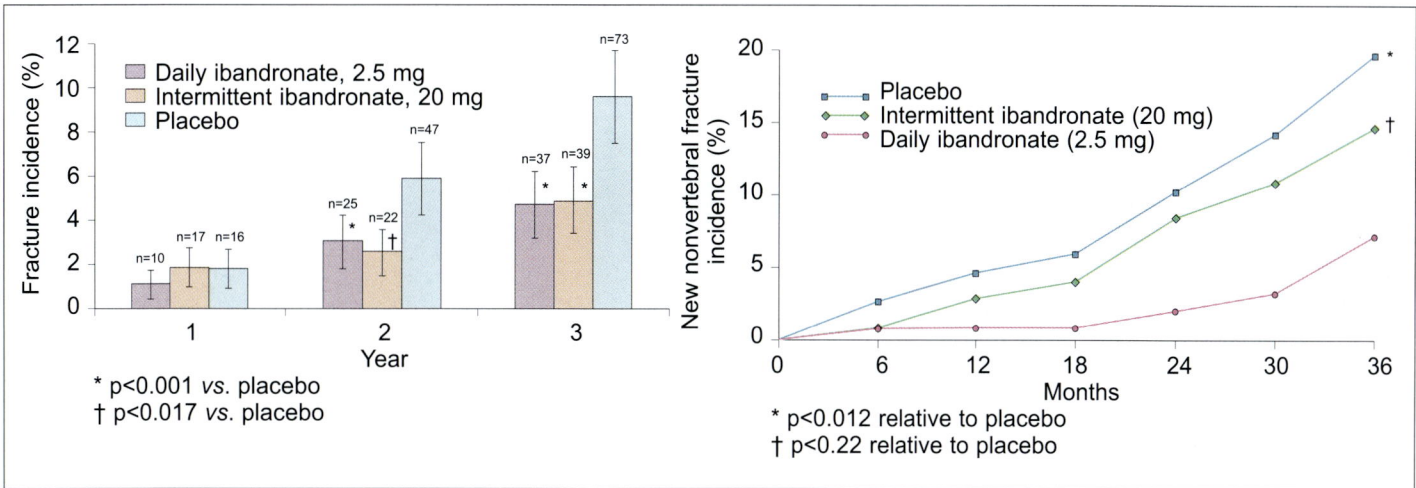

4.32 Ibandronate effect on fracture. (Adapted from Chesnut III CH, *et al.* (2004). Effects of oral ibandronate administered daily or intermittently on fracture risk in postmenopausal osteoporosis. *J Bone Miner Res,* **19**(8):1241–1249.)

during a 3 monthly cycle. The relative risk reduction for incident radiographically identified vertebral fractures was 62% (95% CI 41–75) and 50% (95% CI 26–66) respectively, and both reached significance (p=0.0001, p=0.0006). There was no difference between continuous daily and intermittent dosing. The effect was significant during the second and third year of treatment (**4.32**, left). Close to 60% of the vertebral fractures presented as clinical fractures and the risk reduction for these women was 48–49% but statistically less secure (p<0.05). Nonvertebral fracture risk reduction was not associated with ibandronate treatment. Nevertheless, in a subgroup analysis, nonvertebral fracture risk in those with femoral neck BMD below T-score -3, fracture risk was lower by 69% (p<0.05) (**4.32**, right).

Side-effects

Ibandronate will have a place in the therapy of osteoporosis, not from daily but from intermittent dosing and the benefits that are associated with dosing intervals of one or several months. From the perspective of convenience, it will not only be beneficial for the postmenopausal woman with an active lifestyle, but also for the very elderly where the disadvantage from complex dosing is even more evident. In this respect, side-effects are also of importance. These include gastrointestinal problems (30%), most commonly dyspepsia, musculoskeletal (27%), or general (25%)[77]. However, the side-effects and safety profile are comparable between all different dosing regimens and are no more common than in the placebo group. Intravenous administration may cause transient acute phase reaction, and a higher incidence of arthralgia and myalgia is reported[78].

Zoledronate

The development of more potent bisphosphonates has also prompted the evaluation of their use in treating osteoporosis. Oral bisphosphonates have issues of compliance as well as problems of gastrointestinal tolerance, both of which have implications for their efficacy. Potent bisphosphonates which can be administered parenterally may avoid these issues.

Bisphosphonates are administered intravenously in patients with malignant hypercalcaemia and in those with Paget's disease. Intermittent intravenous administration reduces skeletal events in breast cancer patients, with zoledronate associated with the largest risk reduction (RR 0.59, 95% CI 0.42–0.82)[79]. Zoledronic acid is the most potent bisphosphonate, 100–850-fold more potent than pamidronate. Like other nitrogen-containing bisphosphonates, it binds to the mineral phase of bone where it is internalized by osteosteoclasts, inhibiting farnesyl disphosphate synthase in the mevalonate pathway. The exact molecular mechanism of action is not clear; however, acidification is an absolute prerequisite[80]. Zoledronate is administered as an infusion over 15 minutes.

The majority of studies on zoledronate have been performed in patients with malignant conditions; however, intravenous bisphosphonates have also been used to alleviate pain in patients with Paget's disease and to inhibit progression of the associated bone pathology. In a study comparing intravenous zoledronate with oral risedronate, the 6 month response rate was 96% in those receiving zoledronate and 74% in those receiving oral risedronate, as evaluated by change in alkaline phosphatase (p<0.001)[81].

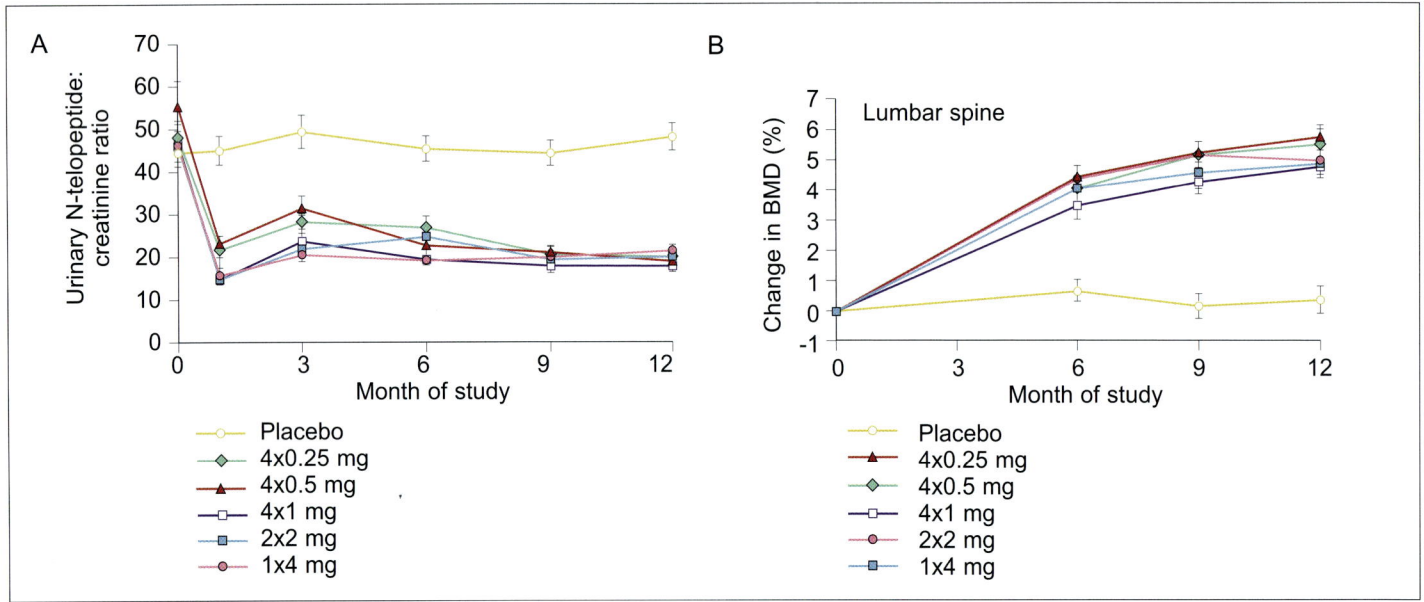

4.33 A Effect of zoledronate on bone markers. (Adapted from Reid IR, *et al.* (2002). Intravenous zoledronic acid in postmenopausal women with low bone mineral density. *N Engl J Med*, **346**(9):653–661.) **B** Effect of zoledronate on BMD. (Adapted from Reid IR, *et al.* (2002). Intravenous zoledronic acid in postmenopausal women with low bone mineral density. *N Engl J Med*, **346**(9):653–661.)

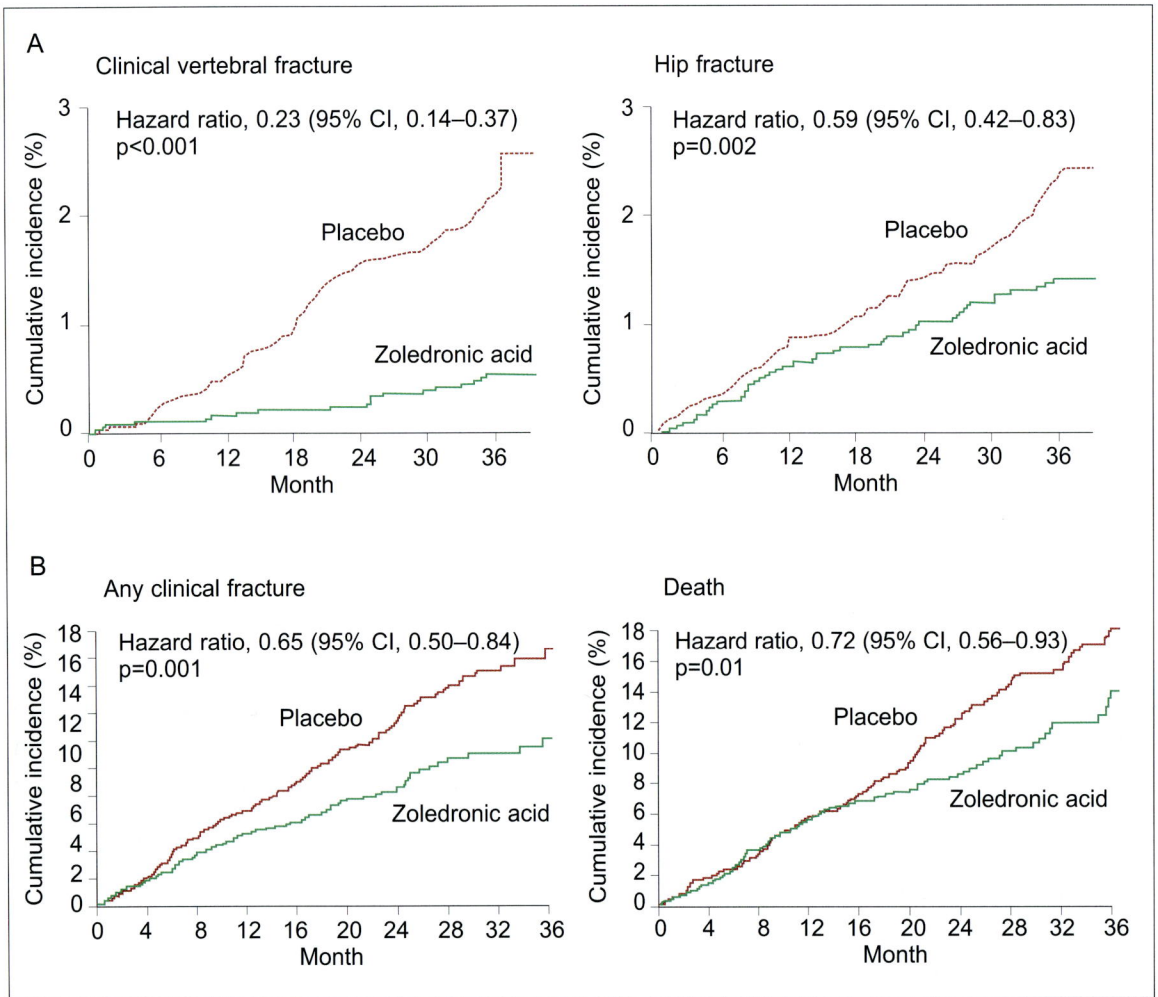

4.34 Effect of Zoledronate on fracture. (**A** Adapted from Black DM, *et al.* (2007). Once-yearly zoledronic acid for treatment of postmenopausal osteoporosis. *N Engl J Med*, **356**(18):1809–1822. **B** Adapted from Lyles KW, *et al.* (2007). Zoledronic acid and clinical fracture and mortality after hip fracture. *N Engl J Med*, **357**(18):1799–1809.)

Effect on bone turnover

A first study on the use of zoledronate in postmenopausal osteoporosis included 351 women, assigned to four different dosing regimens or placebo and lasting for 12 months, used change in BMD as a primary end-point and bone markers as a secondary end-point[82]. The effect on bone turnover markers follows a pattern comparable to that of other potent bisphosphonates; most pronounced for resorption markers and to a lesser extent for formation markers, with resorption markers rapidly suppressed with a maximum decrease at 1 month; serum C-telopeptide decreased by a median of 65–83% and urine N-telopeptide by 50–69% (**4.33A**)[82].

Effect on BMD

The protocol of the initial study included a single yearly dose of 4 mg or a divided dose of 2 mg, two times over a year. Four different dose regimens of zoledronate produced similar effects on bone density (4.3–5.1% at the lumbar spine) after 12 months. Notably, the single annual intravenous dose of 4 mg zoledronic acid gave the same increase as more frequent dosing 82 (**4.33B**). Clearly, it was possible to administer one yearly dose or biannual doses of a potent bisphosphonate and still achieve significant effects. This was later confirmed, where annual infusions of zoledronic acid lead to BMD increases of 5–7% over 3 years[83].

Effect on fracture

To evaluate the effect on fracture, a large-scale randomized controlled study has been performed in women with postmenopausal osteoporosis (n=3889)[83]. With a mean age of 73 years, this is a population at somewhat higher risk compared to similar studies of oral bisphosphonates. After 3 years of annual 5 mg zoledronic acid infusions, the relative risk of clinical vertebral fractures was reduced by 77% (p<0.001), and nonvertebral fractures, all clinical fractures, and hip fracture by 25%, 33% and 41% respectively (**4.34A**). In absolute terms 2.5% (n=88) in the placebo group and 1.4% (n=52) in the treated group suffered a hip fracture.

Hip fracture patients have a high risk of recurrent fractures; in a randomized, double-blinded, placebo controlled study including 1065 hip fracture patients, zoledronic acid was given 90 days after fracture[84]. A 35% reduction of any clinical fracture was evident (p=0.001), as was a 46% decrease in clinical vertebral fractures (p=0.02) (**4.34B**). Furthermore, mortality was reduced by 28% among those treated with zoledronic acid (p=0.01).

Side-effects

Among side-effects, the major difference in all reported studies, is the experience of influenza-like symptoms, e.g. acute phase reaction within the first 3 days after intravenous administration – in postmenopausal women 32–54% and in hip fracture patients 7%. Common complaints included musculoskeletal pain, fever, and nausea and most occurred during the first time administration of the drug, while to a much lesser extent at subsequent infusions. A nonexplained increase in atrial fibrillations was seen in postmenopausal women, but not in hip fracture patients[83, 84].

In summary, current data on zoledronate for the treatment of osteoporosis support a beneficial effect on BMD and a significant reduction in both vertebral and nonvertebral fractures.

Tiludronate is a third generation, non-nitrogen containing bisphosphonate that can be administered either orally or intravenously and has mainly been used in the treatment of Paget's disease; after initially promising results, it has not been further developed for use in osteoporosis.

Hormone replacement therapy

Oestrogen is important both for skeletal development and structural maintenance of bone. The balance between bone resorption and bone formation in adulthood is in part dependent on intact oestrogen levels, and bone loss during the initial years after menopause is linked to oestrogen withdrawal. Oestrogen exhibits its effect on both osteoblasts and osteoclasts through several mechanisms, but action via the oestrogen receptors (ER) is probably most important. Two ERs are identified, and ERα appears to be the main receptor associated with bone.

The rapidly decreasing oestrogen levels at menopause may lead to increased activation frequency, that is the number of active resorption sites increase while the capacity to refill the site with new bone diminishes, causing bone loss. By substituting for oestrogen loss or manipulating the ER activity, the rate of bone turnover should remain in balance. This is the rationale for the use of oestrogen replacement therapy (ERT) and for the development of new drugs that modify the ER.

Oestrogen replacement

Oestrogen replacement therapy (ERT) has been widely used for many years to alleviate postmenopausal symptoms related to oestrogen withdrawal, with the additional effect on bone turnover and bone mass. The effect on fracture by ERT has been evaluated in meta-analysis of randomized trials finding a reduction in nonvertebral fractures of 27%[85] and in vertebral fractures of 33%[86]. The effect was less clear in older women. There is an offset of benefit; thus the advantages of taking hormone replacement therapy (HRT) while the woman is in her 50s on fracture risk at the peak age of 70–80 years is unclear. The recent Women's Health Initiative (WHI) study, which recruited 16,608 healthy postmenopausal women aged 50–79 years, found that ERT reduced the risk of both vertebral and hip fracture. The bone density was unknown at the start of the study.

The major concern for the role of ERT in the prevention of osteoporosis and fracture is the increased risk of breast cancer, endometrial cancer, ovarian cancer, stroke, and venous thromboembolism (*Table 4.6*). The risks and benefits and individual circumstances, therefore, have to be carefully considered when recommending ERT, and the duration of treatment should stay within 5 years for a postmenopausal woman in most circumstances.

It is common practice to use ERT in premature oestrogen deficiency to ensure adequate levels up to the expected age of menopause as these women may otherwise be at increased risk of future fracture. However, there is little evidence for the long-term benefits of this approach. Oestrogen should be given opposed with either cyclic or continuous gestagen to women with an intact uterus, as there is otherwise an increased risk of endometrial cancer.

Table 4.6 Summary of risks and benefits associated with using HRT

Condition	Age of woman (years)	Number of cases/1000 nonHRT users		Extra number of cases in 1000 HRT users for 5 years HRT use over the same period*	
Cumulative cancer risk over 5 years				*Oestrogen only*	*Combined HRT*
Breast cancer Million Women Study	50–64	14[a]		1.5 (±1.5)	6 (±1)
		CEE[b]	CEE + MPA[b]		
WHI	50–79	15	16	No significant effect	4 (±4)
Endometrial cancer	50–69	3[b]		5 (±1)[c]	Cannot be estimated[d]
Ovarian cancer	50–69	3		1 (±1)	Not known
Cardiovascular risks over 5 years					
		CEE[b]	CEE + MPA[b]		
Stroke	50–59	8	3	2 (±2)	1 (±1)
	60–69	15	11	6 (±4)	
VTE	50–59	6.5	3	1 (±1)	4 (±2)
	60–69	11.5	8	4 (±4)	9 (±5)
Benefits over 5 years				*Reduced number of cases in 1000 HRT users over the same period*	
		CEE[b]	CEE + MPA[b]		
Colorectal cancer	50–59	6	3	No significant effect	1 (±1)
	60–69	10	8		3 (±2)
Fracture of neck of femur	50–59	0.5	1.5	0.3 (±0.51)	0.3 (±1)
	60–69	5.5	5.5	3 (±2)	3 (±2)

Numbers are best estimates (± approximate range from 95% CI)
* All values are from the WHI trial unless otherwise stated
[a] CA cumulative risk of 14 cases/1000 non-HRT users over 5 years has been used to facilitate comparison of the MWS and the WHI studies
[b] Estimates from the placebo group of the WHI trial
[c] Relative risk associated with 5 years' use of oestrogen-only HRT (RR = 2.8 (2.3–3.5) from metaanalysis)
[d] Risk cannot be reliably estimated – the addition of a progestogen for at least 12 days per month greatly reduces the additional risk of endometrial cancer due to unopposed oestrogen, but the magnitude of the reduction is poorly defined at present

Selective oestrogen receptor modulators

Oestrogen plays an important role in the maintenance of skeletal integrity in women and probably also in men. Oestrogen exhibits agonistic effects, whereas selective oestrogen receptor modulators (SERMs) have both agonistic and antagonistic effects in tissues responsive to oestrogen. SERMs are nonsteroidal ligands that produce agonistic effects in bone, similar to those of oestrogen, but antagonistic effects in, for example, breast tissue. Raloxifene has been evaluated in major trials for treatment of osteoporosis and breast cancer, alongside substudies evaluating the effects on other organ systems.

In addition to the significant antioestrogenic effect on breast tissue from tamoxifen, a pronounced effect was also recognized in uterine tissue, as was a weak agonistic effect on bone. When raloxifene was developed it was discovered that it provided not only a minimal uterine response, but also a significant inhibition of bone resorption[87]. Both tamoxifen and raloxifene bind to the oestrogen receptor, despite different primary structures compared to oestrogen (**4.35**)[88].

Mechanisms of action

Oestrogen binds to the oestrogen receptor, inducing conformational changes of the receptor and forming an oestrogen receptor–oestrogen complex that diffuses into the nucleus[89]. Raloxifene acts as a competitive ligand to oestrogen receptor, blocking the conformational changes of the receptor modulating the gene activation and subsequent protein production. Raloxifene can bind to both oestrogen receptor-α and oestrogen receptor-β, but has a four-fold greater affinity for oestrogen receptor-α[90].

When oestrogen receptor-SERM binds in tissues where a primarily agonistic expression is expected (such as bone for raloxifene), the receptor-ligand complex acts preferentially via a coactiviator enhancing the agonistic effect (**4.36**). When oestrogen receptor-SERM binds in tissues where a primarily antagonistic expression is expected (such as breast for raloxifene), the receptor-ligand complex acts preferentially via a corepressor enhancing the antagonistic effect[91].

Effect on bone turnover

Raloxifene reduces urinary calcium excretion, conferring a positive calcium balance[92] and decreases bone turnover as assessed by bone markers[93]. The decrease in bone markers of between 30–40% indicates that raloxifene is primarily an antiresorptive agent; however, this is a less pronounced de-

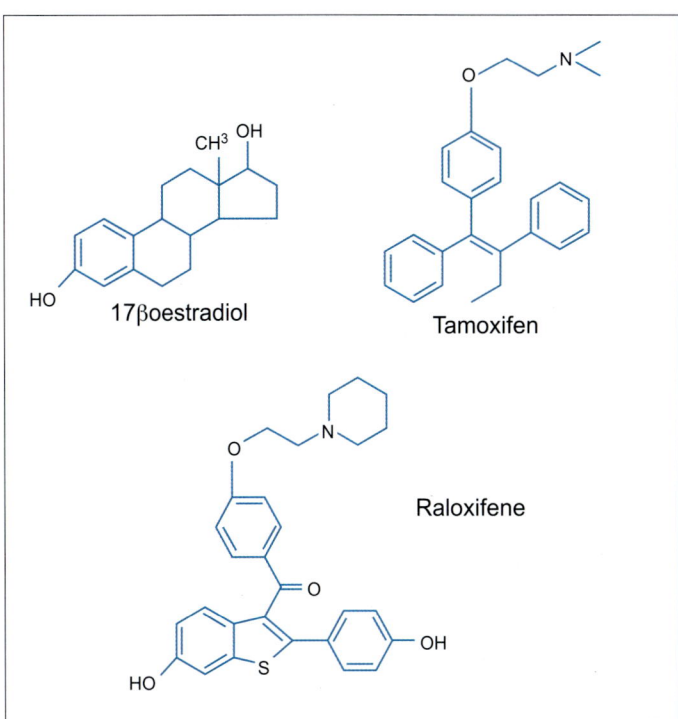

4.35 Structure of oestrogen in relation to raloxifene.

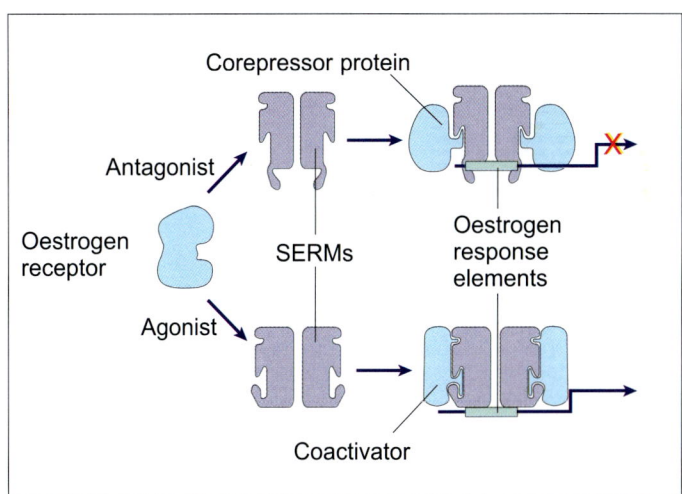

4.36 SERM and mechanisms of action.

crease compared to what is seen with bisphosphonates[94, 95].

Raloxifene inhibits bone resorption as indicated in animal studies; however, the exact mechanism remains to be elucidated. The effect on bone turnover is that of an antiresorptive agent with levels of bone markers decreasing during the first 6–9 months. The change in bone markers over 24 months of raloxifene at three different doses *vs.* placebo is clear[93]. The mean decrease after 24 months of raloxifene treatment was 15–23% for bone formation and

34% for bone resorption in those receiving the 60 mg dose.

In a comparative 1-year study[95], raloxifene 60 mg was compared with alendronate 10 mg daily or a combination of raloxifene and alendronate (**4.37**).

In women with prior alendronate treatment for over 3 years, treatment continued for 2 additional years with placebo, raloxifene, or continued alendronate **4.38**[96]. Bone turnover remain depressed in those continuing with alendronate, whereas it increased within 6 months in those receiving raloxifene or no treatment. After this a new steady state was reached. This indicates that if a change of therapy is required, the antiresorptive effect is maintained with raloxifene after alendronate treatment and include a potential benefit from a less pronounced depression of bone turnover. Bone formation was assessed by PINP and osteocalcin, and bone resorption by CTx. The significance level was p<0.005.

Effect on density

The Multiple Outcome Raloxifene study (MORE) which enrolled 7705 osteoporotic women with and without

vertebral fractures, evaluated the effect of two different doses of raloxifene – 60 mg/day and 120 mg/day – with the 60 mg dose chosen for clinical use[97]. The primary end-point was vertebral and nonvertebral fracture risk, with effects on BMD as secondary outcomes. Bone mass increased significantly by 2.6% in the spine and 2.1% in the femoral neck in the 60 mg of raloxifene group, the now recommended dose, and was only slightly higher in the 120 mg group. The change in BMD is similar when evaluated in a meta-analysis[98].

Figure **4.39** describes the enrolment into the MORE study[94]. The study has also provided data on raloxifene effects on other relevant organ systems. The initial evaluation occurred at 3 years but the cohort was followed allowing for a 4-year evaluation. The study population is divided into two groups: group 1 with BMD below -2.5 T-score and group 2 with at least one vertebral fracture with or without low BMD[97]. This study shows the effect on BMD from the two different raloxifene doses compared to placebo. BMD increased significantly in the lumbar spine by

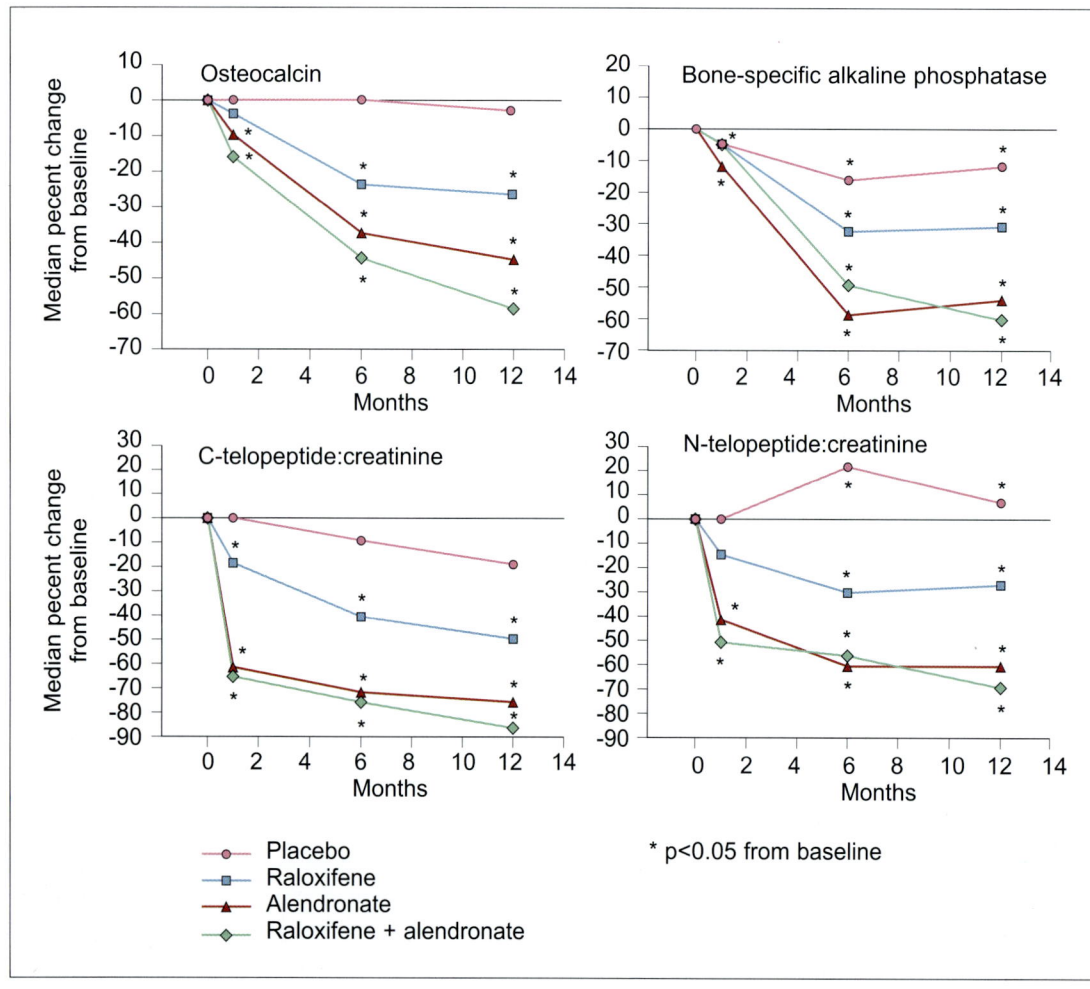

4.37 Raloxifene and bone markers. Bisphosphonates have direct inhibitory effects on osteoclasts, commonly producing a profound decrease in bone resorption. The depression of bone turn-over doubled when alendronate was given and the combined treatment indicated an additive effect on BMD. (Adapted from Johnell O, *et al.* (2002). Additive effects of raloxifene and alendronate on bone density and biochemical markers of bone remodeling in postmenopausal women with osteoporosis. *J Clin Endocrinol Metab*, **87**(3):985-992.)

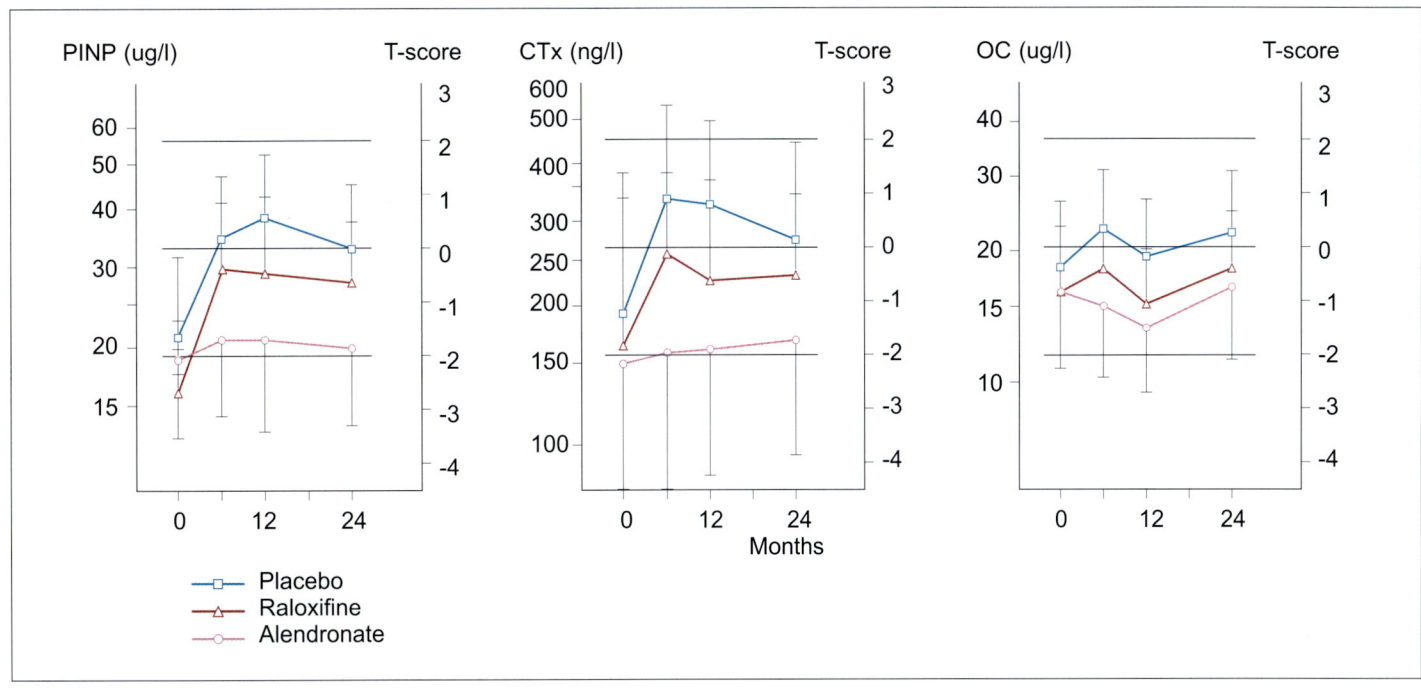

4.38 Raloxifene and bone markers. (Adapted from Michalska D, *et al.* (2006). The effect of raloxifene after discontinuation of long-term alendronate treatment of postmenopausal osteoporosis. *J Clin Endocrinol Metab,* **91**(3):870–877.)

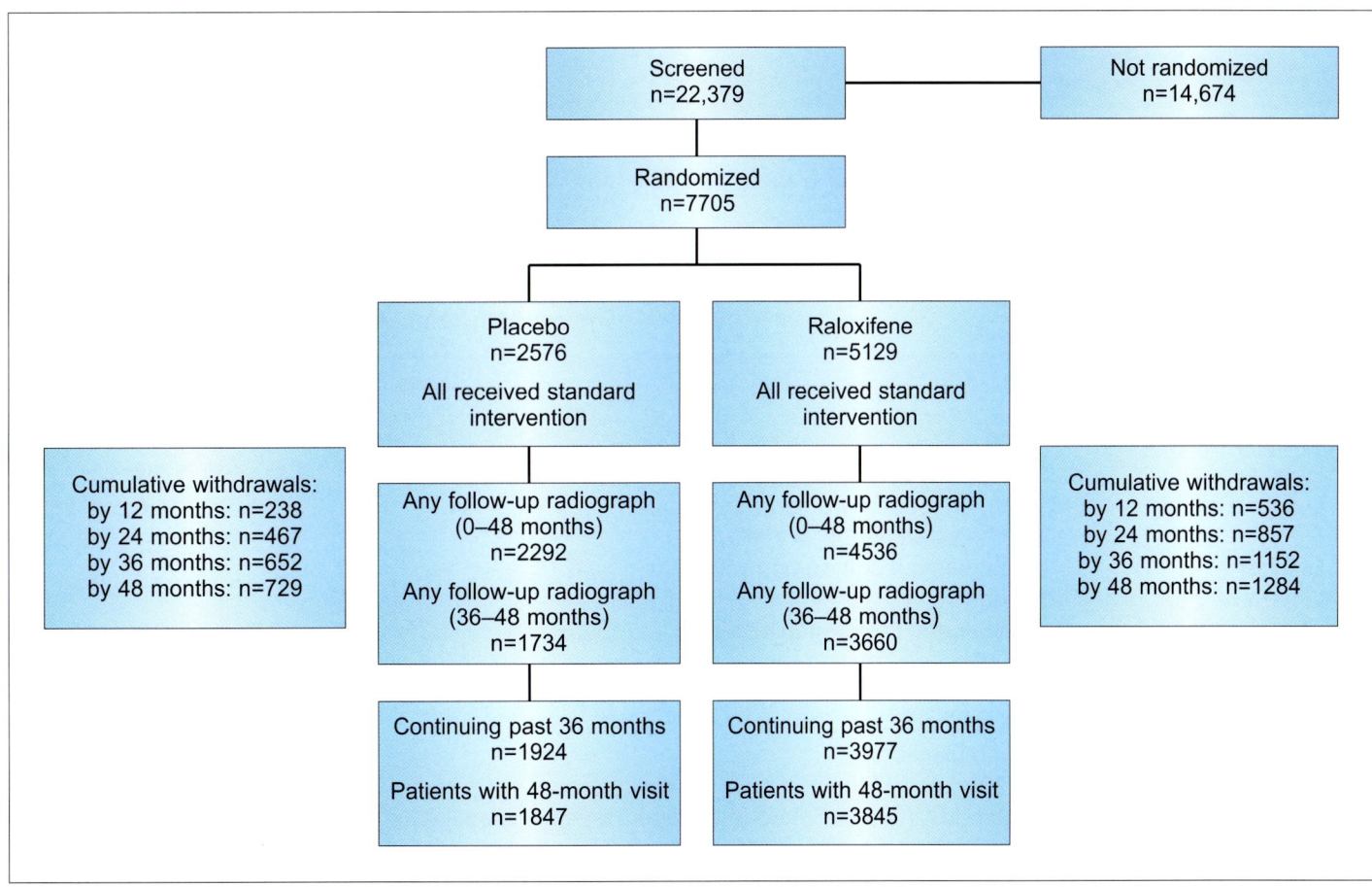

4.39 The design of the MORE study. (Adapted from Delmas PD, *et al.* (2002). Efficacy of raloxifene on vertebral fracture risk reduction in postmenopausal women with osteoporosis: four-year results from a randomized clinical trial. *J Clin Endocrinol Metab,* **87**(8):3609–3617.)

2.6–2.7% and in the hip 2.1–2.4%. In women previously treated with alendronate, continued treatment with combined raloxifene and alendronate appears to have a maintaining and additive effect on BMD in both spine and hip compared to either treatment alone or discontinuation of treatment (**4.40**)[97]. The changes in BMD of the lumbar spine and femoral neck from available trials are compared in *Table 4.7*[91]. The overall change is approximately 2–3% and, therefore, lower than the changes seen during bisphosphonate treatment; nevertheless, the change is associated with a similar decrease in vertebral fracture risk.

Effect on fractures

In the MORE study there was a 30% overall risk reduction of vertebral fractures (RR 0.70, 95% CI 0.50-0.80) with 60 mg/day of raloxifene over 3 years. No effect was seen on nonvertebral fractures. Additional analyses showed that fracture reduction was most pronounced in those with

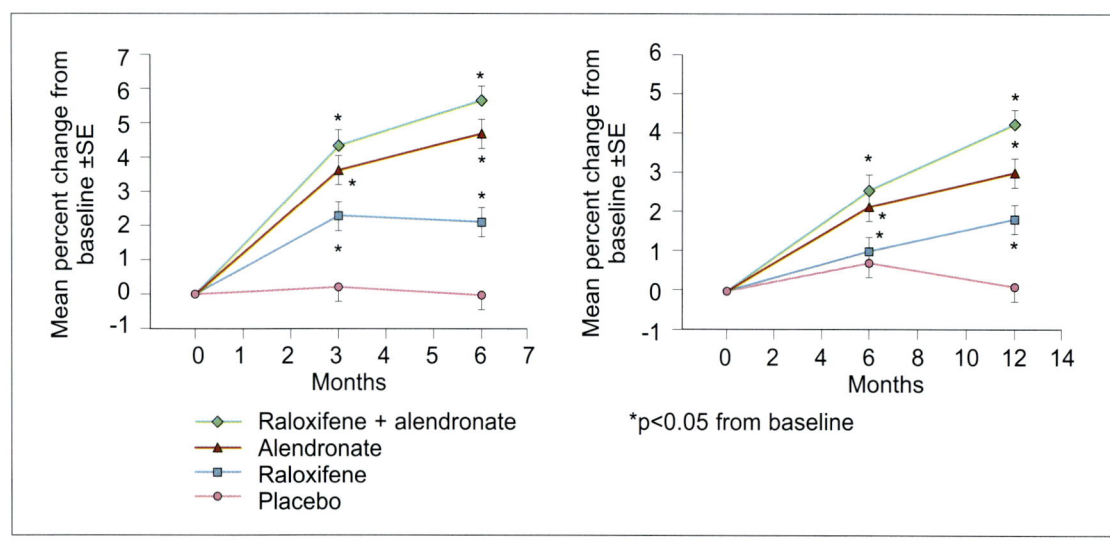

*p<0.05 from baseline

Raloxifene + alendronate
Alendronate
Raloxifene
Placebo

4.40 Raloxifene and BMD. (Adapted from Johnell O, *et al.* (2002). Additive effects of raloxifene and alendronate on bone density and biochemical markers of bone remodeling in postmenopausal women with osteoporosis. *J Clin Endocrinol Metab*, **87**(3):985–992.)

Table 4.7 Results of major randomized clinical trials of SEMs with regard to BMD

Trial	Study subjects	Duration (months)	Change in BMD as compared with placebo group		
			Total-body bone mineral	Lumbar spine	Proximal femur
Raloxifene (60 mg/day)					
Delmas *et al.*	302 normal postmenopausal women	24	2.0*	2.4*	2.4*
Lufkin *et al.*	143 postmenopausal women with osteoporosis and vertebral fractures	12	-0.1	1.8†	1.0†
Ettinger *et al.*	5140 postmenopausal women with osteoporosis	36	–	2.6*	2.1*
Johnston *et al.*	576 health early postmenopausal women	36	1.7*	2.6*	2.5*

* p=0.05 for the comparison with placebo
† p=0.005 for the comparison with placebo

Adapted from Riggs BL, Hartmann LC. (2003). Selective estrogen-receptor modulators – mechanisms of action and application to clinical practice. *N Engl J Med*, **348**(7):618–629

previous severe vertebral fractures with the effect independent of BMD[99, 100]. Fracture reduction was maintained but not augmented during the fourth year of treatment[94].

In Figure **4.41** new vertebral fractures in women who completed a study are shown (n=6828)[97]. The data are presented separately for women with prior fracture and women without prior fracture. Women with prior fracture represent those with a higher risk. Fracture risk was significantly reduced with both raloxifene doses, with a 50% reduction in those with prior fracture and 30% in women without prior fracture for the 60 mg dose.

Raloxifene treatment for 3 years did not reduce the nonvertebral fracture risk[97]. Cumulative incidence of nonvertebral fractures in the total study cohort (n=240/2576 placebo treated and n=437/5129 raloxifene treated) and for the most common types of fractures with wrist fracture being the most prevalent (n=86 placebo and 151 raloxifene groups). It should be noted that the mean age of the study population was 67 years, ranging from 25–80 years, indicating that the study was not powered to evaluate any effect on hip fracture based on the epidemiology of hip fractures where the mean age is above 80 years.

In a reanalysis of the MORE data, excluding the 120 mg treatment arm and including women without prevalent fractures, classification was based on BMD (**4.42**)[100]. Women were defined as osteoporotic (n=2557) or osteopenic (n=635), based BMD measurements. In patients with osteoporosis based on spinal BMD, raloxifene significantly

reduced the risk of vertebral fractures by 69% and clinical vertebral fractures by 84%. The risk of new vertebral fracture also was estimated on BMD T-score total hip (**A**) and T-score femoral neck (**B**). The figures show the almost linear relationship between T-score and fracture risk, indicating

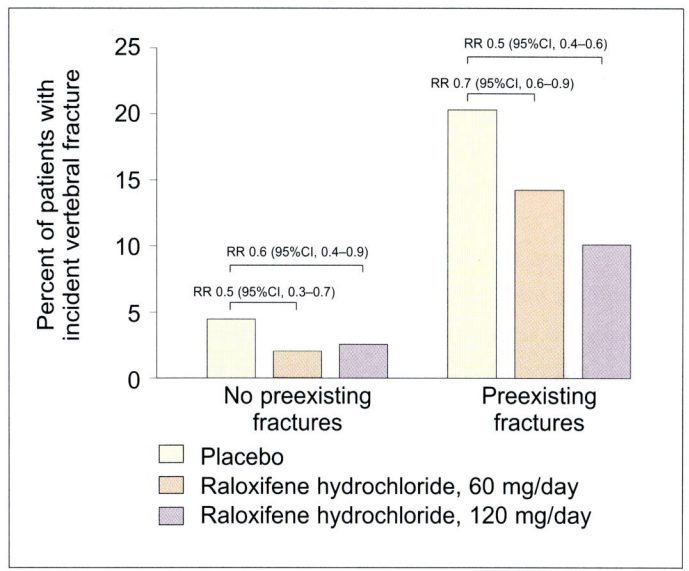

4.41 Raloxifene and fracture. (Adapted from Ettinger B, *et al.* (1999). Reduction of vertebral fracture risk in postmenopausal women with osteoporosis treated with raloxifene: results from a 3-year randomized clinical trial. Multiple Outcomes of Raloxifene Evaluation (MORE) Investigators. *JAMA*, **282**(7):637–645.)

4.42 Raloxifene and fracture. (Adapted from Kanis JA, *et al.* (2003). Effect of raloxifene on the risk of new vertebral fracture in postmenopausal women with osteopenia or osteoporosis: a reanalysis of the Multiple Outcomes of Raloxifene Evaluation trial. *Bone*, **33**(3):293–300.)

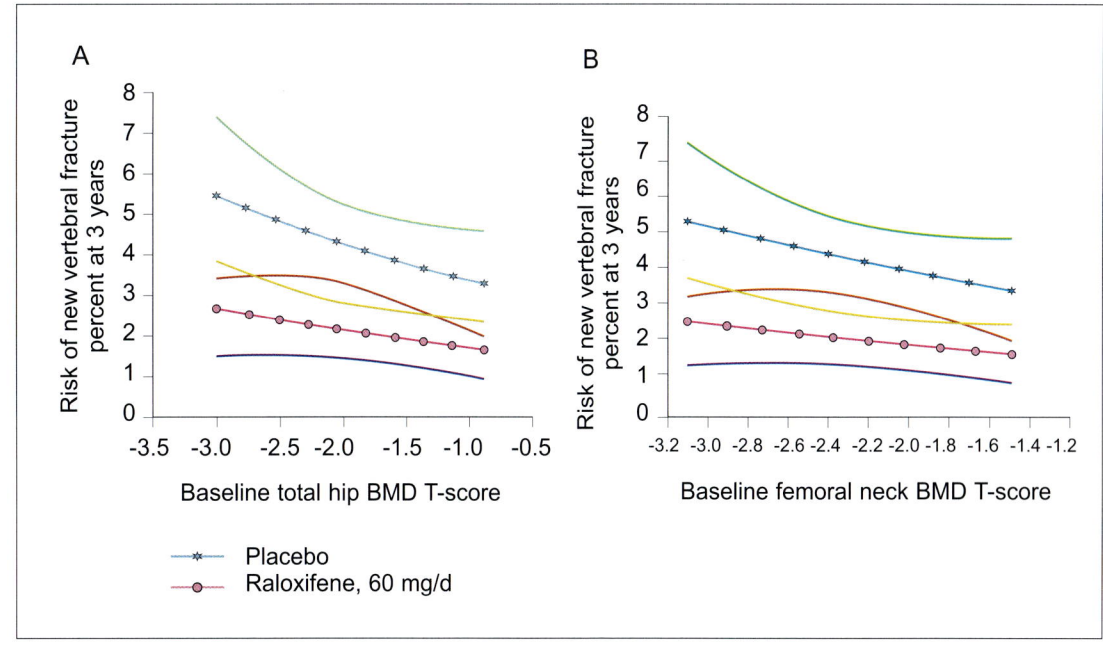

that the risk reduction was independent of baseline BMD but those on raloxifene had a significantly lower risk.

Women with severe prior vertebral fracture had a higher risk of sustaining a new vertebral fracture[99]. In these women the new fracture was more likely to be moderate or severe. Raloxifene 60 mg significantly decreased the vertebral fracture risk in this high risk group (0.74, 95%CI 0.54-0.99), which relates to a number needed to treat (NNT) of 10 over 3 years.

The MORE study was continued during a fourth year in order to evaluate the effect on fracture risk with prolonged duration of treatment. Most interesting is to follow fracture risk in those receiving the 60 mg dose over 4 years, since this is the recommended dose. The data are reported for years 0–3 and for year 4 alone (**4.43**)[94]. The risk reduction during the year 4 is similar to that of the first three years.

The cumulative incidence of new vertebral fractures following 4 years of treatment with raloxifene was sustained but not increased during years 2–4. The risk reduction for the 60 mg dose was 35% in those with prevalent fractures and 48% in those without prevalent fractures; however, the number of fractures was, as expected, higher in those with prevalent fracture. There was no risk reduction over 4 years regarding nonvertebral fractures (11.5% in the placebo group and 10.7% in the pooled treatment groups sustained a nonvertebral fracture, most commonly a wrist fracture).

Safety data and side-effects

Fewer women in the raloxifene treated groups in the MORE study were diagnosed with breast cancer[101], a result indicating a significant effect since the study was not powered to study breast cancer. The risk reduction persisted at 4-year follow up[102]. Among the 5129 women treated with raloxifene, 13 new cases were diagnosed, compared to 27 cases in 2576 women on placebo, giving an overall relative risk of 0.24 (95% CI 0.13–0.44). The risk reduction was most pronounced in those with oestrogen-positive tumours. In a recent study, the STAR trial, with the objective to compare the effect on breast cancer risk from tamoxifen or raloxifene in 20,000 women, a similar risk reduction of incident breast cancer was shown[103]. In addition, patient related outcome was reported to be similar between the treatments[104].

The incidence of new breast cancer was evaluated as a tertiary end-point in the MORE study, albeit such studies

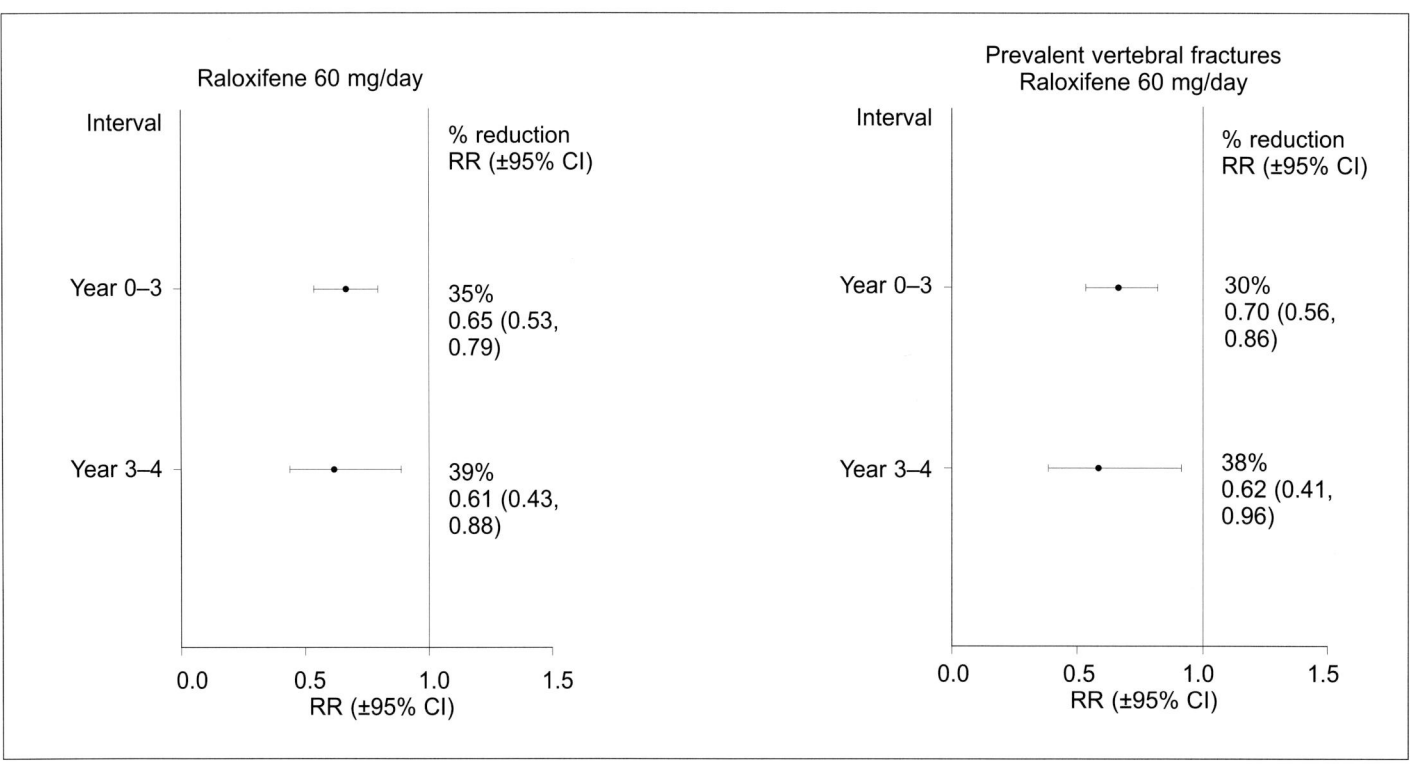

4.43 Raloxifene and fracture. (Adapted from Delmas PD, *et al.* (2002). Efficacy of raloxifene on vertebral fracture risk reduction in postmenopausal women with osteoporosis: four-year results from a randomized clinical trial. *J Clin Endocrinol Metab,* **87**(8):3609–3617.)

usually require a larger study population[101]. The 3-year cumulative incidence of breast cancer in the placebo group (n=2576) and in the combined raloxifene groups (n=5129) are shown in Figure **4.44**. The risk of breast cancer was significantly decreased in those receiving raloxifene by 76% (p<0.001).

The STAR trial was specifically designed to evaluate the preventive effect of raloxifene compared to tamoxifen on women with an increased 5-year risk of breast cancer. 19,747 women of whom 48.9% were 50–59 years were randomized to receive either tamoxifen or raloxifene[103]. Mean follow-up time 3.9 years (1.6 SD). The cumulative incidence of invasive and noninvasive breast cancer over a maximum of 5 years of treatment is shown (**4.45**). The study showed that raloxifene was equally effective in reducing the incidence of breast cancer. In addition the incidence of DVT and cataracts was lower.

Recent studies suggest that the effect on cardiovascular risk from oestrogen treatment is increased. Serum lipids are associated with risk of cardiovascular events, such as stroke. Raloxifene has been reported to change the lipid profile to a more favourable one from a risk perspective[92, 105] (with a decrease in LDL and by an increase in HDL without increasing triglycerides), but the number of cardiovascular events remained comparable to those of placebo[106]. Hence it is not possible to conclude that outcome is affected.

Side-effects were usually mild and mostly short lasting vasomotor symptoms, with only hot flashes significantly influenced during withdrawal from treatment (RR 1.46, 95% CI 1.23-1.74)[107]. The more serious side-effect was thromboembolic events, both deep vein thrombosis and pulmonary embolism, with a relative risk of 3.1 (95% CI 1.5-6-2) in the MORE trial, which corresponds to the risk with HRT[101].

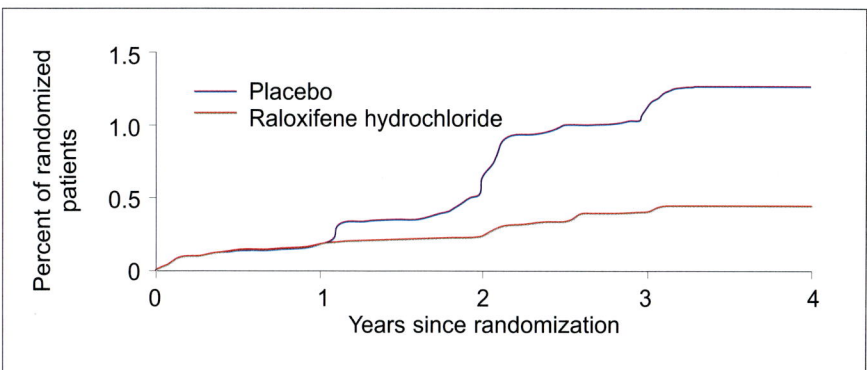

4.44 Raloxifene and risk of breast cancer. (Adapted from Cummings SR, *et al.* (1999). The effect of raloxifene on risk of breast cancer in postmenopausal women: results from the MORE randomized trial. Multiple Outcomes of Raloxifene Evaluation. *JAMA*, **281**(23):2189–2197.)

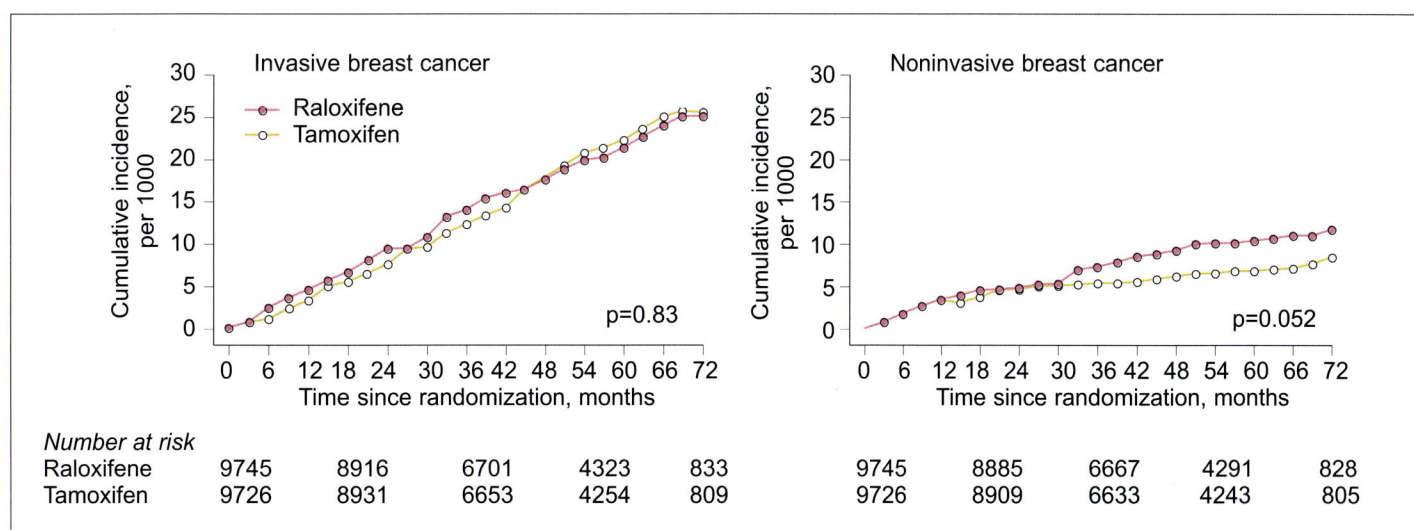

4.45 Cumulative incidence of invasive and noninvasive breast cancer. (Adapted from Vogel VG, *et al.* (2006). Effects of tamoxifen vs raloxifene on the risk of developing invasive breast cancer and other disease outcomes: the NSABP Study of Tamoxifen and Raloxifene (STAR) P-2 trial. *JAMA*, **295**(23):2727–2741.)

During oestrogen treatment an early increase in cardiovascular events has been noted (**4.46**)[106]. Raloxifene treatment over 4 years did not affect the risk of cardiovascular events in the total treatment group but decreased the risk in those women with increased cardiovascular risk. Reported side-effects including influenza symptoms, hot flashes, leg cramps, and peripheral oedema are more common with raloxifene compared to placebo[97]. The effects of raloxifene in relation to oestrogen and tamoxifen are shown in *Table 4.8*[91].

Parathyroid hormone

Treatments for osteoporosis, such as bisphosphonates, oestrogens, selective oestrogen receptor modulators, and calcitonin, all reduce bone resorption with a moderate effect on bone mass and a subsequent moderate reduction of fractures, mainly vertebral fractures. However, none of these agents has the capacity to restore bone structure and skeletal integrity. Anabolic therapies are thus warranted to induce direct effects on bone formation in order to obtain larger

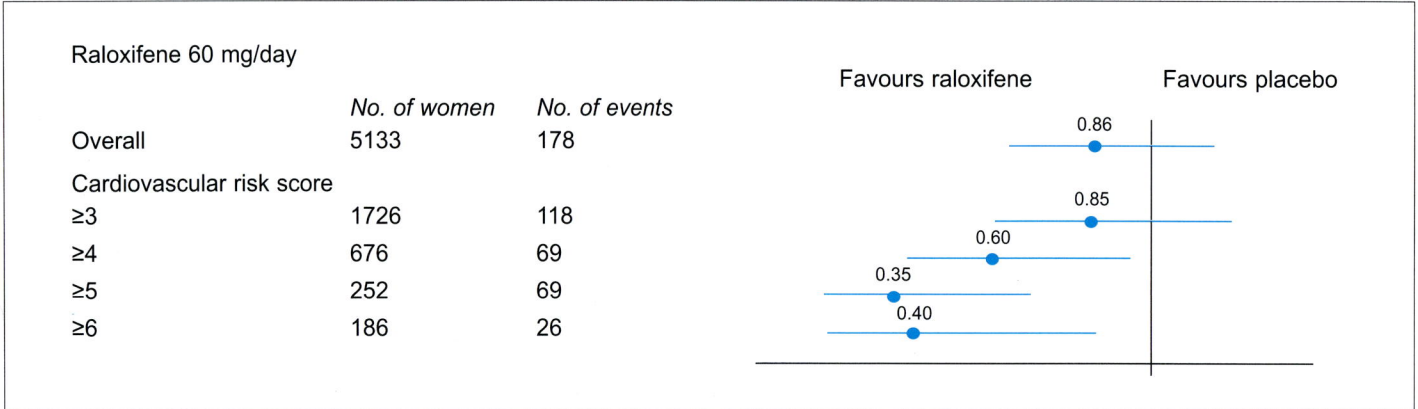

4.46 Raloxifene and cardiovascular risk. (Adapted from Barrett-Connor E, *et al*. (2002). Raloxifene and cardiovascular events in osteoporotic postmenopausal women: four-year results from the MORE (Multiple Outcomes of Raloxifene Evaluation) randomized trial. JAMA, **287**(7):847–857.)

Table 4.8 comparison of selected actions and side-effects of oestrogen and clinically available SERMS

Side-effect	Oestrogen	Tamoxifen	Raloxifene
Hot flashes	↓↓↓	↑*	↑*
Uterine bleeding	↑↑↑	↑	↔
Risk of endometrial cancer	↑↑†	↑	↔
Prevention of postmenopausal bone loss	↑↑↑	↑	↑↑
Risk of breast cancer	↑↑	↓↓	↓↓
Favourable pattern of serum lipids	↑↑↑‡	↑	↑
Venous thrombosis	↑↑	↑↑	↑↑

↑ indicates that the drug increases the effect; ↓ indicates that the drug decreases the effect; ↔ indicates no change; the number of arrows indicates the size of the change
* In perimenopausal women, the action would be ↑↑
† This effect can be prevented by concurrent treatment with a progestin
‡ This effect may be attenuated by concurrent treatment with androgen-derived progestins

(Adapted from Riggs BL, Hartmann LC (2003). Selective estrogen-receptor modulators – mechanisms of action and application to clinical practice. *N Engl J Med*, **348**(7):618–629.)

4.47 Mode of action of PTH. The figure shows that PTH is a key regulator of calcium homeostasis. Parathyroid hormone is released from the parathyroid glands in response to serum calcium changes mediated through the calcium-sensing receptor. The action of PTH is mediated through the PTH receptor in target tissues. PTH acts on the kidney, bone, and intestine. The negative feed-back from vitamin D is not shown. (Adapted from Marx SJ (2000). Hyperparathyroid and hypoparathyroid disorders. *N Engl J Med*, **343**(25):1863–1875.)

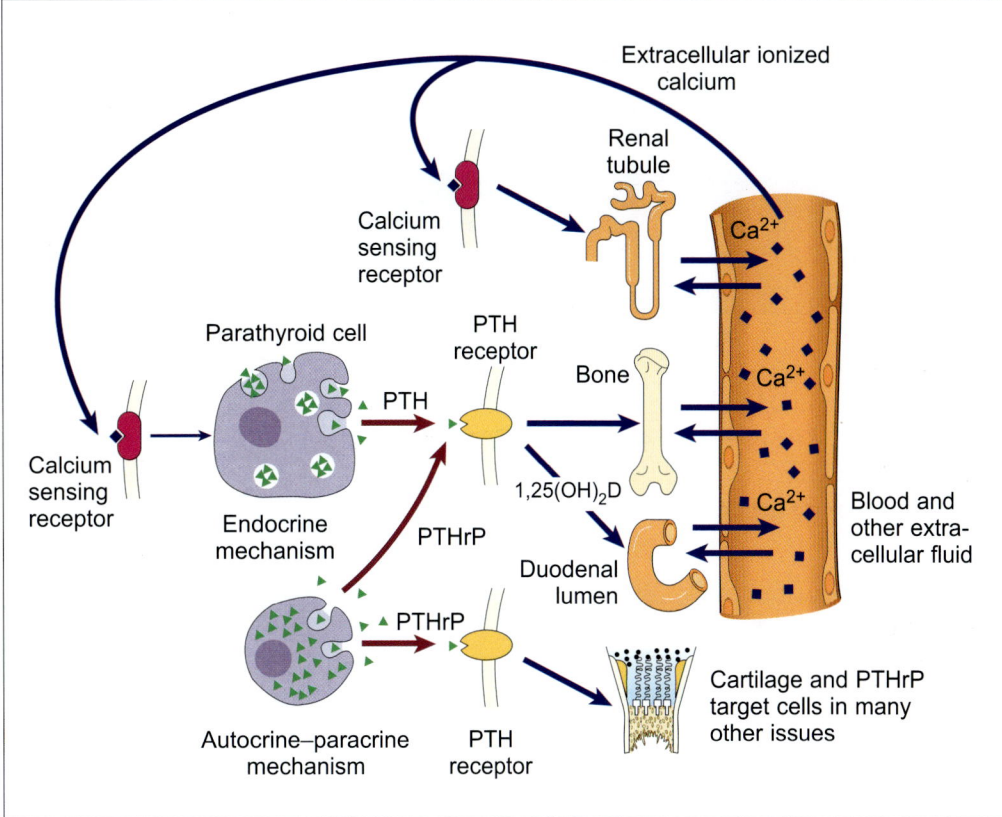

fracture sparing effects in those treated. Such bone anabolic effects of parathyroid hormone (PTH) were first recognized in 1980[108] and since then both PTH and PTH analogs have been evaluated in a number of clinical trials.

Mechanisms of action

The physiological function of parathyroid hormone is to maintain extracellular calcium levels. The effects are either direct on target cells or indirectly mediated through synthesis of 1,25 dihydroxyvitamin D. Serum calcium is closely regulated, with PTH secretion increasing in response to decreasing serum calcium, an effect mediated through the calcium-sensing receptor. The skeleton is the major calcium reservoir of the human body, hence skeletal calcium becomes an important target for PTH action. There is evidence for a dual action on bone, and both osteoblasts and osteoclasts are responsive to PTH. The resorptive effect predominates during continued elevation of PTH, while an anabolic effect on bone is seen with intermittent dosing(**4.47**)[109].

Human PTH consists of a single-chain peptide of 84 amino acids (hPTH1-84), with its sequence and structure well defined (**4.48**). The N-terminal amino acid residues are

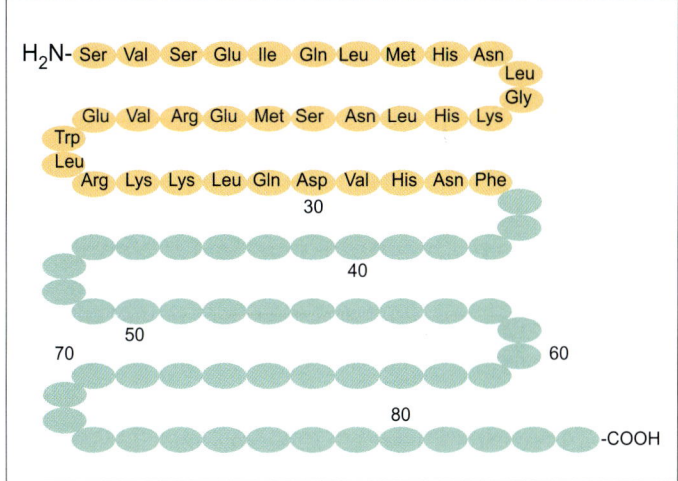

4.48 Human intact PTH 1–84. The first 34 amino acids are high-lighted.

essential for the hormonal activity, with the first two amino acids absolutely required. In clinical trials, intact PTH 1-84 and PTH 1-34 have been evaluated, where PTH 1-34 is now named teriparatide. The bone anabolic properties are thus conserved in PTH 1-34; however, it has been suggested that only the first 31 amino acids are required.

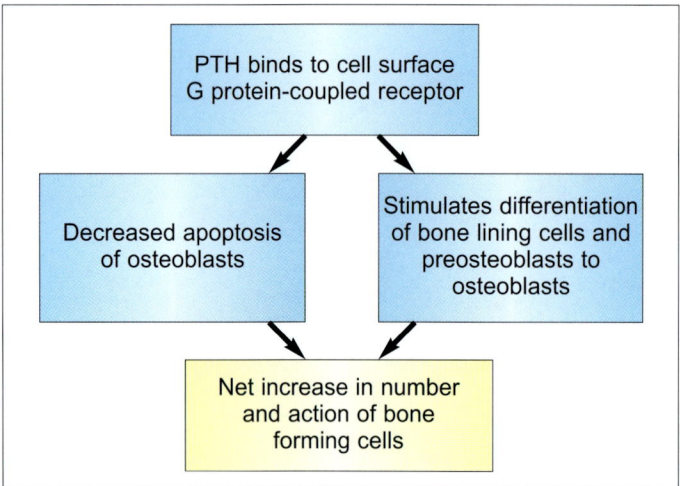

4.49 Mechanism of action of PTH.

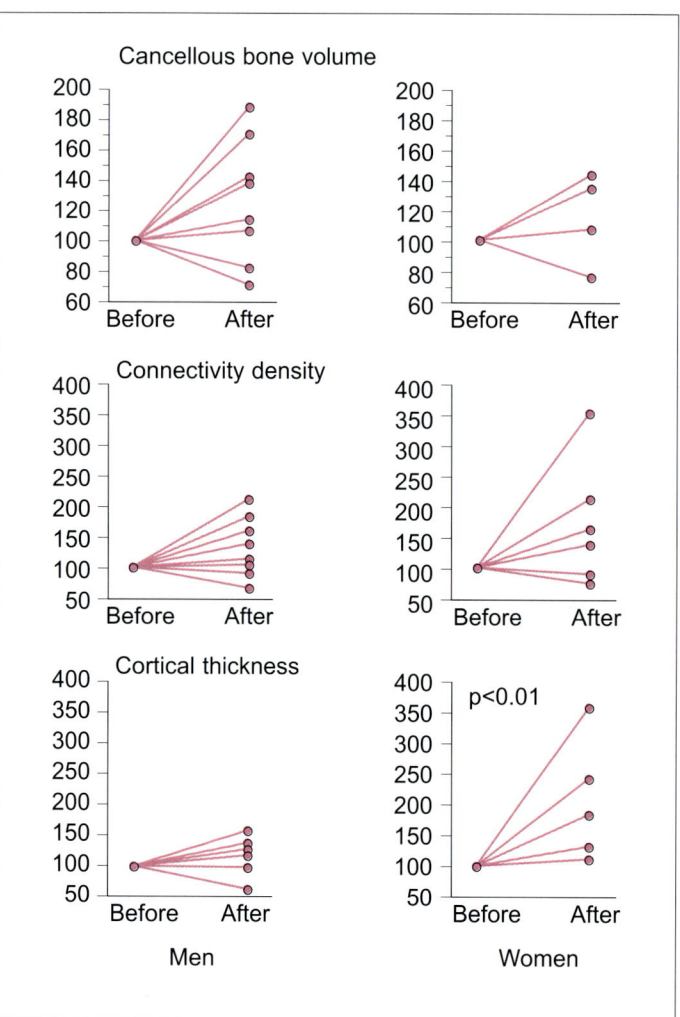

4.50 Paired biopsies in men and women treated for 36 months with PTH. Histomorphometry parameters. (Adapted from Dempster DW, *et al.* (2001). Effects of daily treatment with parathyroid hormone on bone microarchitecture and turnover in patients with osteoporosis: a paired biopsy study. *J Bone Miner Res,* **16**(10):1846–1853.)

Utilizing the anabolic properties of PTH on bone has been an attractive concept in order to obtain larger increases in bone mass than are possible with antiresorptive agents. PTH has been shown to primarily increase the cancellous or trabecular bone, hence the effects are most pronounced on spinal bone density. However, a smaller but clear effect is also seen on the endosteal surface of cortical bone, including increased breaking strength in animal studies[110, 111].

PTH induces an activation of the lining cells, increasing the activated bone surface and the recruitment of osteoblasts without prior bone resorption. Furthermore, osteoblast apoptosis decreases, adding to the enhancement of bone formation. However, bone resorption is increased with delay, indicating that normal bone remodelling is increased.

An increase in trabecular thickness and trabecular connectivity indicate that trabeculae that have been disconnected through increased bone resorption during postmenopausal osteoporosis may be reconstructed. This property alone may mean more in terms of bone strength than any other, and is differentiating this class of drugs from bisphosphonates where inhibition of bone resorption leads to secondary trabecular thickening without improvement of connectivity.

Continuous elevation of PTH, as in hyperparathyroidism, has negative effects on bone in a significant proportion of patients. Contrary to this, intermittent administration of PTH has bone anabolic effects. These effects stem from direct stimulatory effects on the bone surface lining cell, but also effects on preosteoblasts. In addition, the lifespan of osteoblasts increases. The anabolic effect is the result of both increased number of osteoblasts and increased cellular activity (**4.49**).

Cortical remodelling is slower than trabecular remodelling and already in the first study by Reeve *et al.*[108], it was shown that the change in bone mass at cortical sites was smaller or even negative. Additional studies with PTH 1-34 have shown that the intracortical remodelling involves periosteal apposition leading to an increase in bone diameter, which in itself increases the breaking strength of bone[112]. These type of changes are not well detected by DXA but need quantitative methods such as QCT.

Bone histomorphometry is a tool for evaluation and visualization of changes at the tissue level. In a study by

4.51 Biopsy micrographs from a woman – left, before, right, after. (From Dempster DW, *et al.* (2001). Effects of daily treatment with parathyroid hormone on bone microarchitecture and turnover in patients with osteoporosis: a paired biopsy study. *J Bone Miner Res,* **16**(10):1846–1853, with permission.)

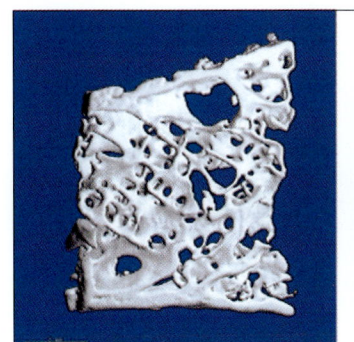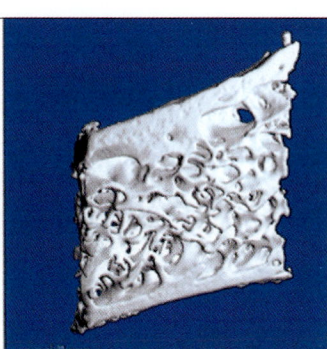

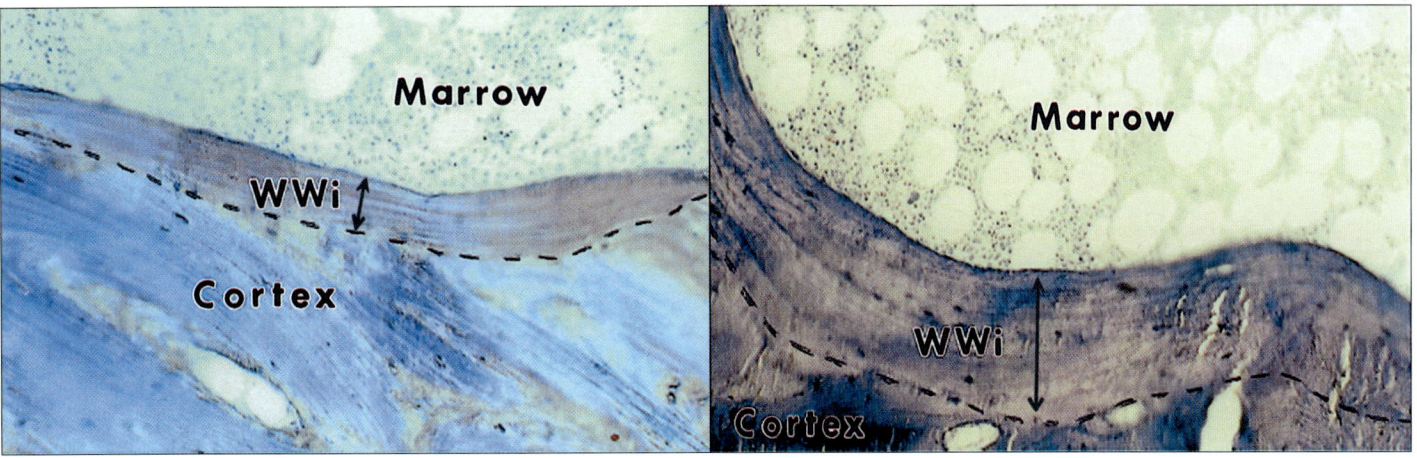

4.52 Endocortex showing the increase in width after PTH treatment – before (top) and after 36 months (bottom). (From Dempster DW, *et al.* (2001). Effects of daily treatment with parathyroid hormone on bone microarchitecture and turnover in patients with osteoporosis: a paired biopsy study. *J Bone Miner Res,* **16**(10):1846–1853, with permission.)

Dempster *et al.*[113], paired biopsies were acquired prior to treatment and after 18 or 36 months of treatment with PTH 1-34 in men and women respectively. The cortical variables in most women increased as is seen in Figure **4.50** and no adverse cortical effects were seen. Their percentage change from baseline is reported. This is confirmedusing microcomputed tomography, where the increase in connectivity and trabecular width are clearly visible. This is illustrated by a micrograph from a biopsy from a woman where the left panel shows before and the right after (**4.51**). The incresed endocortical apposition is also seen (**4.52**) from a male biopsy where the average wall width was increased by 58%.

Clinical trials have evaluated intermittent dosing of both intact PTH 1-84 and PTH 1-34 with regard to bone markers, BMD and fracture. In addition, combination, sequential, and cyclic treatment regimens have been evaluated in both women and men.

Effect on bone turnover

PTH induces rapid changed in bone formation with an increase observed within a month[114–116]. The markers of bone formation increase rapidly, up to 100% and over within 3 months. Markers of bone resorption will increase but with a delay and at a somewhat lower magnitude.

In a study using full-length PTH (1-84) and testing three different doses in osteoporotic women, the markers increased for the first 6 months, where after they levelled off (**4.53**)[117]. The highest dose had the largest effect on bone formation but also on bone resorption. The dose chosen for clinical use is the lowest dose, 50 micrograms, to balance turnover in relation to bone gains.

Biochemical marker of bone formation increases rapidly during PTH treatment as an indication of the anabolic response. A subsequent increase in bone resorption is seen. In a study of 437 men treated with PTH 1-34[118], the bone formation markers bone alkaline phosphatise and PICP

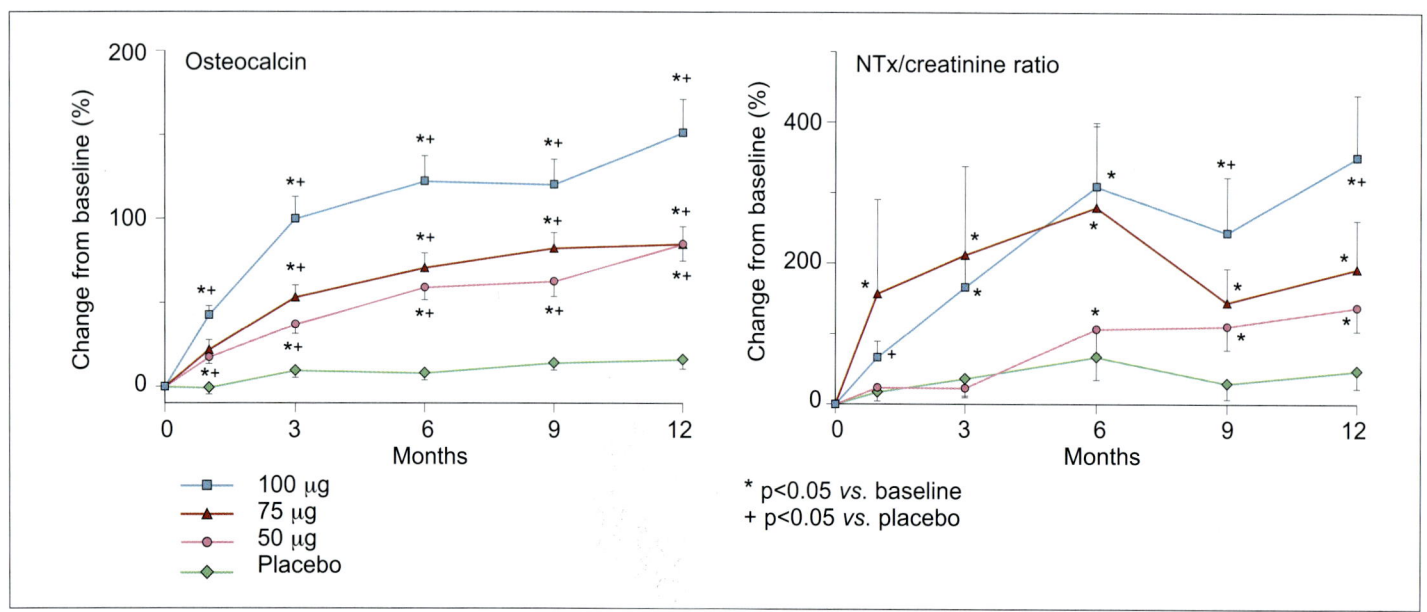

4.53 PTH and bone markers. (From Dempster DW, *et al.* (2001). Effects of daily treatment with parathyroid hormone on bone microarchitecture and turnover in patients with osteoporosis: a paired biopsy study. *J Bone Miner Res,* **16**(10):1846–1853, with permission.)

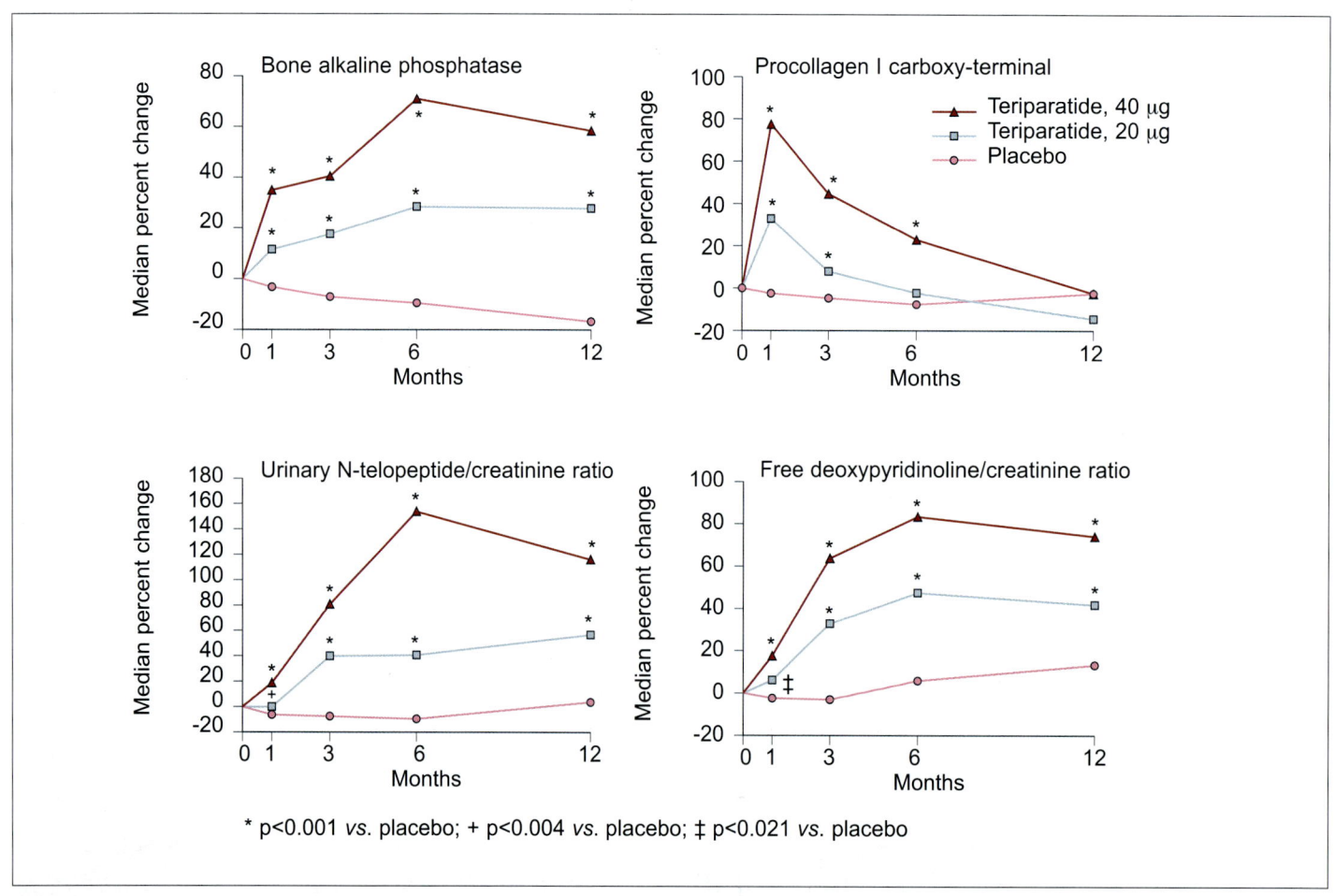

4.54 PTH and bone markers. (Adapted from Orwoll ES, *et al.* (2003). The effect of teriparatide [human parathyroid hormone (1-34)] therapy on bone density in men with osteoporosis. *J Bone Miner Res,* **18**(1):9–17.)

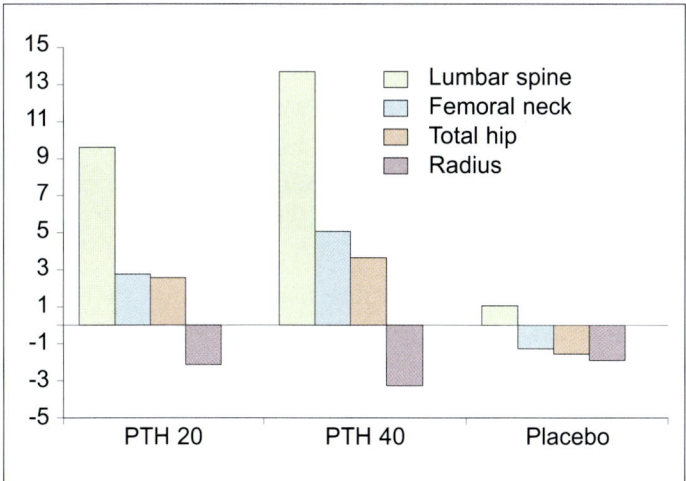

4.55 Fracture reduction after treatment with teriparatide in 1632 women. (Adapted from Neer RM, *et al.* (2001). Effect of parathyroid hormone (1-34) on fractures and bone mineral density in postmenopausal women with osteoporosis. *N Engl J Med*, **344**(19):1434–1441.)

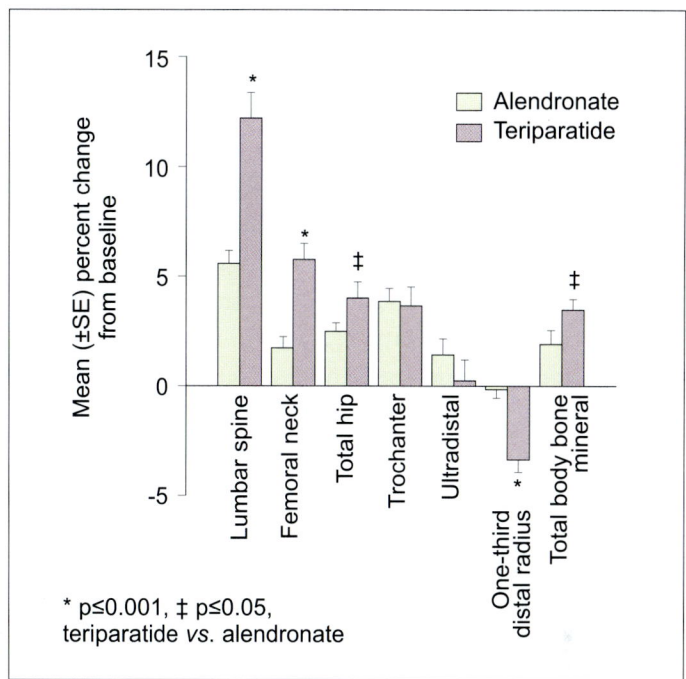

* p≤0.001, ‡ p≤0.05, teriparatide *vs.* alendronate

4.56 Mean change from baseline comparing the effect of teriparatide and alendronate. (Adapted from Neer RM, *et al.* (2001). Effect of parathyroid hormone (1-34) on fractures and bone mineral density in postmenopausal women with osteoporosis. *N Engl J Med*, **344**(19):1434–1441.)

increased within the first month, whereas the bone resorption markers increased at 3 and 6 months. Notably, PICP appears to decrease after the initial increase (**4.54**).

Effect on BMD

The effect of PTH on BMD is dose dependent, as shown in studies of both full-length PTH 1-84 or in truncated forms as in PTH 1-34. The dose finding studies have used two or three different doses in order to optimize the benefits and minimize the less favourable effects.

Using PTH 1-34 there is a dose-dependent increase in spinal and femoral neck BMD of 9–13% and 6–9%, when using 20 or 40 micrograms respectively. Other placebo-controlled studies have shown marked increases in predominantly spinal BMD[117, 119] and suggested reduction in vertebral fractures, particularly when PTH has been combined with agents reducing bone resorption[120, 121]. Furthermore, recombinant human PTH (rhPTH) 1-34 increased both spinal and hip BMD significantly more than did daily alendronate during a 14-month study of osteoporotic women[116].

In a placebo-controlled randomized trial of 1637 women treated with PTH 1-34 (**4.55**, **4.56**)[122], the bone anabolic effect from PTH was most pronounced in the mainly trabecular bone of vertebrae as seen by the large increase in spinal BMD. The effects were also evident in the hip, but to a lesser extent, whereas a negative effect was shown for the

distal radius. The mean duration of treatment was 21 months. The effects were dose dependent with a greater effect from the highest dose (40 micrograms). The 20 microgram dose was chosen for clinical application balancing the desired effects on fracture and BMD versus side-effects.

Effect on fractures

Recombinant human PTH 1-34 given as daily subcutaneous injection has been evaluated for fracture efficacy. Postmenopausal women with prevalent vertebral fractures (n=1637) receiving 20 or 40 micrograms of rhPTH 1-34 experienced a 65–69% reduction in new vertebral fractures and 53–54% reduction in nonvertebral fractures over 21 months[122]. Since most other clinical studies have been too small in number to evaluate fracture efficacy, reported fracture data points in a similar direction with a reduction in mainly vertebral fractures.

A number of studies use BMD as the end-point, which is insufficient from an evidence-based perspective. The study by Neer *et al.*[122] was powered to evaluate fracture efficacy.

The majority of women had established osteoporosis with prevalent vertebral fractures. The number of women suffering new vertebral fractures was significantly lower with PTH 1-34 treatment. Furthermore, those treated reported less back pain (p=0.007) and lesser loss of height (p=0.002).

For most antiresorptive treatments reduction of nonvertebral fractures is not unequivocal but often marginally significant, which probably mirrors the different aetiological factors involved and not reached by pharmacological treatment. In the Neer et al. study[122], nonvertebral fractures were significantly reduced. The estimate uses both total number of fracture and those fractures that are associated with bone fragility. The cumulative incidence of total and fragility nonvertebral fractures indicates a more pronounced difference towards the end of treatment when the maximum effect of PTH was reached (**4.57**).

Table 4.9 compares fracture risk reduction of PTH (for 19 months) and bisphosphonates (alendronate and risedronate for 36 months) in clinical trials of women

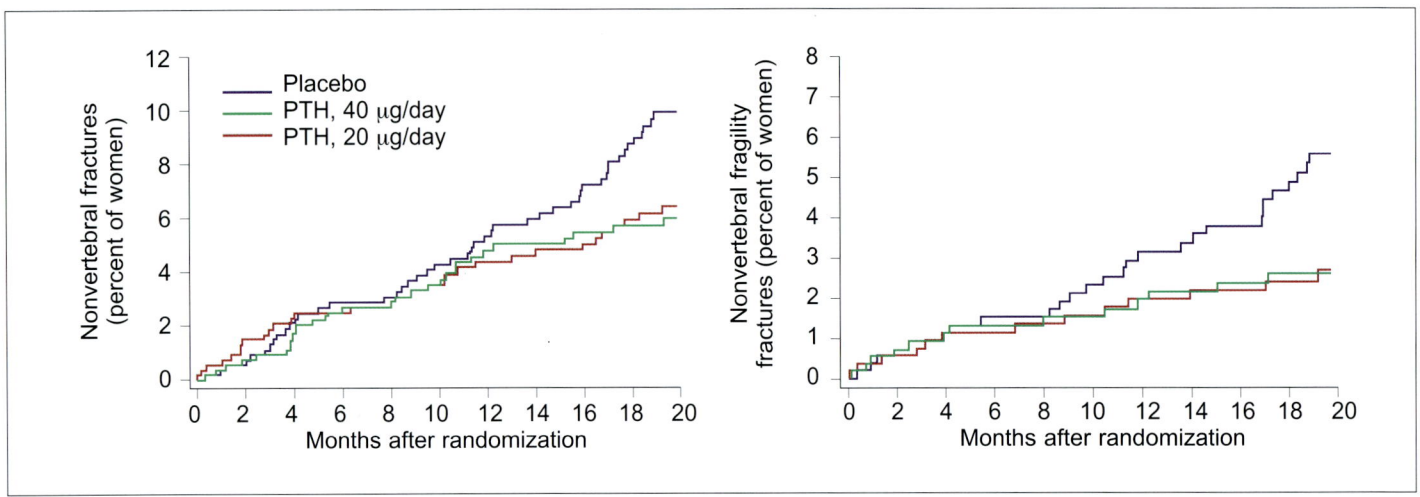

4.57 Fracture reduction after treatment with teriparatide. (Adapted from Neer RM, et al. (2001). Effect of parathyroid hormone (1-34) on fractures and bone mineral density in postmenopausal women with osteoporosis. *N Engl J Med*, **344**(19):1434–1441.)

Table 4.9 Comparison of fracture risk reduction between teriparatide (for 19 months) and bisphosphonates (for 36 months) during the clinical trials in postmenopausal women with at least one baseline incident vertebral fracture

	Teriparatide Neer *et al.*	Alendronate Black *et al.*	Risedronate Harris *et al.*	Risedronate Reginster *et al.*
New vertebral fractures				
Relative risk (95% CI)	0.4 (0.2–0.6)	0.5 (0.4–0.7)	0.6 (0.4–0.8)	0.5 (0.4–0.7)
Placebo incidence rate (%)	14	15	16	29
Absolute risk reduction (%)	9	7	5	11
NNT	11	9	20	10
New nonvertrebral fractures				
Relative risk (95% CI)	0.5 (0.3–0.9)	0.8 (0.6–1.0)	0.6 (0.4–0.9)	0.7 (0.4–1.0)
Placebo incidence rate (%)	6	15	8	51
Absolute risk reduction (%)	3	3	3	15
NNT	34	34	43	20

(Adapted from Hodsman AB *et al.* (2005). Parathyroid hormone and teriparatide for the treatment of osteoporosis: a review of the evidence and suggested guidelines for its use. *Endocr Rev*, **26**(5):688–703.)

treated for osteoporosis and with at least one prevalent fracture. The table includes the number needed to treat for comparison. The number needed to treat is related to the specific study, thus 11 women need to be treated for 19 months with teriparatide to avoid one fracture, whereas 9 need to be treated with alendronate for 3 years to avoid one vertebral fracture.

Use with other osteoporotic therapies

The initial studies on PTH was in combination with oestrogen and indicated that women on oestrogen responded to PTH with a 13% increase in spinal BMD over 3 years, whereas no significant change occurred in women on oestrogen alone[123]. It should be pointed out that the mean duration of prior oestrogen therapy was 7–10 years. The additive effect of PTH with oestrogen deficiency or replacement has also been seen in other studies[124, 125].

Since antiresorptive therapy with bisphosphonates is the established treatment for postmenopausal osteoporosis, it is of importance to evaluate the interaction between bisphosphonates and PTH in clinical practice. The aim of these studies has been to evaluate the therapeutic response (1) in those with prior bisphosphonate treatment, (2) in combination therapy, and (3) after treatment with PTH.

A comparative trial using teriparatide and alendronate clearly showed the incremental increase in bone formation from PTH as compared with alendronate, indicating a larger effect on bone density, mainly at the lumbar spine[116, 126].

Direct comparison between the effects of PTH and bisphosphonates using PTH 1-34 and daily alendronate (10

mg) in postmenopausal women is shown in **4.58**[126]. The changes in bone turnover indicate the different mechanism by which the two different classes of drugs work. The rapid and large increase in bone formation is associated with a larger increase in BMD compared to alendronate (10.3% *vs*. 5.5%).

Similar differences in BMD have been observed in similar studies and showing the differential site dependent response to parathyroid hormone and alendronate, with virtually identical effects in the trochanter but significant positive or negative differences for lumbar spine and distal radius, respectively (**4.56, 4.59**)[116].

To answer whether there is an additive effect from combining a bisphosphonate with PTH, one study suggests a reduced effect from PTH when combined with alendronate[127], whereas another study using a daily or cyclic regimen in women with prior alendronate treatment showed a beneficial effect on bone density[128]. These findings suggest that the different preparations of PTH, different bisphosphonates, and different modes of administration may play a role for the response.

In the Black *et al.*[127] study of 238 postmenopausal women, no synergy was found from PTH 1-84 (100 micrograms) and alendronate (10 mg). There is no difference between alendronate alone or in combination with PTH on spinal bone density assessed by DXA or QCT. As for the hip, a negative balance is seen for PTH using DXA, whereas QCT indicates a positive effect.

In women with prior alendronate treatment, PTH was initiated as a continuous 12-month treatment or as a cyclic treatment with the aim to utilize the initial and rapid

4.58 PTH compared with bisphosphonates. (Adapted from McClung MR, *et al.* (2005). Opposite bone remodeling effects of teriparatide and alendronate in increasing bone mass. *Arch Intern Med*, **165**(15):1762–1768.)

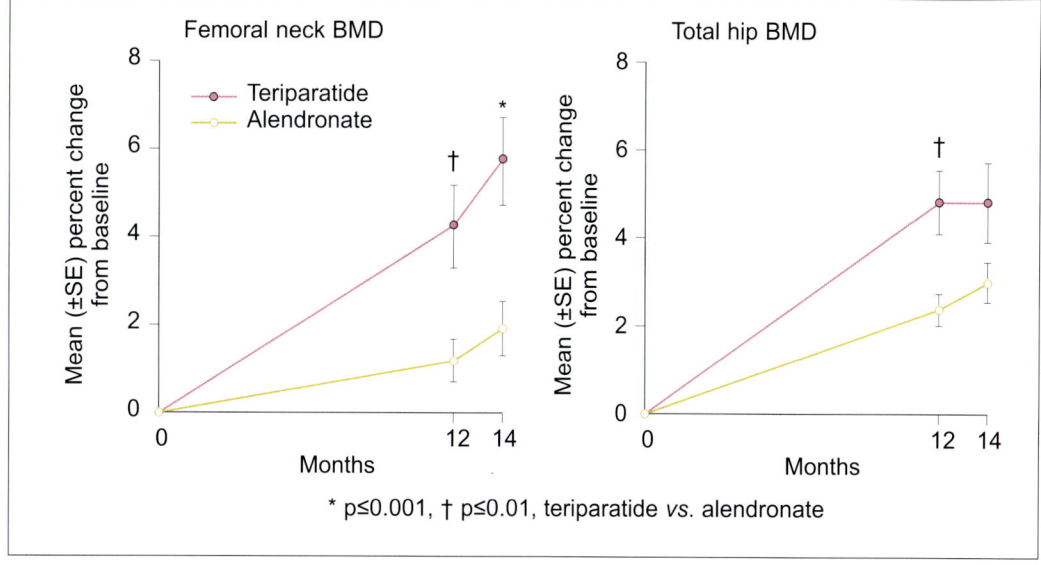

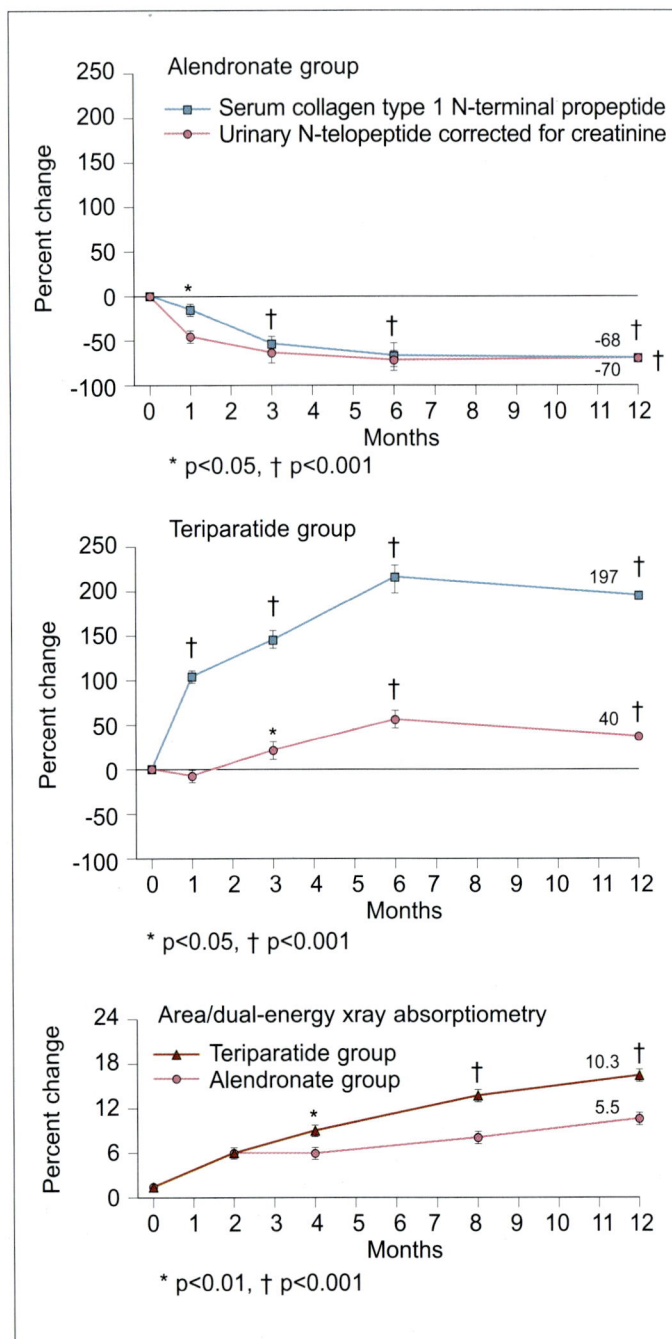

4.59 Head-to-head trial of teriparatide and alendronate in postmenopausal women. (Adapted from Body JJ, *et al.* (2002). A randomized double-blind trial to compare the efficacy of teriparatide [recombinant human parathyroid hormone (1-34)] with alendronate in postmenopausal women with osteoporosis. *J Clin Endocrinol Metab,* **87**(10):4528–4535.)

activation of bone formation from PTH that has been seen in earlier studies. The figure (**4.60**) shows the median changes in bone formation markers (**A–C**) and bone resorption (**D**) for those given daily or cyclic PTH in combination with alendronate or alendronate alone. Spinal bone density increased by 6.1% and 5.4%, respectively, as compared to alendronate alone at 12 months[128]. This increase is somewhat less than in alendronate naïve subjects[122].

The anabolic effects of PTH on the skeleton are not likely to be maintained without additional therapy. Sequential or cyclic treatment regimens have been involved oestrogen but also calcitonin[129] but without additional beneficial effects. Bisphoshonates should have the capacity to maintain the effect by closing down the expanded remodelling space. This concept has been tried with success, when giving alendronate after PTH[121, 130].

After discontinuation of PTH, it is unclear for how long the effect is maintained, but a loss is likely to begin in the metabolically more active trabecular bone of the spine. Subsequently, there is a need to use another agent to maintain the effects. In a study by Black *et al.*[130], women treated with PTH 1-84 (100 micrograms) or alendronate were during year 2 were re-randomized to placebo or alendronate. When PTH was followed by placebo, spine BMD no longer increased (**4.61A**), whereas a significant increase continue when PTH is followed by alendronate. In the hip the change was significantly greater in PTH-alendronate compared to PTH-placebo (**4.61B–C**).

Safety data

The major concern in using PTH was the early reports from animal studies indicating development of osteosarcoma in rats after prolonged exposure of high doses[131]. These reports had the effect that the duration of several of the clinical trials were shortened. The administration of PTH has been limited to 18–24 months as a result of the studies. Currently, no known cases of sarcoma related to PTH administration exists, but PTH should not be given to patients with a history of prior skeletal exposure to, for example, irradiation.

A number of side-effects are reported in the clinical trials. Hypercalcaemia is an observation but the major studies indicate no clinical difference in hypercalcaemia in those treated with PTH 1-34[122, 126]. Nevertheless, careful selection of patients is recommended in order not to treat patients with decreased kidney function, which could be common in the very elderly.

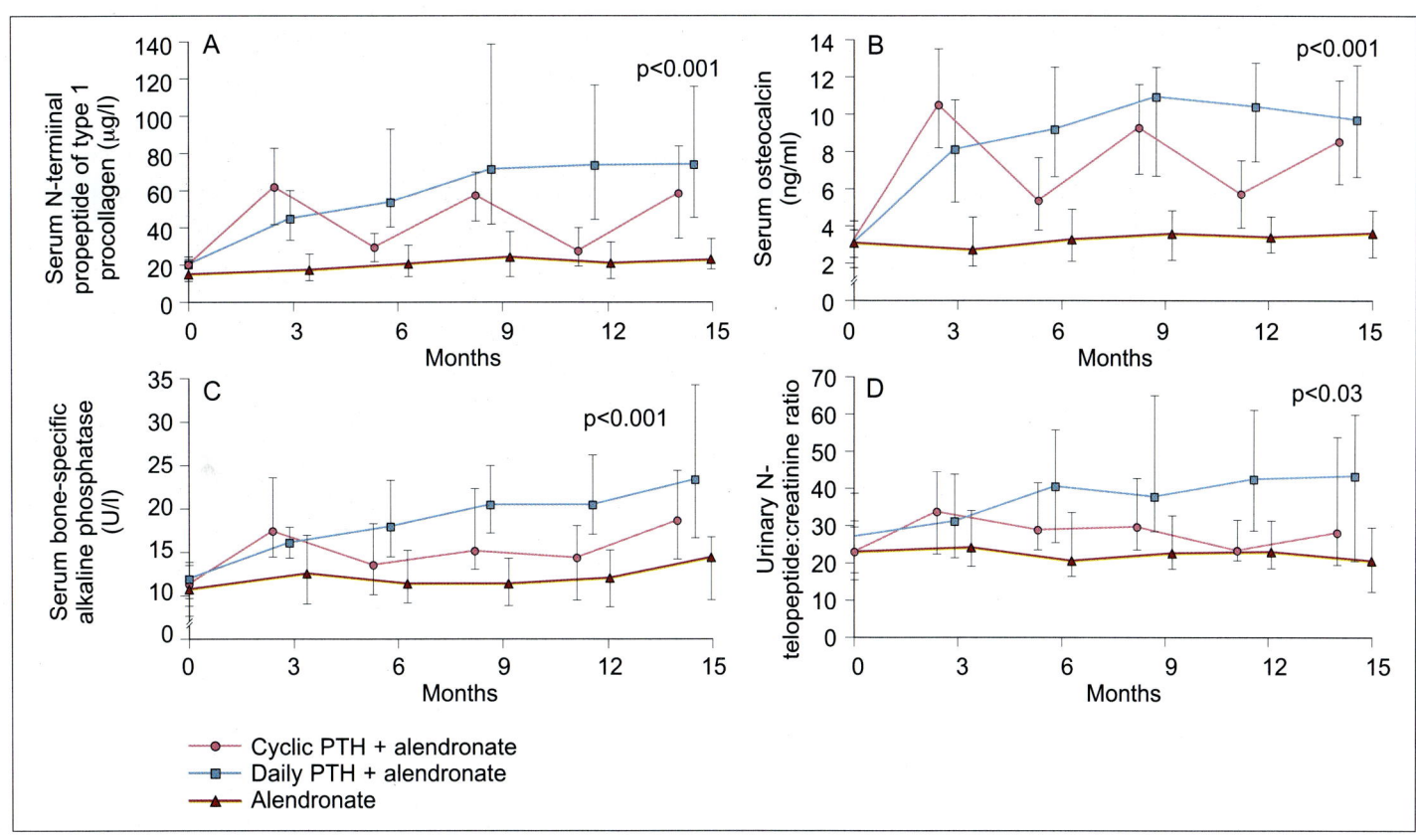

4.60 PTH and bisphosphonates combined. (Adapted from Cosman F, *et al.* (2005). Daily and cyclic parathyroid hormone in women receiving alendronate. *N Engl J Med,* **353**(6):566–575.)

4.61 PTH and alendronate combined. (Adapted from Black DM, *et al.* (2005). One year of alendronate after one year of parathyroid hormone (1-84) for osteoporosis. *N Engl J Med,* **353**(6):555-565.)

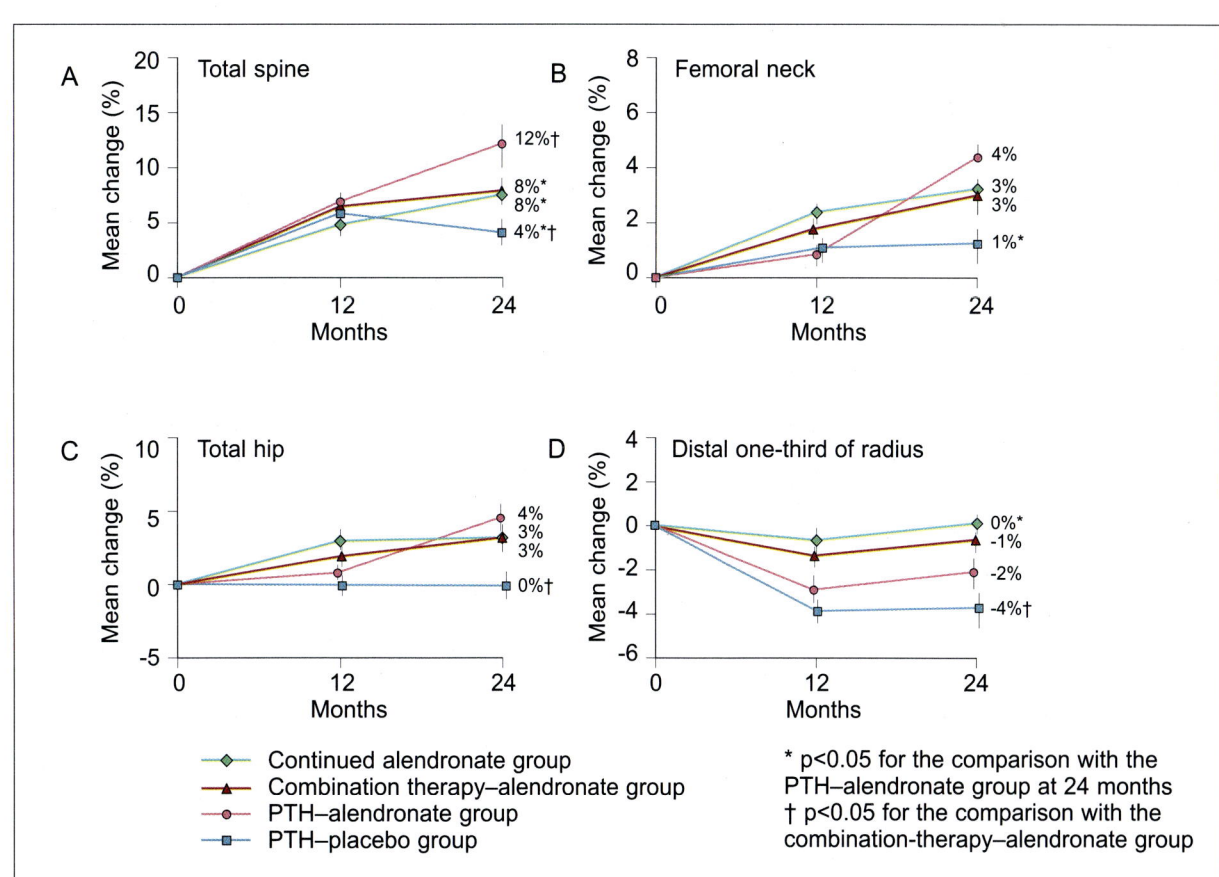

In clinical studies, over 80% of the participants reported at least one side-effect, regardless of whether they were treated with a placebo or an active substance. The most common adverse events reported for teriparatide are shown in *Table 4.10*. Most of them subside after an initial period. Hypercalcaemia commonly occurs within the first 4–6 hours after injection and is normally without significance. However, caution is warranted when a patient has decreased kidney function and when given a too high dose of calcium.

Glucocorticoids may induce rapid bone loss. In a study by Lane *et al.*[132], women on long-term prednisone treatment for various rheumatic disorders received PTH 1-34 for 12 months. All women were using oestrogen and a significant additive effect was noted in the central skeleton. The results show PTH treatment can reverse corticosteroid-induced osteoporosis.

PTH may be used for severe male osteoporosis and the effects appear similar. In the Finkelstein *et al.* study[133], 83 men between the ages of 46–85 were randomized to alendronate daily, PTH (1-34) daily or both. Treatment with PTH was for 24 months; the total duration was 30 months. The effect was similar to that seen in women, but with a slightly greater increase also in the hip. The anabolic effect of PTH appeared attenuated when alendronate was used concurrently[118, 133, 134].

Anabolic agents to counteract severe bone loss in osteoporosis are highly desirable. Treatment with PTH is producing incremental increases, particularly of cancellous bone in the vertebrae, even after short periods of treatment. PTH seems to offer new treatment options especially for severe cases of osteoporosis, unresponsive to other agents or possibly when side-effects prohibit their use.

Table 4.10 Reported side-effects for teriparatide

	Treated (%)	Placebo (%)
Hypercalcaemia	11.0	2.0
Musculoskeletal pain	10.0	9.0
Leg cramps	3.6	2.7
Headache	7.7	7.4
Nausea	8.5	6.2
Dizziness	8.0	5.2
Depression	4.1	2.5

Calcitonin

Calcitonin is an endogenous hormone involved in calcium homeostasis. Calcitonin acts as an endogenous inhibitor of bone resorption by suppressing osteoclasts, a property that has led to its use in the treatment of osteoporosis.

Mechanisms of action

Calcitonin is a 32 amino acid peptide secreted by thyroid C-cells, with 5 of 9 residues in the N-terminal end identical in all species. It has not been possible to identify a specific region determining the biological activity as, for example, compared with PTH. The biological effects are mediated via the calcitonin receptor (CTR), which is highly expressed in osteoclasts, but also in cells of the central nervous system[135]. Calcitonin is rapidly secreted in response to acutely increased levels of serum calcium, but does not seem to play an important role in the long-term regulation of calcium. Osteoclasts appear to be the main biological target, with exposed osteoclasts immediately shrinking and losing their ruffled boarder[135], yet with prolonged exposure to hypercalcaemia, secretion and effect appear to wear off[136]. The exact role of calcitonin in normal physiological processes thus remains to be fully established, but the antiresorptive effects have been utilized in treatment of osteoporosis.

Calcitonin from nonmammalian species is more potent than normally produced human calcitonin, with salmon calcitonin being about 10 times more potent. Salmon calcitonin has sufficient homology to bind to the CTR and is the most commonly used preparation, available as an injectable substance or as nasal spray.

Figure **4.62** illustrates the structure of human calcitonin, a 32 amino acid peptide with a disulphide bridge between the two cysteins at residue 1 and 7.

Effect on fractures

Several studies have shown the effect of calcitonin on BMD in postmenopausal women taking calcitonin, while the fracture effect is less well studied. The PROOF (Prevent Recurrence of Osteoporotic Fracture) trial has been undertaken with the intention to investigate the effect on fracture risk[137]. This 5-year clinical trial involved 1255 women, of whom approximately 80% had prevalent vertebral fractures. Salmon calcitonin was administered as intranasal spray at three different doses; 100 IU, 200 IU and 400 IU and compared with placebo. New vertebral fractures were reduced by 33% (RR 0.67, 95% CI 0.47-0.97, p<0.05) in postmenopausal women despite a small effect on lumbar BMD, when salmon calcitonin was administrated at a dose of 200 IU daily (**4.63**). The 200 IU/day dose is now the recommended dose for clinical use. This has been interpreted as a quality effect of antiresorptive agents beyond the effect on BMD[138] and corresponds to a number needed to treat of 13 (95% CI 7-77). When analysing the group of women with the highest baseline risk, those with 1–5 prevalent fractures, risk reduction was virtually identical (34%). There was no significant reduction in nonvertebral fractures.

The interpretation of the results of this study is not without problems, since the discontinuation rate was high and only 41% completed the study. A meta-analysis has been performed to review the effects of calcitonin on fracture risk and BMD. Treatment included both intranasal and subcutaneous calcitonin; however, the majority received the drug as nasal spray. The meta-analysis showing a pooled relative risk reduction for vertebral fractures of 0.46 (95% CI 0.25-0.87, p=0.02, n=1404) (**4.64**)[139]. Also, according to the meta-analysis the risk of nonvertebral fracture

remained comparable to the nontreated. The meta-analysis evaluating the effect on nonvertebral fractures included three trials. The pooled data indicates that calcitonin treatment does not influence or diminish the risk of nonvertebral fracture (**4.65**)[139].

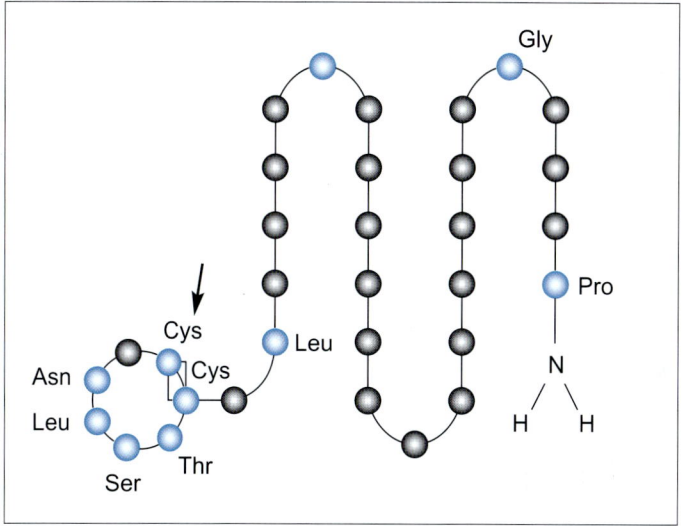

4.62 Structure of human calcitonin.

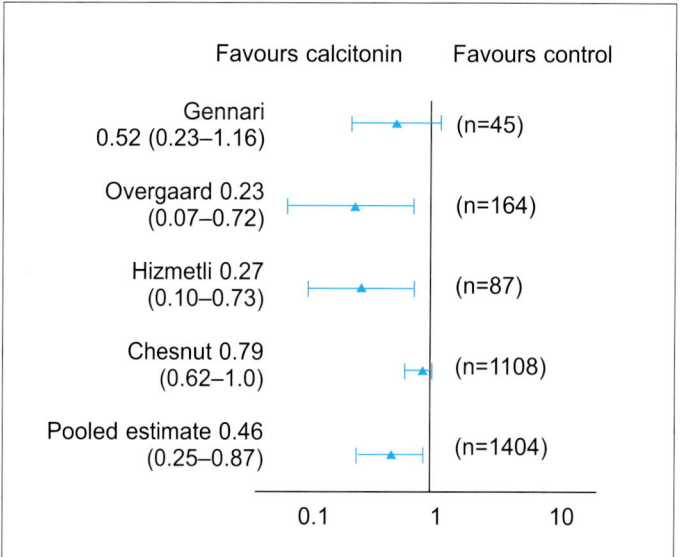

4.63 Calcitonin effect on fracture. Vertebral fractures were significantly reduced by 33% from the third year of treatment. The cumulative percentage of at least one new vertebral fracture per year for each dose is shown. (Adapted from Chesnut CH, III, *et al.* (2000). A randomized trial of nasal spray salmon calcitonin in postmenopausal women with established osteoporosis: the prevent recurrence of osteoporotic fractures study. PROOF Study Group. *Am J Med*, **109**(4):267–276.)

4.64 Calcitonin and fracture – meta-analysis evaluating the effect on vertebral fractures. (Adapted from Cranney A, *et al.* (2002). Meta-analyses of therapies for postmenopausal osteoporosis. VI. Meta-analysis of calcitonin for the treatment of postmenopausal osteoporosis. *Endocr Rev*, **23**(4):540–551.)

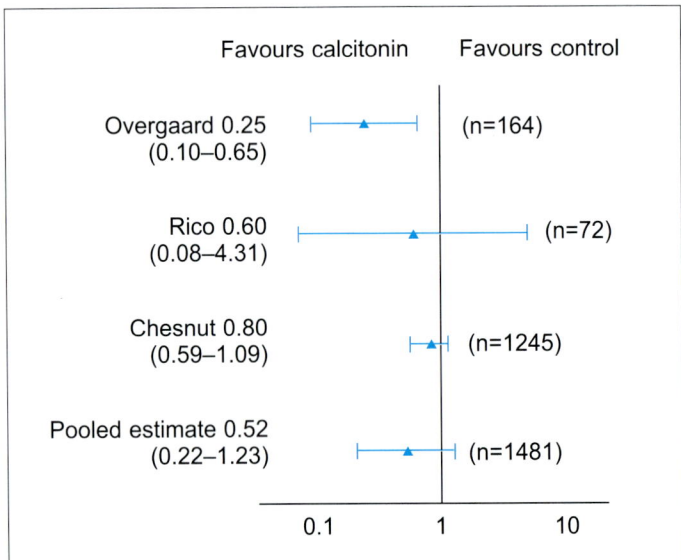

4.65 Calcitonin and fracture – meta-analysis evaluating the effect on nonvertebral fractures. (Adapted from Cranney A, *et al.* (2002). Meta-analyses of therapies for postmenopausal osteoporosis. VI. Meta-analysis of calcitonin for the treatment of postmenopausal osteoporosis. *Endocr Rev*, **23**(4):540–551.)

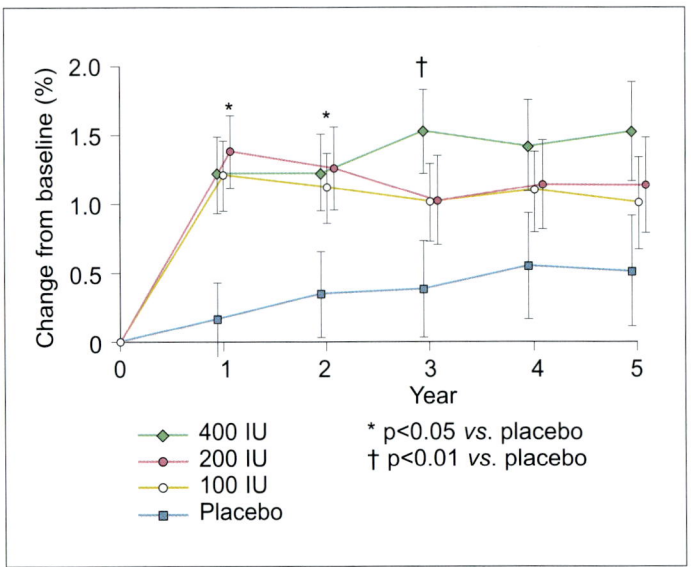

4.66 The effect of calcitonin on BMD. (Adapted from Chesnut CH, III, *et al.* (2000). A randomized trial of nasal spray salmon calcitonin in postmenopausal women with established osteoporosis: the prevent recurrence of osteoporotic fractures study. PROOF Study Group. *Am J Med*, **109**(4):267–276.)

Effect on BMD

BMD is consistently increased in the lumbar spine with calcitonin treatment; however, the magnitude of increase is small 1–2%. The changes in hip BMD are in the range of 0.5–1.5%. A slightly greater increase has been noted using cyclic intermittent treatment together with active vitamin D, demonstrating a potential for combination therapy in selected cases[140].

In routine clinical practice, changes below 2% cannot be differentiated from the technical precision error of the measurement device. This is cause for a clinical dilemma: is the patient responding or not responding if no bone density gain can be detected? A pragmatic possibility is to regard the absence of bone loss as suggestive of a positive effect, since the normal yearly loss is in the order of 0.5–2%. Furthermore, bone density follow-up is not meaningful within a time frame of 2 years, but could well be extended to 4 years if treatment is well tolerated, a strategy equally relevant when using other antiresorptive treatments.

In the Chesnut *et al.* study[137], BMD of the lumbar spine was significantly different from baseline after the first year of treatment but with no additional increase during the following years (**4.66**). The increase was evident for all doses of calcitonin, thus there was no obvious dose response effect.

A comparative study of calcitonin and alendronate has been performed in 299 postmenopausal women who were randomized to either calcitonin 200 IU or alendronate 10 mg/day for 12 months[141]. The predetermined outcome was the effect on BMD and bone turnover. Alendronate produced larger changes in BMD at all sites compared to calcitonin, evident already at 6 months (**4.67**). The mean percentage changes (+/-SE) in the lumbar spine (5.2 *vs.* 1.6%), trochanter and femoral neck (2.8 *vs.* 0.6%).

Effect on bone turnover

Calcitonin exerts its effects on osteoclasts and bone resorption, as assessed by bone resorption markers, is persistently decreased from the baseline and when compared to a placebo; however, the degree of suppression is significantly less than that of other antiresorptive agents and compared to bisphosphonates in particular. The degree of suppression may be indicative of the limited change in BMD, while the reduction in vertebral fracture risk is evident in spite of this.

Bone marker levels decreased at all time points in the PROOF study (**4.68**)[137]. Serum C-telopeptide (S-CTx) was used to evaluate the effect on bone resorption and was over

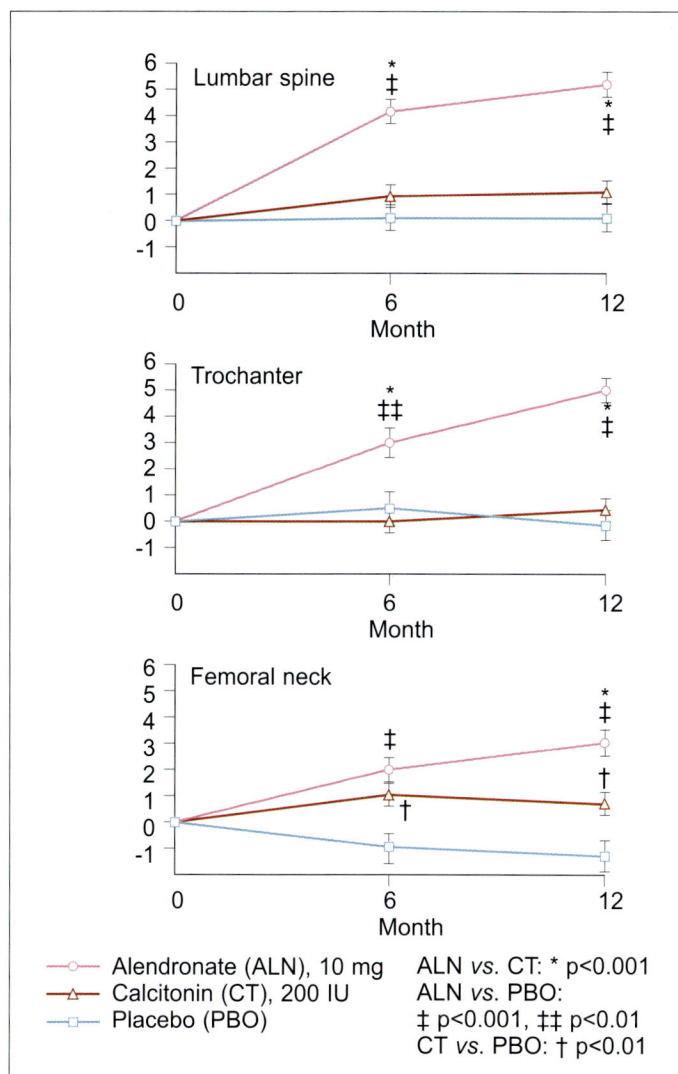

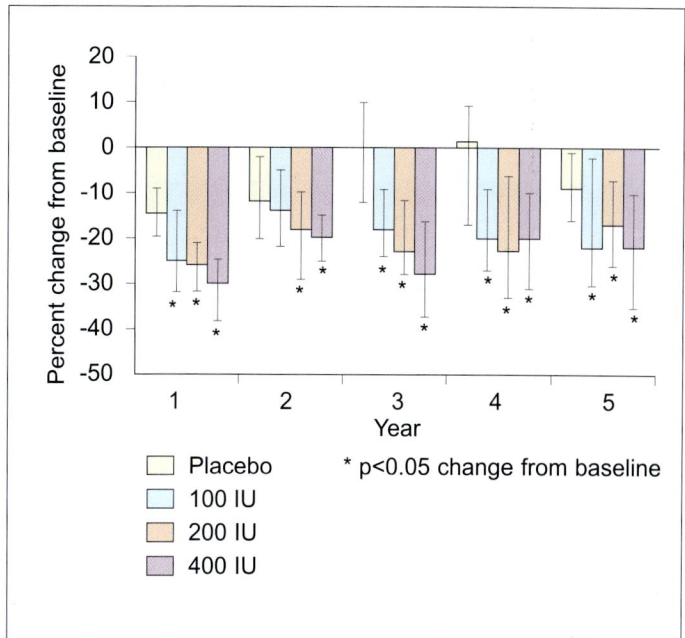

4.68 Effect of calcitonin on bone markers. Median percentage change in S-CTx from baseline. (Adapted from Chesnut CH, III, *et al.* (2000). A randomized trial of nasal spray salmon calcitonin in postmenopausal women with established osteoporosis: the prevent recurrence of osteoporotic fractures study. PROOF Study Group. *Am J Med*, **109**(4):267–276.)

4.67 Calcitonin and BMD. (Adapted from Downs RW, Jr., *et al.* (2000). Comparison of alendronate and intranasal calcitonin for treatment of osteoporosis in postmenopausal women. *J Clin Endocrinol Metab*, **85**(5):1783–1788.)

all decreased by 12% in the 200 IU group.

In the comparative study with alendronate[141], the 6- and 12-month change in bone markers was evaluated using bone specific alkaline phosphatase (BALP) and urinary N-telopeptide (NTx). As expected, bone turnover depression was significantly more pronounced with alendronate treatment (**4.69**).

Side-effects

Side-effects from nasal or injectable calcitonin are only briefly reported. Nasal calcitonin can cause nasal irritation; rhinitis was reported in 22% in the treated group *vs.* 15% in

the placebo group in the PROOF study[137]. In contrast, headache was less frequently reported by treated women (4%) compared to nontreated (7, p=0.03), which may be related to the analgesic properties of calcitonin.

Calcitonin given subcutaneously is associated with facial flushing, nausea and sometimes vomiting in up to 50% of patients, but often subsiding with continued treatment. Antibodies develop in approximately 30% of treated women; however, the relationship to the degree of resistance to treatment is weak.

Additional effects – analgesia

A calcitonin analgesic effect has been described in a number of randomized controlled trials[142–144]. The mechanism explaining the analgesic effect of calcitonin is still unclear. It may be related to the presence of CTR in the central nervous system, or to a rapid postexposure increase in b-endorphine levels, but other explanations are equally plausible, such as inhibition of prostaglandin synthesis. The analgesic effect of calcitonin is rapid and peaks after about 90 minutes. A 200 IU intranasal dose is equivalent to 100

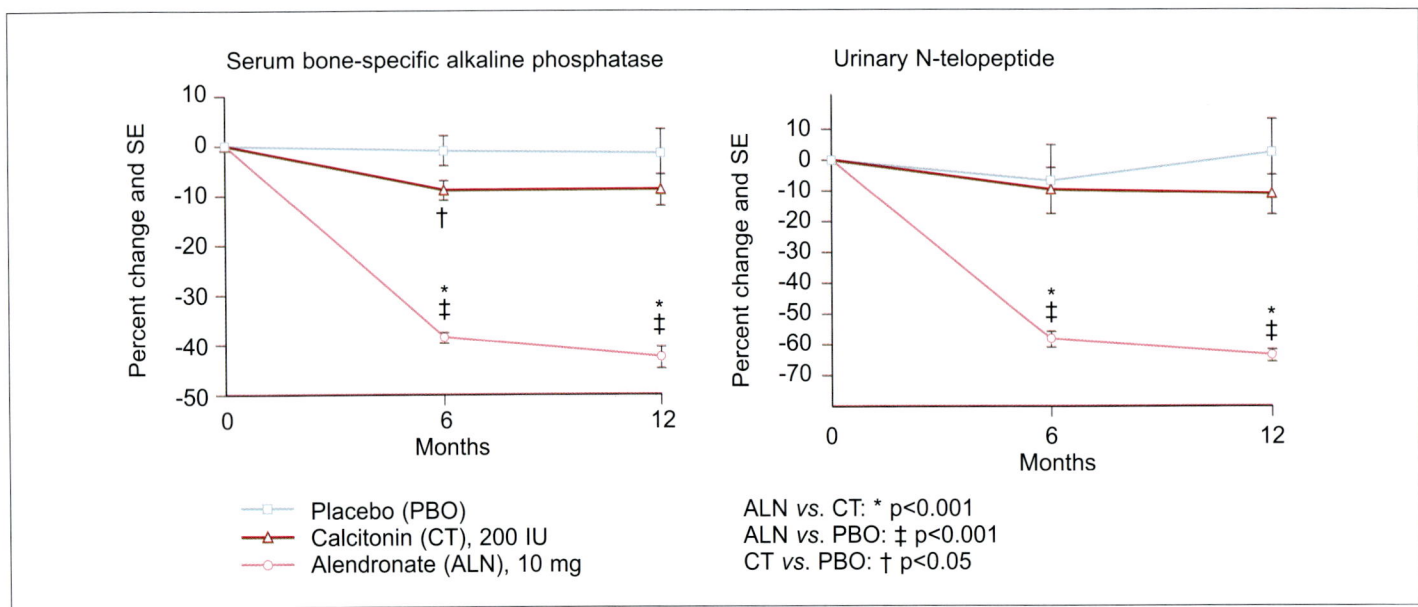

4.69 Effect of calcitonin on bone markers. (Adapted from Downs RW, Jr., *et al.* (2000). Comparison of alendronate and intranasal calcitonin for treatment of osteoporosis in postmenopausal women. *J Clin Endocrinol Metab*, **85**(5):1783–1788.)

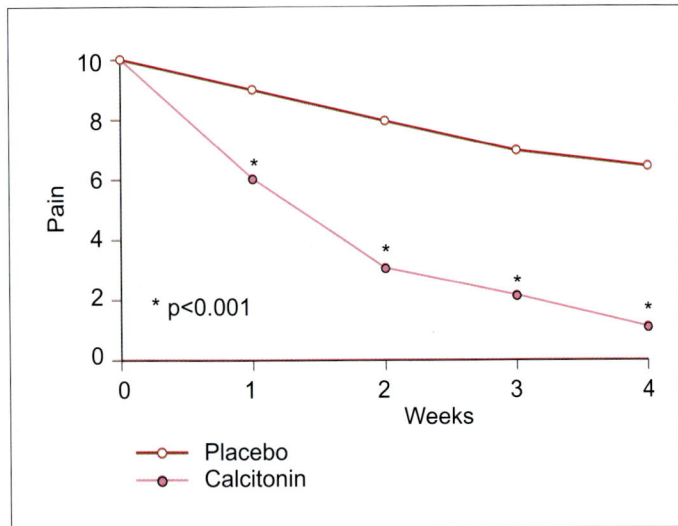

4.70 Analgesic effect of calcitonin. (Adapted from Lyritis GP, Trovas G. (2002). Analgesic effects of calcitonin. *Bone*, **30**(5 Suppl):71S-74S.)

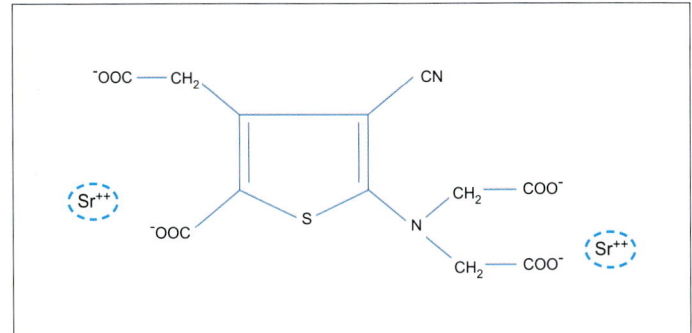

4.71 Structure of strontium ranelate.

IU given subcutaneously and approximately equipotent to 10 mg of morphine[145]. This advantageous effect of calcitonin is most prominent during the first weeks after a vertebral fracture. The effect is also associated with a decreased need for other analgesics, which is beneficial particularly in the elderly[143, 146].

In a study of women hospitalized because of acute vertebral fracture, the analgesic effect of calcitonin was compared to placebo (both groups were allowed to consume regular analgesics [paracetamol]) (**4.70**)[147]. Women receiving calcitonin experienced a significantly faster decrease in pain. The positive effect was also evident as improved mobility and lower consumption of paracetamol[144].

Strontium

Strontium is an alkaline earth element that is taken up by the skeleton, leading to its development as a treatment for osteoporosis. It is poorly absorbed when taken orally but 50–80% is taken up by calcified tissues and areas of active osteogenesis. To make it more palatable, 2 atoms of stable strontium are combined with organic ranelic acid to form strontium ranelate (**4.71**).

Mechanisms of action

Strontium atoms are adsorbed onto the surface of hydroxyapatite crystals without affecting mineral structure. It exchanges with calcium in bone mineral and may remain in the skeleton for a long time. Deposition in newly formed bone will increase apparent values of bone density, as strontium has a higher atomic number than calcium. Strontium appears to result in uncoupling of bone remodelling and increases bone formation as well as inhibiting bone resorption (**4.72**)[148]. It stimulates preosteoblast replication and there is increased matrix synthesis. There is inhibition of osteoclast differentiation and resorbing activity. An increase in trabecular bone mass, trabeculae numbers and thickness, and overall improvement in bone strength has been shown in animal studies.

Effect on BMD and fractures

The benefits on markers of bone turnover, bone density, and prevention of vertebral and nonvertebral fractures has been demonstrated in 2 large studies, SOTI (Spinal Osteoporosis Therapeutic Intervention Study)[149] and TROPOS (Treat-ment of Peripheral Osteoporosis Study)[150]. In SOTI, 1649 women over 50 years (average age 69 years) with low bone density and previous vertebral fracture were studied over 3 years, and were randomized to receive either 2 g sodium ranelate daily or placebo; all participants received calcium and vitamin D to ensure sufficiency. End-points were vertebral fracture prevalence, bone density in the hip and spine, and bone markers (**4.73–4.75**). TROPOS, 4932 women with low bone density and either 70–74 years with an additional fracture risk factor or 74 years or older were studied over 5 years with main analysis at 3 years. They were randomized to receive either 2 g sodium ranelate daily or placebo, and all received calcium and vitamin D to ensure sufficiency. Yearly vertebral fracture analysis were performed in a subgroup of 3640 patients. The effects on nonvertebral and vertebral fracture were the end-points of this study (**4.75**, *Table 4.11*). The occurrence of fractures was also analyzed in a high-risk fracture subgroup who were 74 years or over and had a femoral neck bone density T-score of -3 or lower.

In the SOTI study, at the end of the first year of treatment, the risk of new vertebral fracture was halved in the strontium ranelate group (RR over 12 months was 0.51, 95% CI 0.36–0.75; p<0.001) and over the whole 3 years of the study the risk of new vertebral fracture in the treatment group was reduced by 41% (RR over 36 months 0.59, 95% CI 0.48–0.73; p<0.001). Over the 3 years of the study, measured BMD in the strontium ranelate group had increased from baseline by 12.7% at the lumbar spine, 7.2% at the femoral neck, and 8.6% at the total hip and the

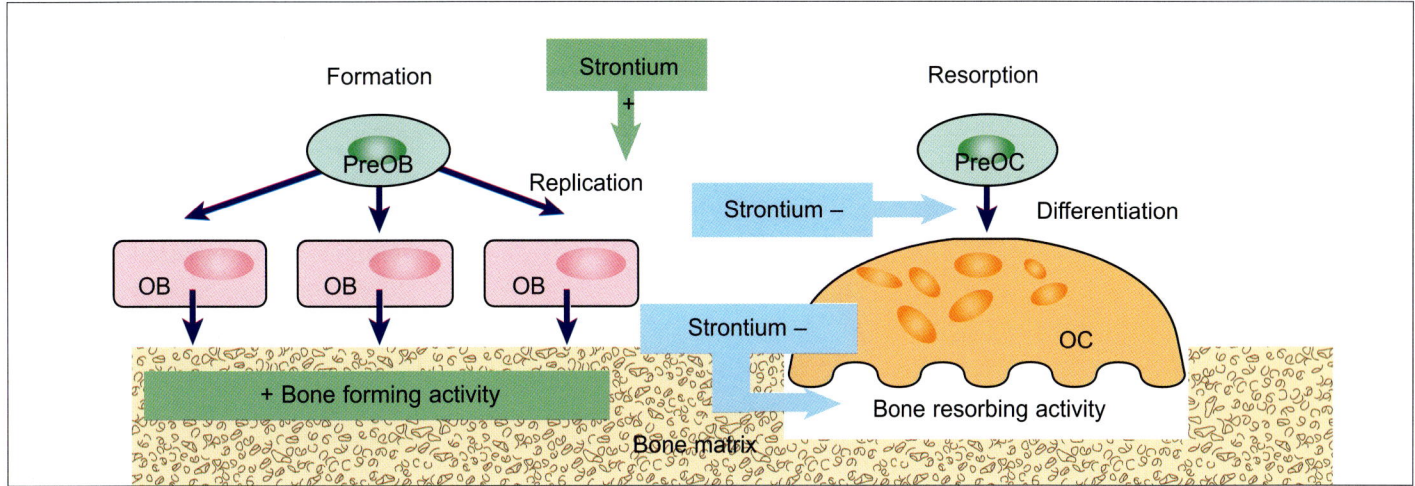

4.72 Mode of action of strontium.

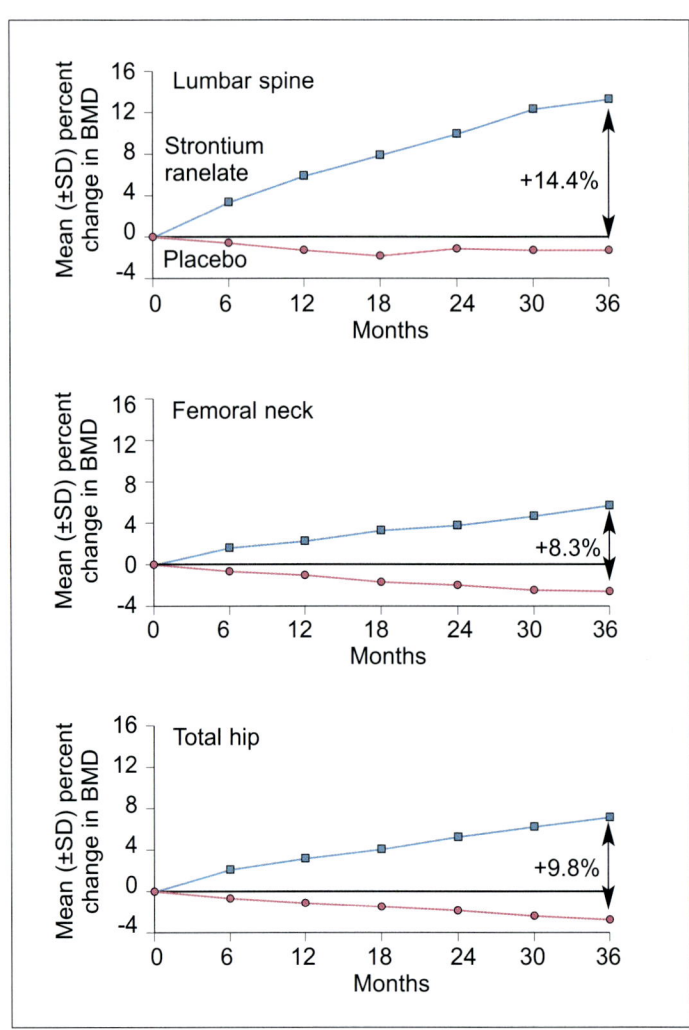

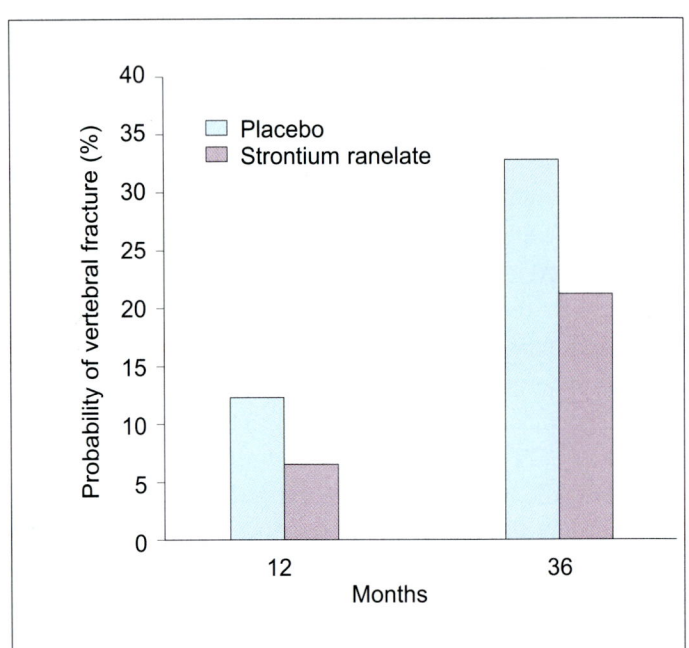

4.73 Proportion of patients who had one or more new vertebral fractures. (Adapted from Meunier PJ, *et al.* (2004). The effects of strontium ranelate on the risk of vertebral fracture in women with postmenopausal osteoporosis. *N Engl J Med*, **350**(5):459–468.)

4.74 Effects of strontium ranelate on BMD in all patients receiving 2 g a day of oral strontium ranelate. (Adapted from Meunier PJ, *et al.* (2004). The effects of strontium ranelate on the risk of vertebral fracture in women with postmenopausal osteoporosis. *N Engl J Med*, **350**(5):459–468.)

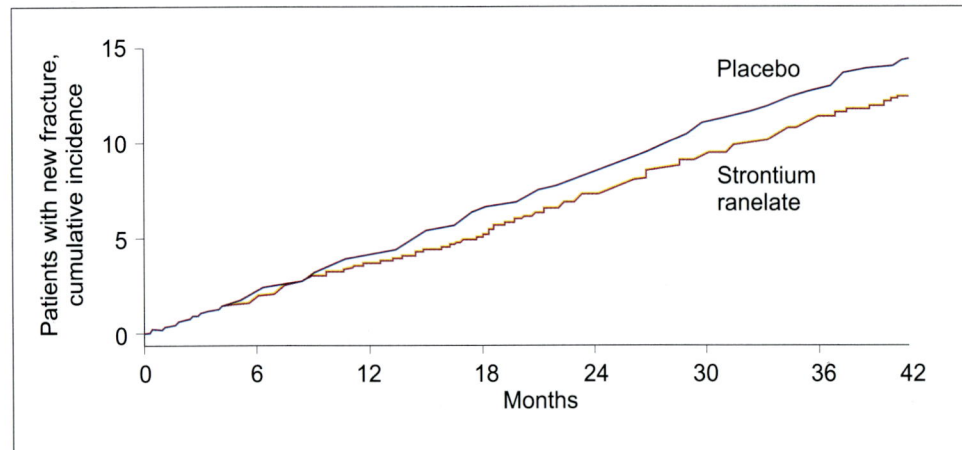

4.75 Nonvertebral fracture incidence in patients with at least one incident of osteoporosis-realted nonvertebral fracture. (Adapted from Reginster JY, *et al.* (2005). Strontium ranelate reduces the risk of nonvertebral fractures in postmenopausal women with osteoporosis: Treatment of Peripheral Osteoporosis (TROPOS) study. *J Clin Endocrinol Metab*, **90**(5):2816–2822.)

Table 4.11 TROPOS Study

Number entered into study	Average age (years)	End point	Relative risk of fracture (95% CI)
Whole study population			
4932	77	Nonvertebral – all	0.84 (0.702–0.995)
		Nonvertebral – major osteoporotic	0.81 (0.660.98)
		Nonvertebral – hip	NS
High-risk fracture subgroup (≥74 year with femoral neck BMD T-score ≤ -3)			
1977	80	Nonvertebral – hip	0.64 (0.412–0.997)
Vertebral fracture study subgroup (nonmandatory annual vertebral xrays)			
3640	77	Vertebral fractures (new)	1 year: 0.55 (0.39–0.77) 3 year: 0.61 (0.51–0.73)
		Vertebral fractures (first fracture during observation period)	0.55 (0.42–0.72)
		Vertebral fractures (had pre-existing)	0.68 (0.53-0.85)

(Adapted from Reginster JY, *et al.* (2005). Strontium ranelate reduces the risk of nonvertebral fractures in postmenopausal women with osteoporosis: Treatment of Peripheral Osteoporosis (TROPOS) study. *J Clin Endocrinol Metab*, **90**(5):2816–2822.)

differences between the placebo and the treatment groups were 14.4%, 8.3%, and 9.8% respectively. However, the strontium content will result in an overestimate of the increase in bone density. When bone density was adjusted for the strontium content, the increase over the baseline value was 6.8% in the strontium ranelate group in contrast to a decrease of 1.3% in the placebo group (p<0.001), i.e. a treatment-related increase of 8.1%.

In the TROPOS study there was a reduction in relative risk of all nonvertebral fractures over 3 years of 16% (RR 0.84, 95% CI 0.702–0.995; p=0.04). These studies show that strontium ranelate reduces the risk of new vertebral and nonvertebral fractures in postmenopausal women with osteoporosis, with or without prevalent vertebral fractures.

Effect on bone turnover

The changes in bone markers indicate both an effect on bone formation and resorption (**4.76**). The changes in bone

markers indicate that the mechanism of action of strontium ranelate is different from other drugs. When compared with the placebo group, there is an ongoing increase in bone formation, on the basis of serum concentrations of bone-specific alkaline phosphatase, and an ongoing decrease in bone resorption, on the basis of serum concentrations of C-telopeptide cross-links. The changes in biochemical markers of bone resorption and formation were most pronounced during the first 6 months; the dissociation between the bone markers was noted throughout the study.

Side-effects

Strontium ranelate is well tolerated and adherence to treatment was good in the studies. The commonest adverse events are nausea and diarrhoea, usually in the first few months. A small increase in venous thrombotic events (RR 1.42, 95% CI 1.02–1.98) was found.

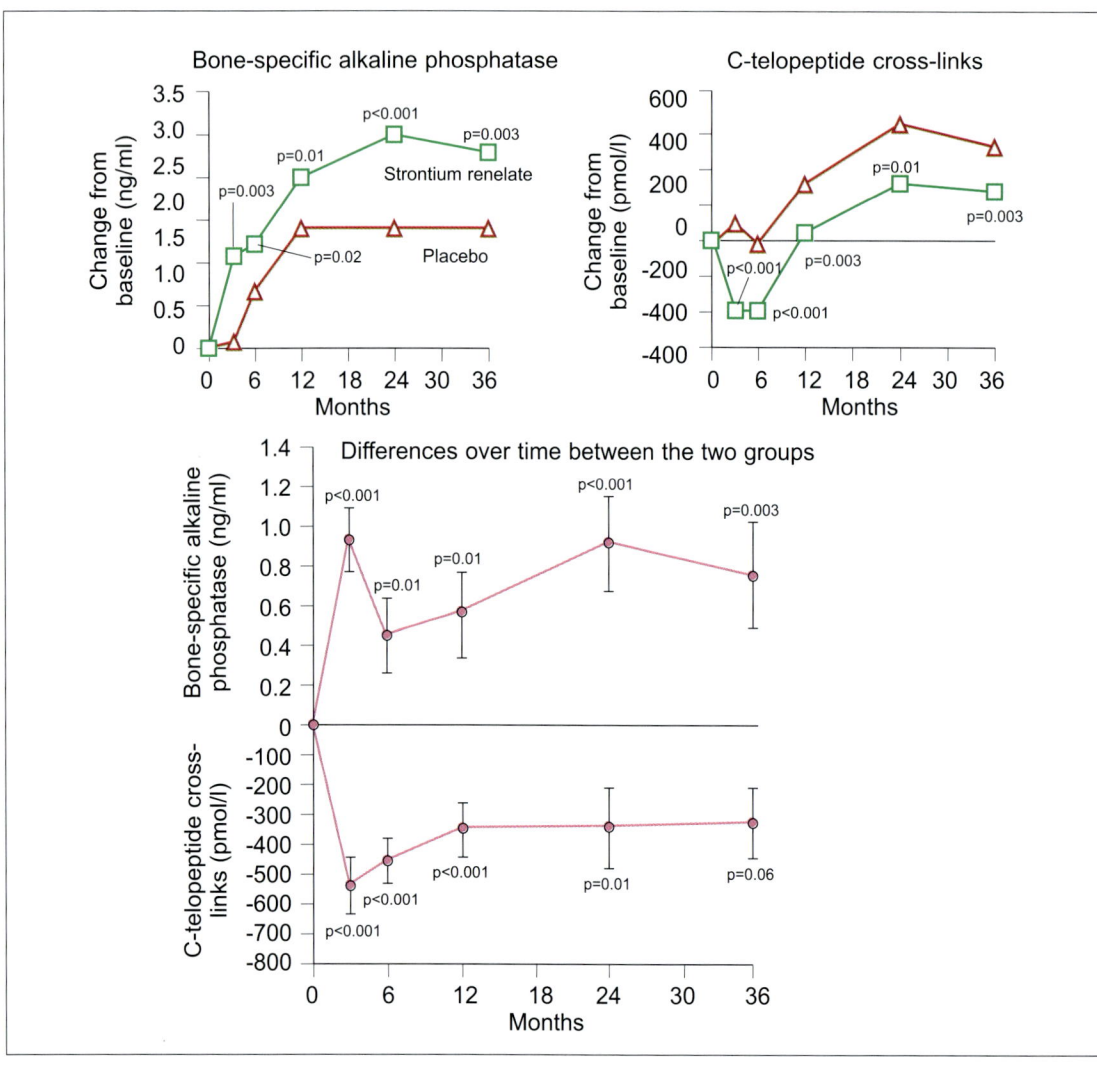

4.76 Strontium renelate-induced changes in serum biochemical markers of bone metabolism. (Adapted from Meunier PJ, *et al.* (2004). The effects of strontium ranelate on the risk of vertebral fracture in women with postmenopausal osteoporosis. *N Engl J Med*, **350**(5):459–468.)

Emerging therapies

Osteoclasts have an unique ability to dissolve and degrade bone tissue. In addition to factors influencing osteoclast development, the production of numerous substances both for mineral dissolution and the enzymatic degradation of matrix have been the primary targets for prospective drug research. However, development of bone anabolic agents would in reality be even more attractive, but so far the clinical utility of potent anabolics beyond PTH, such as growth hormone and androgens, have not achieve expected efficacy.

Identification of factors acting on receptors for osteoclast attachment or function, such as the RANKL (receptor activator of nuclear factor kB ligand), the soluble ligand osteoprotegerin, $\alpha_v\beta_3$integrin, or cathepsin K are currently the most promising avenues as new treatment alternatives.

RANKL/RANK/OPG

The essential function of bone turnover is to maintain skeletal integrity and this requires a balance between bone resorption and bone formation, i.e. a coupling between the processes. The RANKL/osteoprotegerin (OPG) system has emerged as an important regulator of bone resorption and a strong candidate as a mediator of the coupling process.

RANKL, a members of the tumour necrosis factor (TNF) family and expressed on osteoblasts, activates its receptor, RANK, which is expressed on the surface of osteoclasts. The association between RANKL and RANK promotes the recruitment of osteoclast precursors, osteoclast activity, and suppresses osteoclast apoptosis. OPG is a soluble receptor and acts as decoy, competitively blocking the binding of RANKL to RANK on osteoclasts and subsequently it has an inhibitory effect on osteoclast induced bone resorption[151].

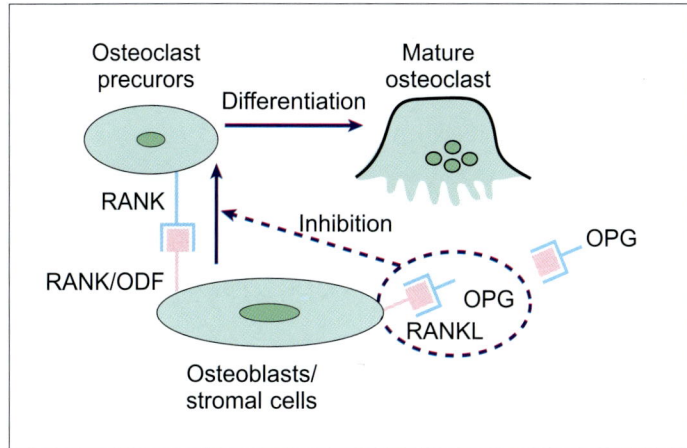

4.77 Mode of action of RANK/RANKL/OPG.

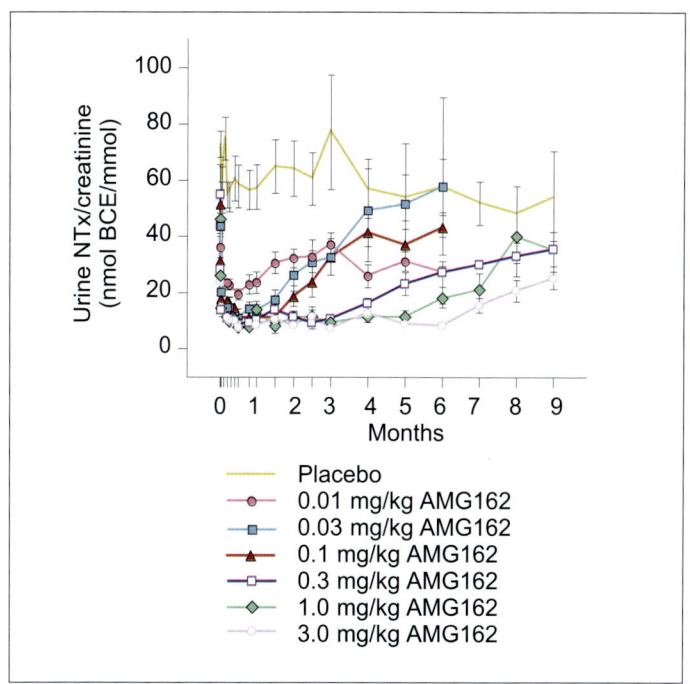

4.78 The effect of AMG 162 on bone markers. (Adapted from Bekker PJ, *et al.* (2004). A single-dose placebo-controlled study of AMG 162, a fully human monoclonal antibody to RANKL, in postmenopausal women. *J Bone Miner Res*, **19**(7):1059–1066.)

In Figure **4.77**, the interaction RANK/RANKL stimulates osteoclast differentiation leading to increased bone resorption. As a soluble receptor that acts as a decoy receptor for RANKL, OPG leads to decreased RANKL/RANK interaction and by this inhibiting osteoclast differentiation. OPG secretion is stimulated by the presence of oestrogen (17β-estradiol), whereas RANKL expression is suppressed, hence as a consequence of menopause OPG decreases allowing for increased RANKL/RANK mediated bone resorption.

Theoretically, RANKL activity could be reduced by suppressing its expression or blocking its action, blocking RANK binding or blocking competitive binding by increasing OPG. A fully human monoclonal antibody to RANKL has been developed that prevents its binding to RANK and thus acts as a potent antiresorptive agent. This antibody, denosumab (AMG 162), mimics the activity of OPG but without structurally resembling OPG, which should reduce the risk of generating antibodies against endogenous OPG[152, 153].

Suppression of bone resorption occurs within the first 24 hours and is sustained over time but is dose dependent. Figure **4.78** illustrates the effect of a single dose of AMG 162 on bone resorption reflected by changes in second morning void urinary NTx over time. Data are presented as mean and SEM. The line without a symbol is placebo, whereas the others are describing different doses. The decrease in bone resorption was evident already after 12 hours. The cohorts receiving the largest doses were followed for 9 months. In those receiving the lower doses the effect

was not sustained at the maximum level but a return towards baseline occurred.

Denosumab has been tested in a phase 2 dose-finding study evaluating the effects on BMD and bone turnover over 12 months[154]. Figure **4.79** illustrates the study design. Recruited to the study were postmenopausal women with a mean age of 63 years and with osteopenia or osteoporosis. Fracture as an outcome was not included. Denosumab was administered by subcutaneous injections and in this study either every third or sixth month. The 3-month protocol included three different doses and the 6-month protocol four different doses. Both placebo and alendronate (70 mg/week) served as comparators. BMD increased up to 6% with the largest response in the lumbar spine (**4.80**). Markers of bone resorption decreased rapidly, within 3 days, and remained suppressed at the same level as with weekly alendronate. The rapid effect on bone resorption has in safety studies been observed already within 12 hours. In the lowest doses the suppression subsided over time, indicating reversibility with discontinuation.

BMD at the hip increased with denosumab treatment by 1.9–3.6% as compared with 2.1% for alendronate and a loss

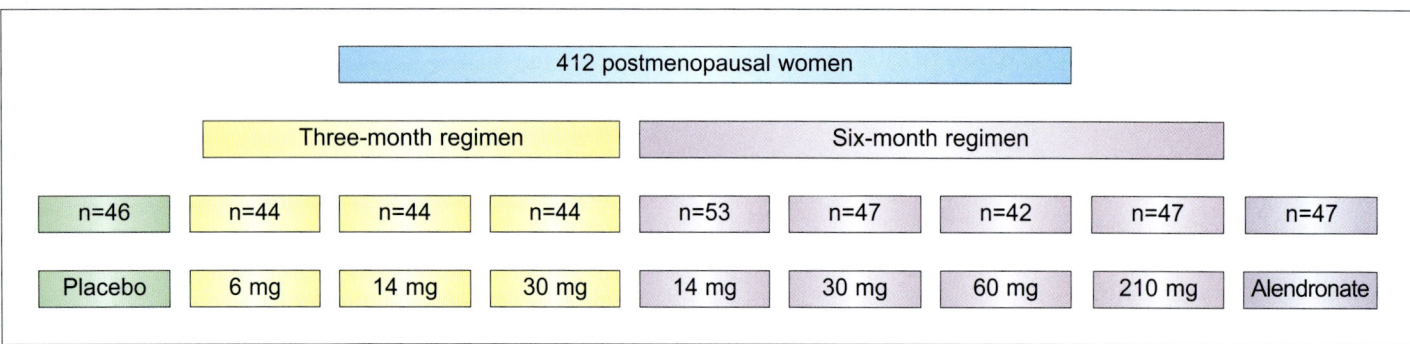

4.79 The design of the clinical phase 2 study in menopausal women. In this dose-finding study women were treated either every third or sixth month. The new treatment was compared to both placebo and alendronate.

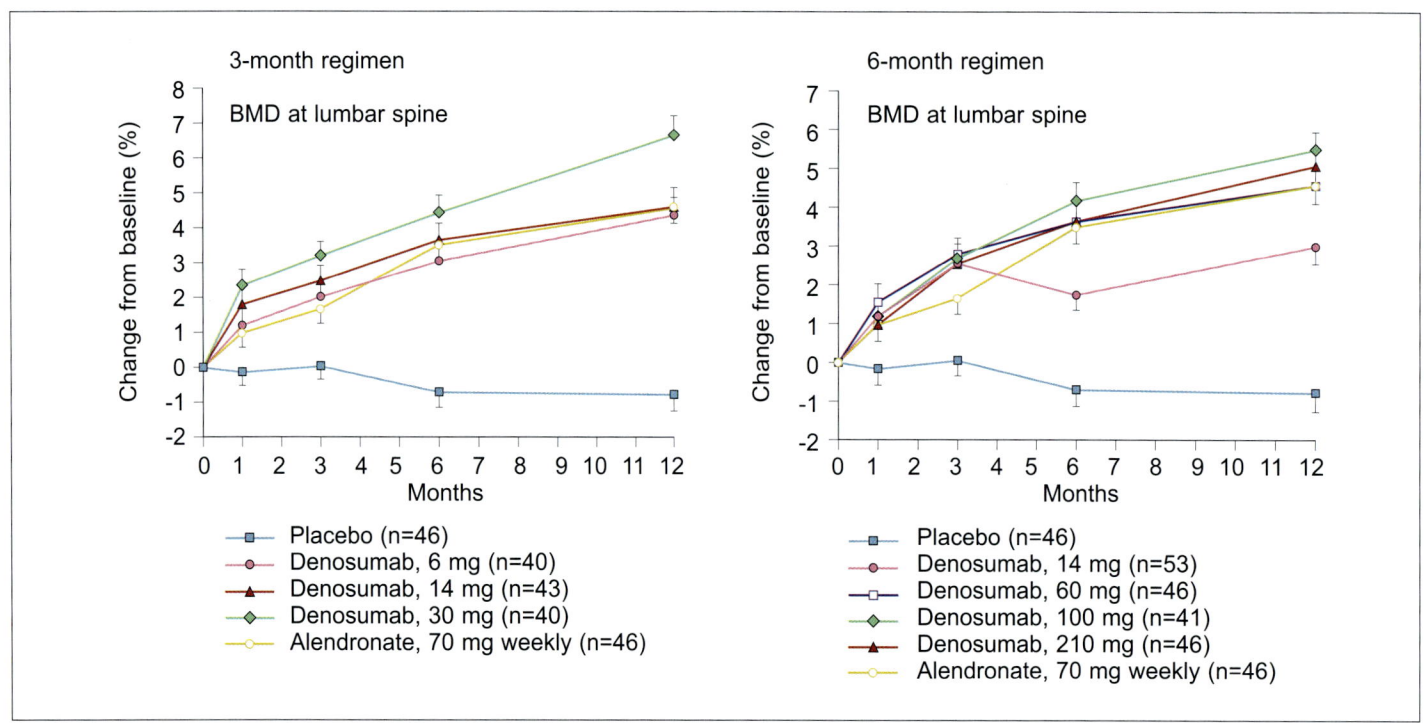

4.80 Increase of BMD at lumbar spine with denosumab treatment. (Adapted from McClung MR, *et al.* (2006). Denosumab in postmenopausal women with low bone mineral density. *N Engl J Med*, **354**(8):821–831.)

of 0.6 % with placebo (**4.81**). BMD was also measured at the distal radius and total body and the results similar but the percentage change between 1% and 2.5%.

Biochemical markers of bone turnover were assessed monthly. CTx as a marker of bone resorption decreased in all denosumab groups with a maximum mean percentage of 88%. The effect was rapid and obvious after 3 days of treatment, which was the first time-point for assessing bone markers. In the denosumab groups receiving the lowest doses (6 mg/3 months or 14 mg/6 months) an increase was

noted indicating a reversible effect. In the placebo group the change in CTx was only 6% (**4.82**). Bone formation was decreased in the denosumab groups as assessed by BALP, however, with a delay of 1 month (**4.83**).

Denosumab has also been given to women with metastases from breast cancer or with multiple myeloma and compared to pamidronate[155, 156]. Denosumab was well tolerated and reduced bone resorption for at least 84 days. The changes in bone resorption were similar to those of pamidronate.

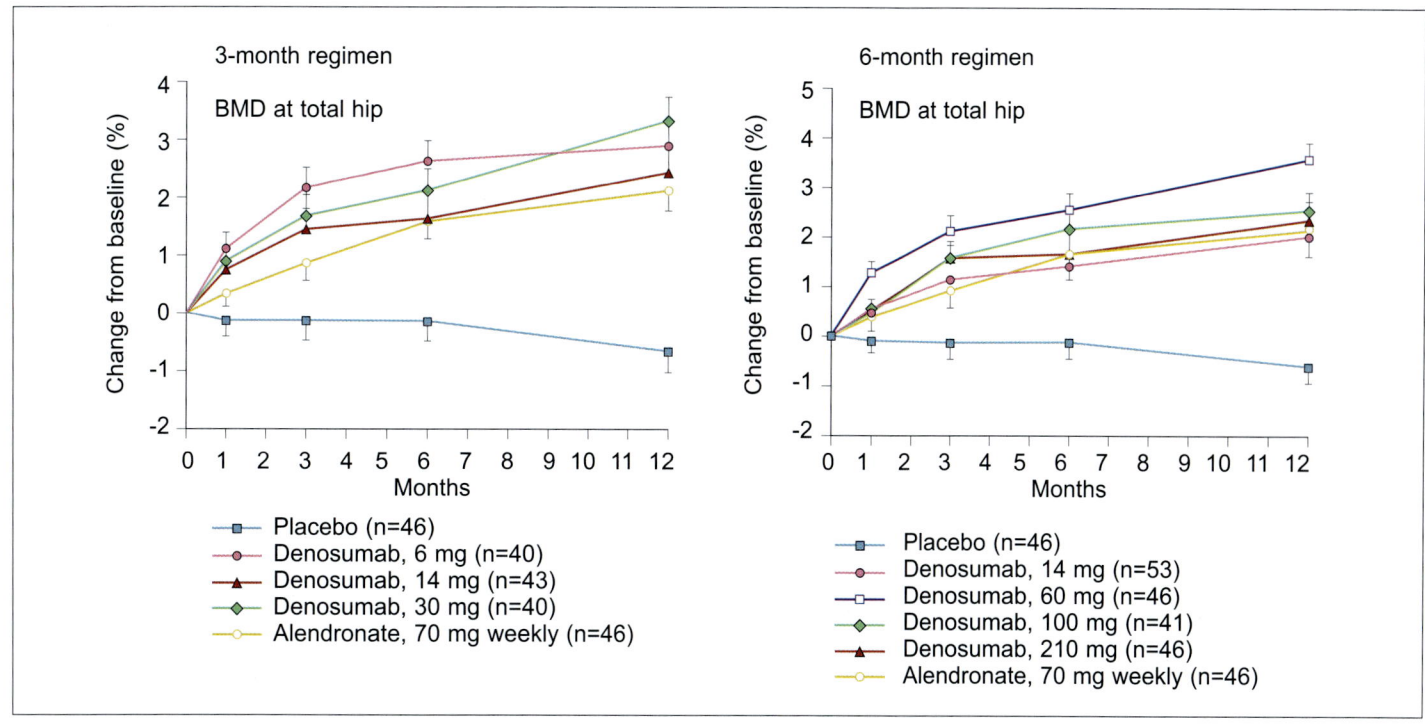

4.81 Increase of BMD at total hip with denosumab treatment. (Adapted from McClung MR, *et al.* (2006). Denosumab in postmenopausal women with low bone mineral density. *N Engl J Med*, **354**(8):821–831.)

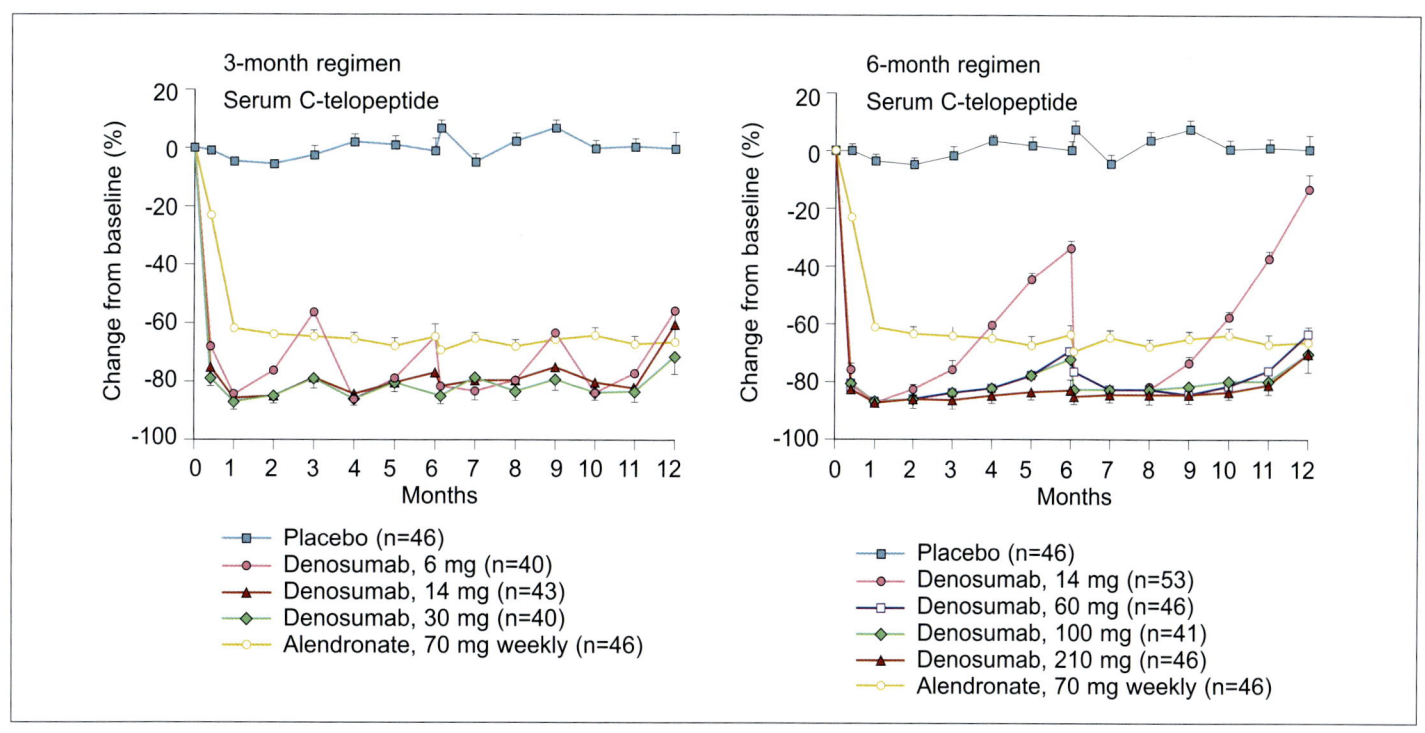

4.82 Assessment of bone turnover using C-telopeptide as a marker of bone resorption. (Adapted from McClung MR, *et al.* (2006). Denosumab in postmenopausal women with low bone mineral density. *N Engl J Med*, **354**(8):821–831.)

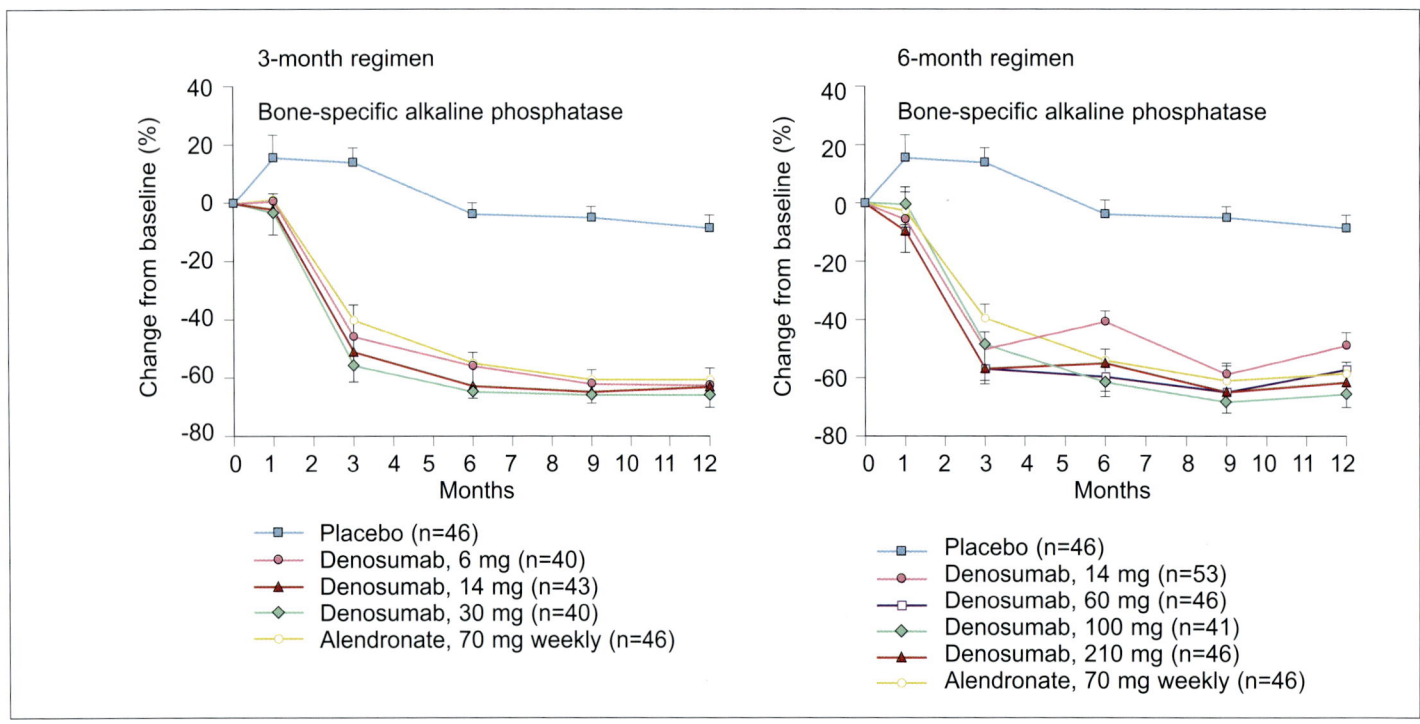

4.83 Decrease in bone formation as assessed by BALP. (Adapted from McClung MR, *et al.* (2006). Denosumab in postmenopausal women with low bone mineral density. *N Engl J Med*, **354**(8):821–831.)

Cytokines

Current knowledge on cell differentiation and cell activity shows that cytokines are important regulators at the local level. Most cytokines are implicated as enhancers of osteoclast activity and subsequently bone resorption. Inhibition of cytokine activity by inhibitory antibodies, such as antiTNFα, have proved extremely successful in the treatment of rheumatoid arthritis. Such treatment may have additional effects on bone turnover, since TNFα has been shown to be one of the more important cytokines that modify bone resorption. Bone resorption markers significantly decrease in patients with RA treated with infliximab[157]. This may allow for development of inhibitors to other bone active cytokines, such as IL-1 or IL-6. The relative nonspecificity and subsequent effects on other organs may, however, limit the usefulness.

Cathepsin K

The degradation of bone matrix is mediated by cathepsin K, an osteoclast protease which appears to specifically act on bone collagen[158]. Animal models confirm the important effect of cathepsin K and deletion of the cathepsin K gene results in an osteopetrotic bone in mice[159]. An inhibitor of cathepsin K may be of potential use as an antiresorptive drug, but has only been tested in animal models[160]. Various integrins mediate the attachment of osteoclast to the exposed bone surface, an integrin antagonist would block osteoclast adhesion and osteoclast-mediated bone resorption. An orally bioavailable $\alpha_v\beta_3$ integrin antagonist has been shown to have dose-dependent antiresorptive effects[161].

Pharmacogenetics

Speculation on future therapeutics may also include genetic modification and pharmacogenetics, utilizing the increasing knowledge of genetics of bone diseases. A number of candidate genes have been associated with osteoporosis and fracture, albeit with inconsistent results. Variations in the collagen, oestrogen and vitamin D receptor genes merits mentioning as they have been associated with bone mass and fracture in elderly women, with implications of functional importance for collagen polymorphism[162].

Collagen is the major organic component of bone matrix. Bone collagen consists of two α-chains and one β-chain. A functional variation in the collagen gene alters the collagen structure and may thus influence bone strength (**4.84**). Variation in the collagen gene contributes to low bone mass

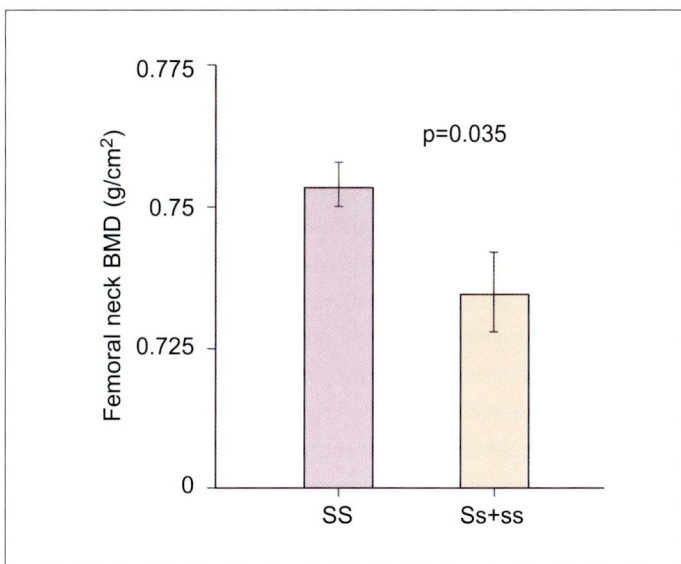

4.84 Effect of variation in the collagen gene. (Adapted from Gerdhem P, *et al.* (2004). Association of the collagen type 1 (COL1A 1) Sp1 binding site polymorphism to femoral neck bone mineral density and wrist fracture in 1044 elderly Swedish women. *Calcif Tissue Int,* **74**(3):264–269.)

in elderly women. Women carrying the 's' risk allele had 2.7% lower bone density of the hip and a more than doubled risk of wrist fracture OR = 2.7 (1.1–6.8). This type of finding may indicate certain gene variations which may not only influence risk but also response to treatment.

NONPHARMACOLOGICAL INTERVENTIONS

Fall prevention

Fall prevention is central to the prevention of osteoporosis as two-thirds of older people with femoral neck osteoporosis have fall-related risk factors and 90% of hip fractures result from a fall. The general risk of falling in the older population needs to be reduced by targeting extrinsic risk factors in the home and community, as well as reducing intrinsic factors which mostly relate to impaired physical and cognitive function as well as development of comorbidities (*Tables 1.4, 2.9*). 'Frail' older people who look older than their chronological age have poor gait, poor balance, low muscle strength, low activity level, and a high risk of falling[163].

People therefore need to maintain their physical activity into later life. It is also important and most effective to target those elderly at most risk of falls or fracture[164]. Their individual risk factors that can be modified need to be identified. How to identify those at most risk has been considered in Chapter 3. The easiest to identify are those older people (especially if they are not living independently) who have already had a fall or have poor balance, poor mobility, or difficulty getting into and out of a chair. The challenge is to prevent further falls and consequent fractures. There have been numerous studies looking at different approaches to fall prevention. At best, a one-third reduction in falls can be achieved, but is more difficult in those at highest risk. There is, however, little evidence that preventing falls translates into the prevention of fracture. A problem is the size of study that is required to demonstrate such a benefit as not all falls will result in a fracture.

There is no single all-encompassing approach to prevent falls. An individualized multifaceted approach to assessing the risks and prevention, with interventions targeted at those specific risk factors is recommended[165]. This approach has been shown by meta-analysis[166] to be effective in older people from an unselected population (four trials including 1651 participants; pooled RR 0.73, 95% CI 0.63–0.85), in those with a history of falling or selected because of known risk factors (five trials including 1176 participants, pooled RR 0.86, 95% CI 0.76–0.98), and in older people in residential care facilities (one trial including 439 participants, cluster-adjusted incidence rate ratio 0.60, 95% CI 0.50–0.73).

Muscle strengthening and balance training is recommended and needs to be part of the multifaceted approach in higher risk people. It should be individualized, home-based, progressive, and maintained or the benefits will be lost. Such programmes have been shown to reduce the risk of falls by 20%[166]. Specific programmes may include Tai Chi which has been found to prevent falls[166]. It is also important to assess the home for any hazards and modify where needed, along with reviewing the person's medication and stopping any psychotropic drugs if possible. A danger of exercise programmes is an increase in the risk of falling and fracture and this was found in a study of unsupervised brisk walking, which is therefore not recommended for those at high risk of falls. Group approaches to exercise do not appear to be effective if they are not individualized, or if given alone and not part of a multifaceted approach.

Over two-thirds of a Falls Clinic population have been shown to be vitamin D deficient and vitamin D supplementation reduces the risk of falls[167]. Vitamin supplementation should therefore be considered if deficiency is likely due to lifestyle factors such as reduced mobility and not going out into daylight.

It is therefore important to remember the role of falls in osteoporotic fractures, identify those at highest risk, and ensure they have an individualized assessment for risk and for modifiable risk factors so that an individualized programme can be developed around these (*Table 4.12*). Strengthening exercises and balance retraining are core parts of any programme and will most likely benefit older people living in the community with a history of recurrent falls and/or balance and gait difficulties. Those older people who are no longer living independently and have risk factors for falls are more likely to need additional interventions.

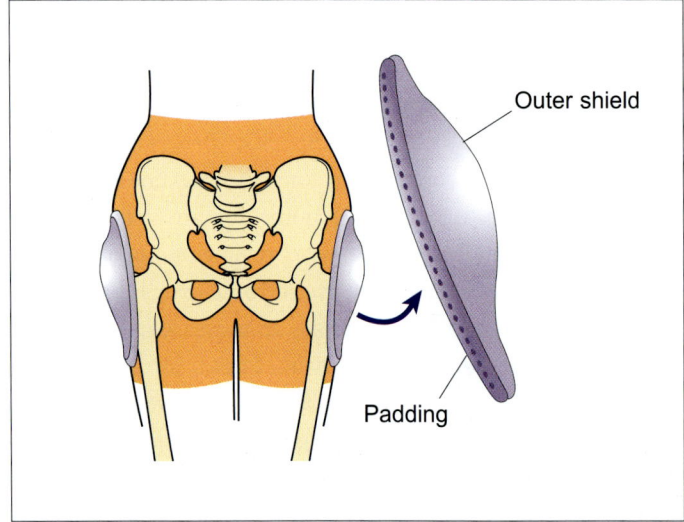

4.85 Hip protectors.

Hip protectors

Hip protectors are designed to both absorb and transfer the energy of a fall onto the hip (**4.85**). The impact of a fall is normally reduced by protective responses and the attenuation of the soft tissues overlying the greater trochanter. The loss of these protective responses and the often reduced forward momentum when an older person falls combined with the loss of soft tissue padding overlying the hip results in a high risk of fracture. Thus a logical approach is to try to protect the hip. The protectors are integral to special underwear, either fitting into pockets over the greater trochanter or are nonremovable.

Initial studies in nursing home residents showed a dramatic reduction in numbers of hip fractures[168], which was also shown in frail but ambulatory elderly people either in geriatric long-stay or supported home living (**4.86**)[169]. Many studies have since been performed. A Cochrane review (**4.87**)[170, 171] found marginally statistically significant reduction in hip fracture incidence for people in nursing homes or residential care wearing hip protectors compared to controls (11 studies including 9859 participants, RR 0.77, 95% CI 0.62–0.97). No reduction in hip fracture incidence was seen for people living in the community (three studies including 5135 participants, RR 1.16, 95% CI 0.85–1.59).

Compliance with wearing the hip protectors has been a problem in all studies, often falling below 40% by the end of the study, due to discomfort, the extra effort needed to wear the protector, urinary incontinence, and physical difficulties/illnesses[171]. This is an unfortunate drawback as few hip fractures have occurred in these studies if the hip protectors are actually being worn correctly; a reduction to one-third was demonstrated if protected falls were compared to unprotected falls in high-risk nursing home residents[172]. Hip protectors should be considered for frail elderly people with a high risk of falls and fracture who are living under supervision, so that assistance and encouragement are given to ensure appropriate and regular use.

FRACTURE MANAGEMENT

Fracture management in not limited to the actual treatment of the fracture but involves a chain of interventions. Optimal fracture management commences at the scene of the fracture event and ends with rehabilitative measures and

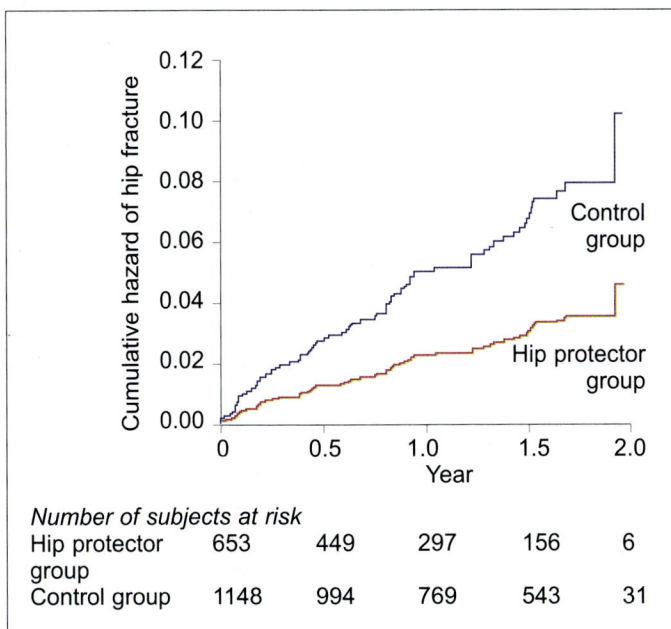

restoration of function. However, the actual treatment of the fracture is the key step in the process, and without optimal fracture treatment the outcome is hampered, leaving the patient with unnecessary functional limitations. Hence fracture management relies on team work, beginning in the ambulance where skilled personnel should initiate pain control and primary stabilization of the fracture, and continuing through orthopaedics to physio- and occupational therapy when needed. Furthermore, in those at middle-age and above, osteoporosis may be an underlying cause and the person should be evaluated accordingly.

Fracture treatment

The principles of fracture treatment depend on the structural damage and the location of the fracture. Classification systems are available for most types of fracture in order to evaluate severity and to give guidance to treatment. The major classifications relate to the location in the bone: diaphyseal or metaphyseal; if it involves the joint:

4.86 Prevention of hip fracture in elderly people with the use of a hip protector. (Adapted from Kannus P, *et al.* (2000). Prevention of hip fracture in elderly people with use of a hip protector. *N Engl J Med*, **343**(21):1506–1513.)

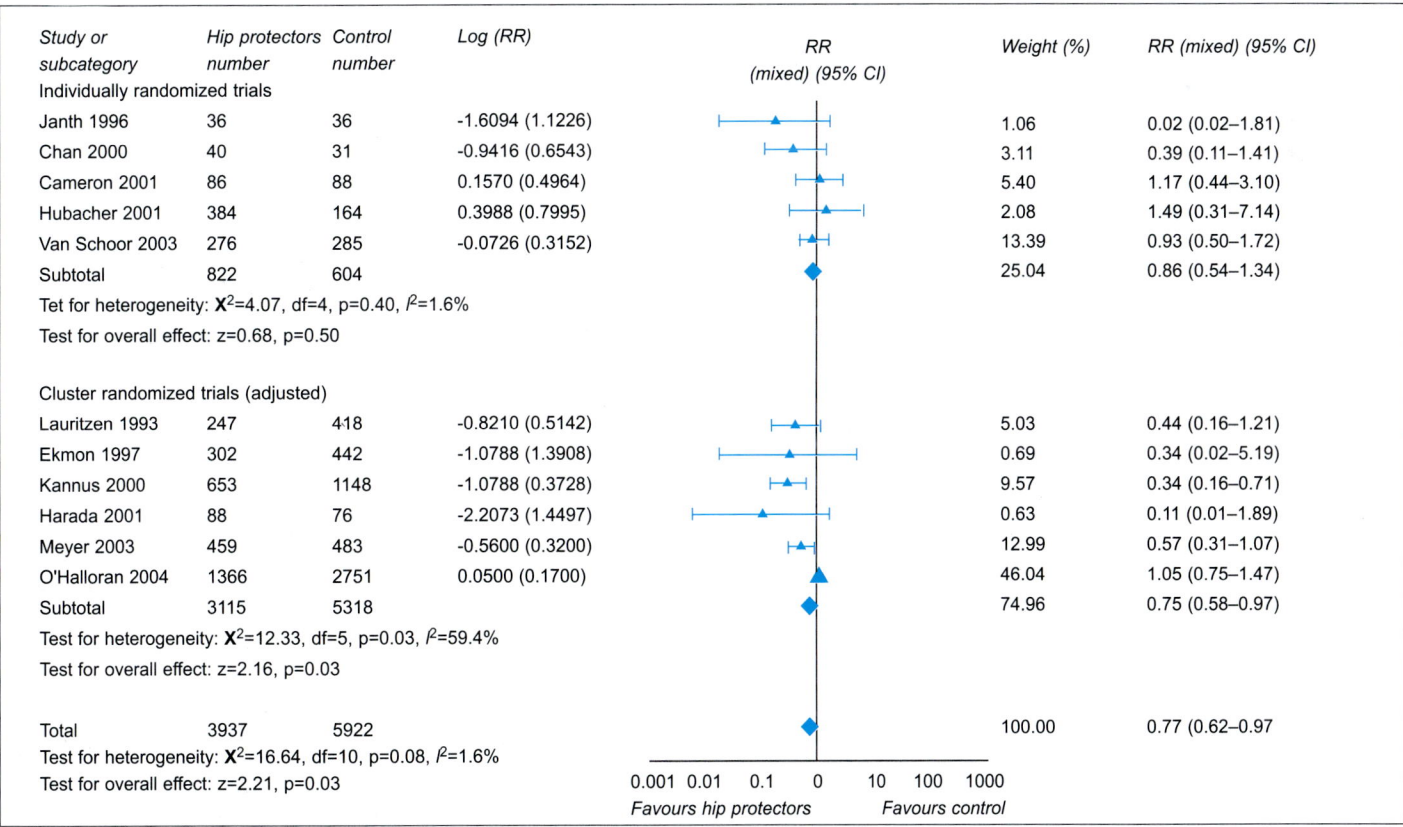

4.87 Meta-analysis showing reduction of hip fracture incidence. (Adapted from Parker MJ, *et al.* (2006). Effectiveness of hip protectors for preventing hip fractures in elderly people: systematic review. *BMJ*, **332**(7541):571–574.)

intra- or extra-articular; if the fracture is open or closed; and to the degree of comminution and dislocation. Certain types of fracture are more common with low-energy trauma, whereas others commonly occur in those sustaining high-energy trauma.

The purpose of treatment is to obtain anatomical realignment supporting future function and to stabilize in order to maintain alignment, diminish pain, and to promote fracture healing. The choice of treatment is to use external stabilization, e.g. casts when possible. However, modern treatment devices and infection control have improved to such an extent that open surgery and internal fixation is used when technically possible. The advantage of surgical treatment is a higher degree of stability which leads to earlier mobilization, earlier weight-bearing, and better function.

Distal forearm fracture

Distal forearm fractures (**4.88**) are classified according to the degree of dislocation: undisplaced, moderately displaced, or severely displaced. In addition, intra-articular involvement may influence the choice of treatment. A stable distal forearm fracture is best treated with a plaster cast. The principles of casting for this type of fracture include stabilization of the fracture, but also free range of motion for the fingers (**4.89**). It is of utmost importance that soft

padding is closest to the skin when applying a cast to avoid pressure sores over bony protrusions, such as the styloid process of the ulna, at the edges of the cast near the elbow, or close to the metacarpal heads. The patient should be instructed to move the shoulder joint, the elbow, and the fingers and to keep the hand elevated when resting. These instructions should be both written and given at an appointment with the physiotherapist during the first week following the fracture. Normally the cast is applied for 4 weeks, with X-ray follow-up after 1 week. Postfracture follow-up should always include assessment of distal status for sensitivity and other indicators of nerve injury.

Dislocated distal forearm fractures are common in women with postmenopausal osteoporosis. This fracture may also be an indicator of future fracture risk. A dislocated fracture should always be reduced as close to the anatomical position as possible. If only dislocated in the anterior-posterior direction and without intra-articular involvement, then closed reduction is often sufficient and the fracture is stabilized with the same type of cast as if the fracture had been undislocated. However, forearm fractures with initial dislocation which require reduction are much more susceptible to re-dislocation and the radiographic follow-up within 1 week is strongly advocated. If re-dislocation occurs, it is still within the time frame to perform secondary surgery.

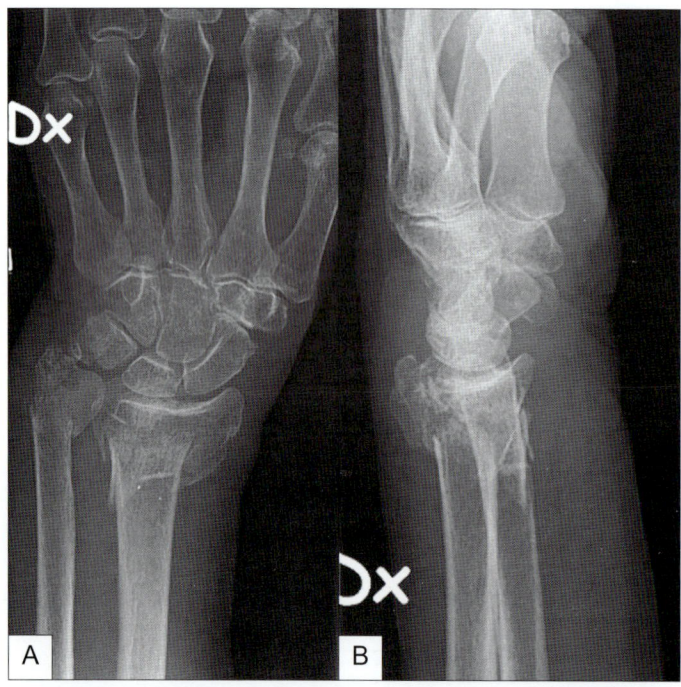

4.88 A, B Distal forearm fracture. The fracture is severely displaced with dorsal angulation and axial compression.

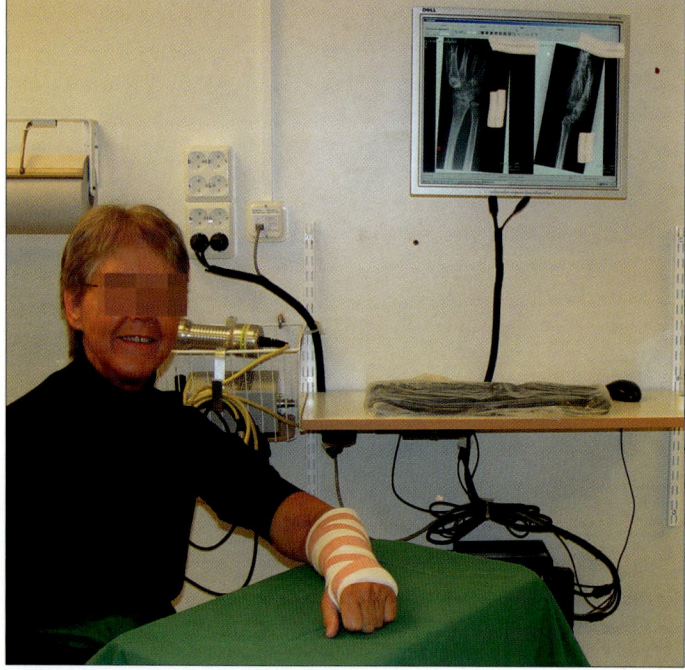

4.89 Distal forearm fracture cast.

If the fracture is highly unstable, intra-articular, or dislocating during the first week, then the most common choice of treatment is application of an external fixation device (**4.90**). Pins are inserted in the second metacarpal bone and in the distal diaphysis of the radius. The pins serve as connection sites for the rods distracting the fracture. In fractures involving the joint it may sometimes be advantageous to fixate the intra-articular fragment with a wire, pin, or a small plate, to secure the joint surface. Fracture follow-up is similar to that of those with nondisplaced fracture, but the fixation time is most often prolonged, reaching 5–6 weeks. Regardless whether the fracture requires surgery or not, postfracture physiotherapy is essential to obtain a favourable outcome both in terms function and pain and to avoid shoulder–hand syndrome.

Proximal humerus fracture

Fractures of the proximal humerus are commonly associated with osteoporosis. The fracture is most often stable and requiring only a sling for relief of pain during the first week or two (**4.91**). If the head of the humerus has dislocated, surgery is advocated and the dislocation reduced and fixed with intramedullar rods or with a plate. Multifragmented fractures are associated with a much more pronounced functional deficit. The anatomy of shoulder joint makes it more difficult to replace the joint with an artificial joint.

However, joint replacement is undertaken in those with the head of the humerus fractured into four fragments, since the possibilities for healing are poor. The outcome after the procedure is related to the age of the person and to the quality of the bone.

Since the shoulder joint has the greatest range of motion of all joints, a fracture virtually always leads to decreased range of motion. Hence, it is important to inform the patient clearly and at an early stage of the outcome and the goals of treatment. Mobility training is initiated at 2–3 weeks, before the fracture is healed, and often needs to be continued for 2–3 months.

Elbow fracture

The supra-condylar fracture of the elbow is one of the more serious fractures in children, because of the high risk of concomitant nerve and vessel injury. Fractures of the elbow in the elderly are often associated with osteoporosis, leading to multifragmentation and dislocation. In the elderly and severely osteoporotic, it may not even be possible to treat these fractures surgically and it is commonly referred to as 'bag of bones' (see **1.41**). It is left to heal as it is, but initially with a supporting cast. The same multifragmented supra-condylar fracture without surgical treatment is shown in **4.92**, initially and at 3 months when healing is on its way.

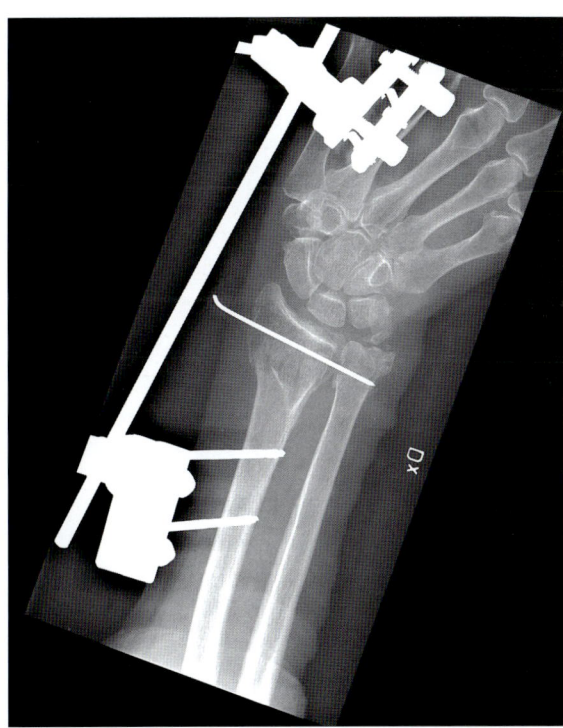

4.90 Distal forearm fracture external fixation.

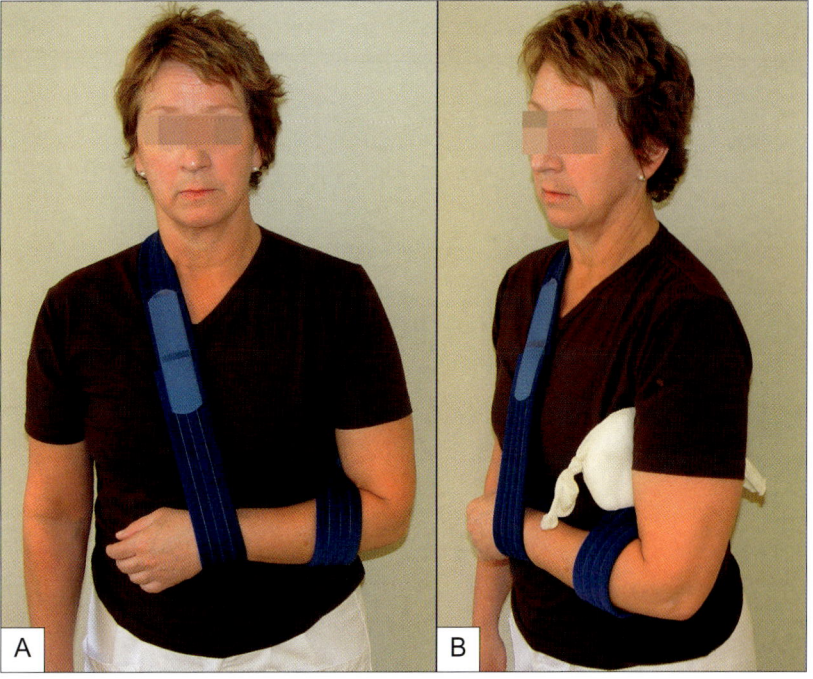

4.91 A, B Proximal humerus fracture treated with a collar-n-cuff sling.

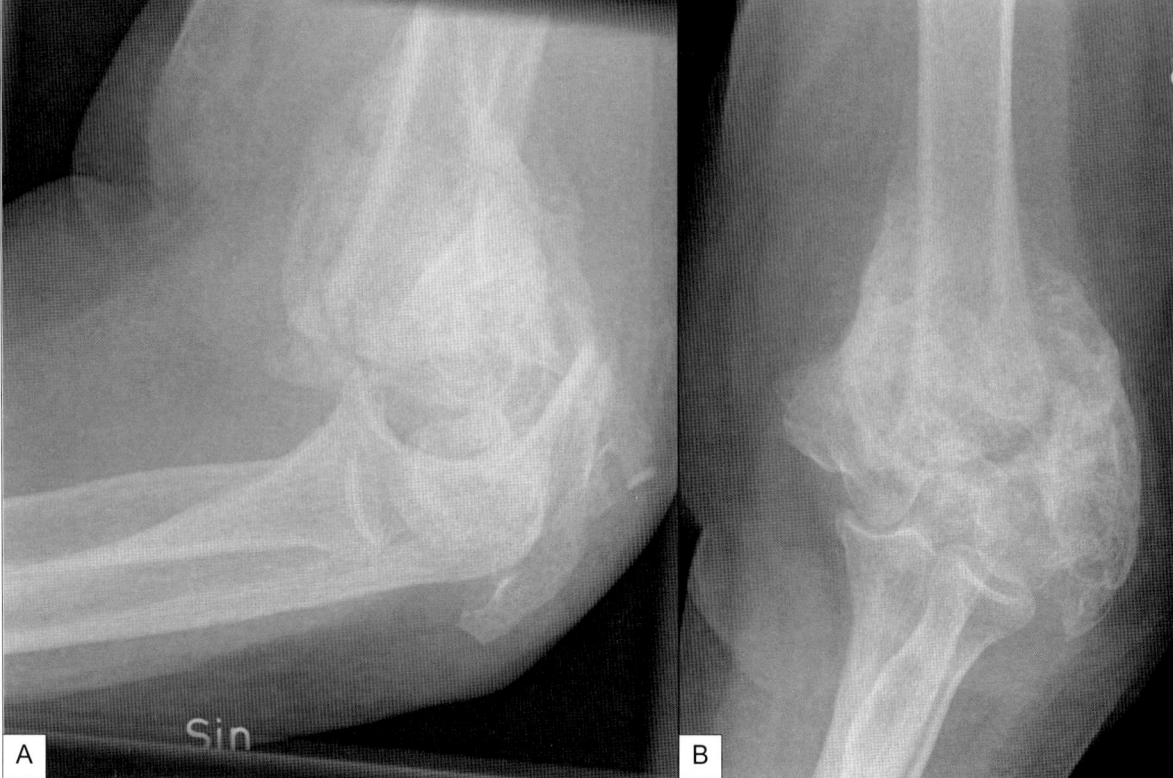

4.92 Healing of a multifragmented elbow fracture (impossible to treat surgically) in an elderly person (see also **1.41** for the acute state).

Vertebral fracture

Deformities of the vertebrae or minimally compressed vertebral fractures are treated when they cause pain with the aim of controlling pain, but not, as with most other fractures, to restore the bone. In recent years, an invasive method to restore vertebral height in severely compressed vertebras has been developed – kyphoplasty. During this procedure a needle is inserted into the vertebral body using the transpedicular approach. A balloon catheter is inserted through the needle and placed centrally in the vertebra. It is slowly filled with fluid and, through this pressure, lifts the crushed bone. The fluid is then exchanged with bone cement. The alternative procedure, vertebroplasty, does not involve trying to lift the vertebra but only to inject bone cement.

Complications include the relatively benign transient increase in pain occurring in 4–23%, to extravertebral leakage of cement which seem to be more common with vertebroplasty (29%) compared to kyphoplasty (8.4%)[174]. Occurrence of new fracture at the adjacent vertebral levels have also been described in up to 16% according to a systematic review[175]. The indications for intervention are vertebral compression fractures with severe pain resistant to regular analgesic therapy and when there is continuing vertebral collapse[176]. Figure **4.93** shows the X-ray of a 76-year-old woman with multiple vertebral fractures, treated at two levels with kyphoplasty.

Lower extremity fractures
Hip fracture – cervical

Cervical or intracapsular hip fractures are challenging to treat, despite there being normally only a single fracture line. The challenges are instead associated with the degree of displacement and the possible interruption of blood supply to the femoral head. The most benign type of undisplaced cervical fracture may even be difficult to identify on a plain X-ray immediately after the trauma, and is only obvious when the metabolic reaction related to the fracture has begun. Previously, these patients often had to stay in hospital at least 1 week in order for a fracture to be identifiable on a bone scan, but with modern magnetic resonance imaging (MRI) fracture oedema is visible within the first day.

Undisplaced fractures are preferably treated with pins. For biomechanical reasons it is necessary to use at least two pins to lock rotation. Subsequently, the pins are placed so that maximum support is obtained either from the posterior or lateral cortex (**4.94**). When dislocated cervical hip

4.93 Vertebral fracture treated at two levels with kyphoplasty.

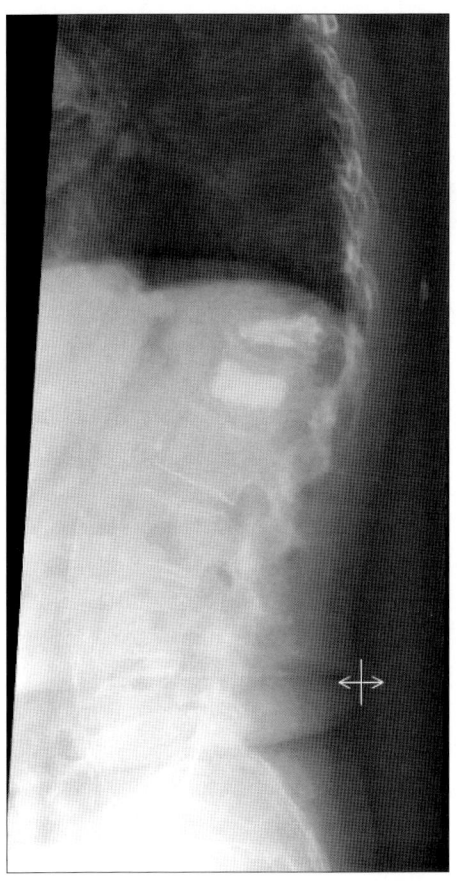

fractures are treated with pins, the failure rate and the subsequent need for secondary surgery reaches 21–57%[177]. The causes of failure are pseudoarthrosis, redislocation, and avascular necrosis within the femoral head. Poor results in this elderly and frail population lead to a devastating functional outcome and for the patient long-term pain, providing a rationale for a change in the treatment paradigm to arthroplasty, preferably unipolar.

The poor outcome in those with dislocated cervical hip fracture has long been known; however, using total hip replacement is not an obvious choice in this population. The arguments against total joint replacement have included: increased risk of luxation of the head from inability to follow postoperative instructions; increased risk of infections from patients touching the wounds or have urinary tract infections; and secondary fractures adjacent to the implant that subsequently are more difficult to treat than common fractures. An increasingly favoured treatment option is to use hemiarthroplasty in the elderly; the acetabulum is not replaced in this procedure and the femoral head implant is larger compared to that used in total hip arthroplasty (**4.95**). The advantages include shorter operating time, which is beneficial in an elderly population with comorbidity, and

4.94 Cervical hip fracture treated with pins.

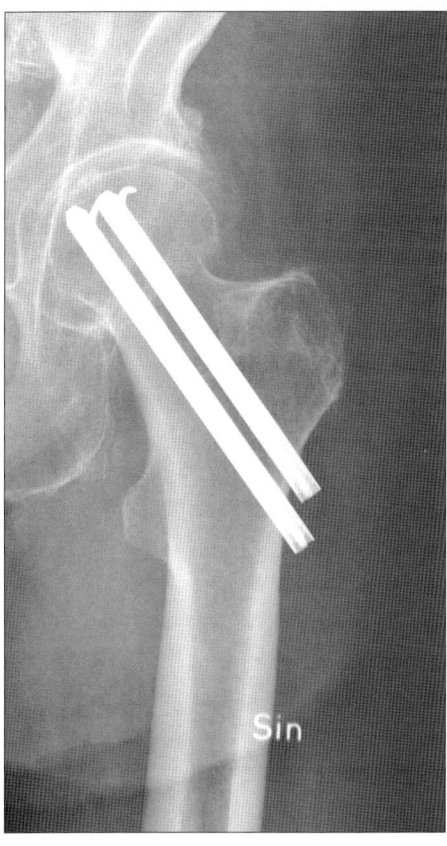

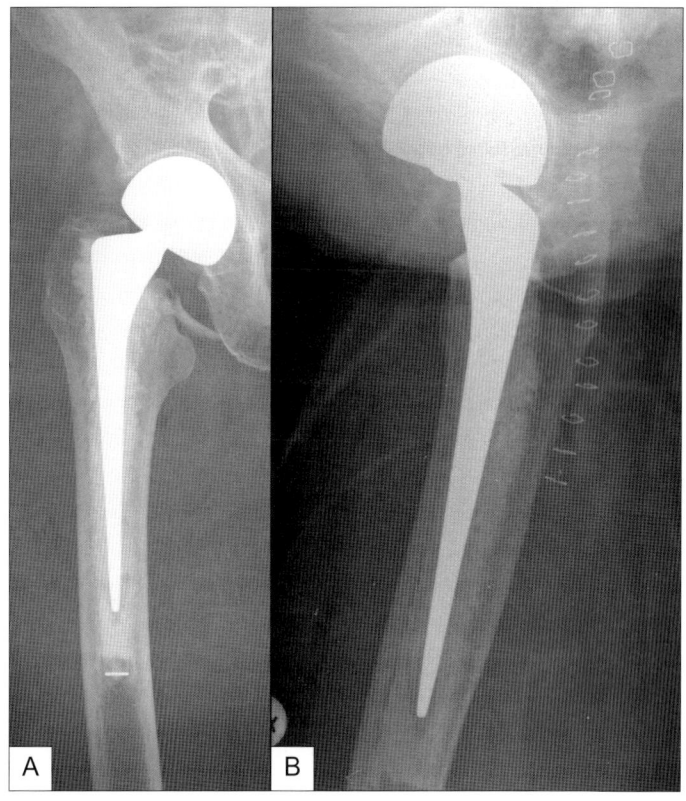

4.95 A, B Cervical hip fracture – unipolar arthroplasty.

decreased risk of luxation from the larger femoral head.

In a RCT, also including patients with dementia, hemiarthroplasty improved walking ability and decreased the need for secondary joint replacement in patients with cervical hip fracture[178]. Similar studies have shown improved quality of life in those primarily treated with joint replacement[179]. Guidelines should therefore, suggest hemiarthroplasty in the elderly, for example those over age 80, and total hip replacement in younger persons with dislocated cervical fractures.

Dislocated fracture of the femoral neck occurring in younger patients with hip fractures is also associated with similar risk of failure when treated with internal fixation such as pins or screws. Despite being associated with osteoporosis, hip fracture in middle-aged patients is commonly associated with better BMD and bone quality than in those of advanced age. In addition, comorbidity and dementia are less common, factors that predispose to complications if total hip replacement is used. Thus, total hip replacement is to be considered in those aged between 60–80 years and the recommended treatment for those in good health or as a secondary procedure if pin osteosyntheses fails in this age group rather than a hemiarthroplasty (see above) (**4.96**). In this group, outcome is clearly improved as is shown in a RCT where those

treated with hip replacement had a complication rate of 4% over 4 years and those with internal fixation 42%[180].

Hip fracture – trochanteric

Trochanteric fractures run from the proximal and lateral part of the major trochanter and obliquely towards the minor trochanter. The fracture primarily runs through cancellous bone, consequently healing is much better compared to that of cervical fractures. Based the structure of the proximal femur and the cancellous bone content, trochanteric fractures are well suited for treatment with a plate and screws (**4.97**). A central screw is placed in the femoral head and the plate is slid over, when it is fixated with transcortical screws. The sliding screw allows for compression when load is put on the leg, thus pushing the fracture surfaces closer together and further improving bone healing. Hence, weight bearing is allowed immediately.

Hip fracture – subtrochanteric

The subtrochanteric fracture is considered a more complex fracture. It is a fracture of the proximal femur and is described as either transverse, oblique, or spiral, sometimes comminute, and often signifying severe osteoporosis. Depending on the nature of the fracture, several treatment options are available. In general terms, if the fracture is best

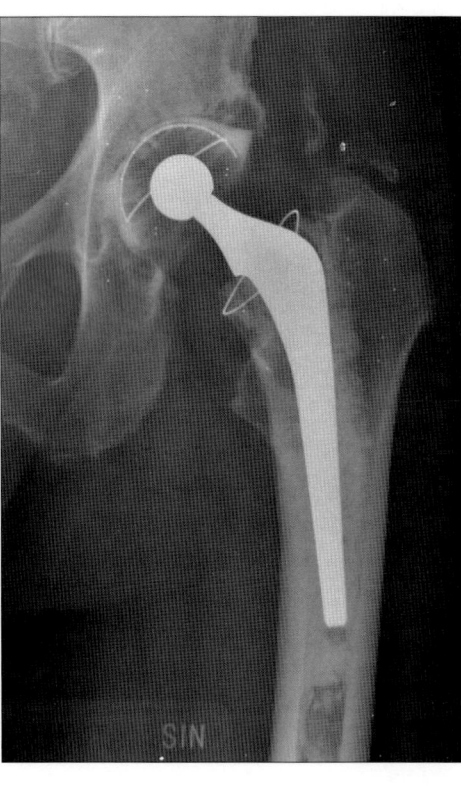

4.96 Cervical hip fracture – bipolar arthroplasty.

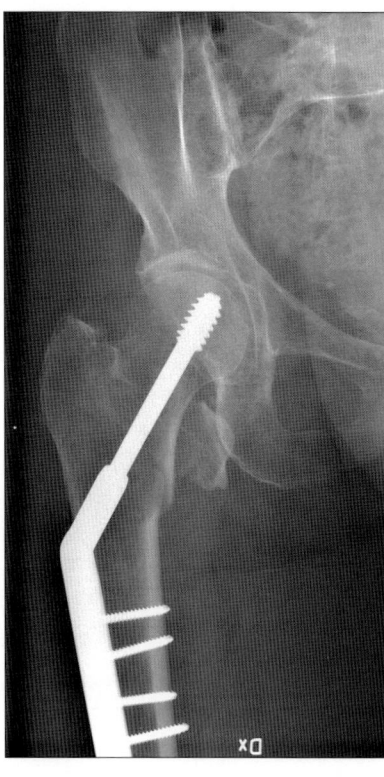

4.97 Trochanteric fracture – dynamic hip screw and plate (see also **1.46** for acute state).

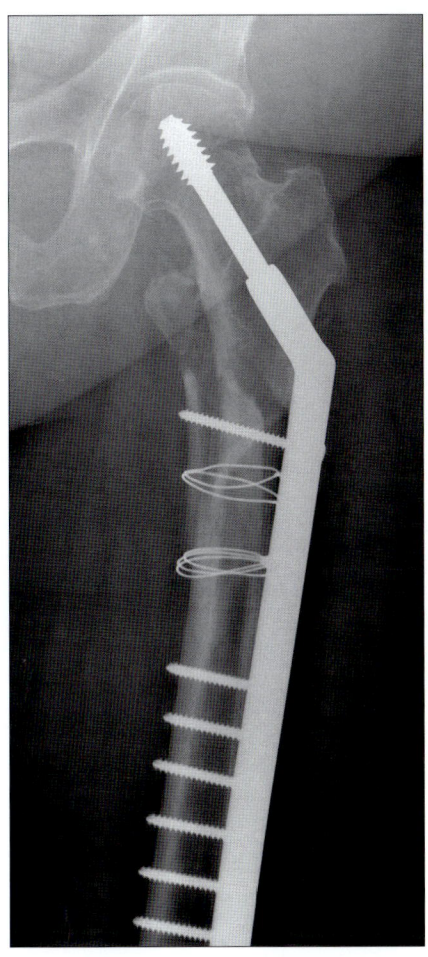

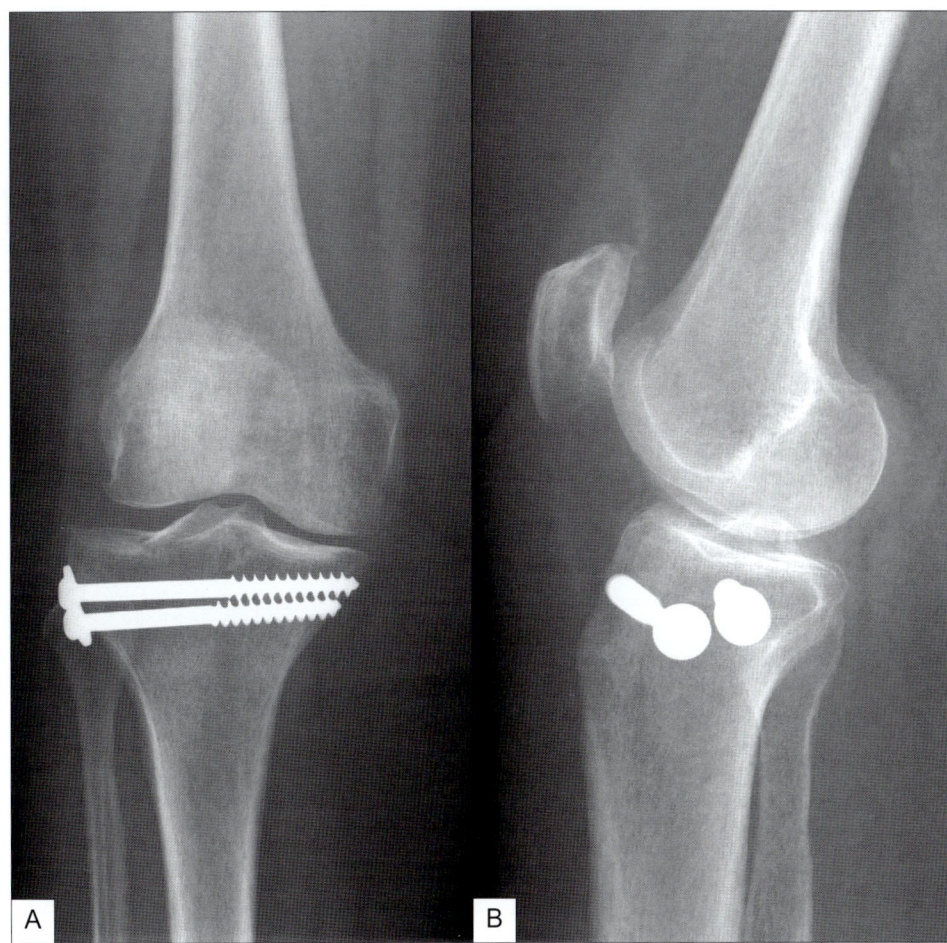

4.98 Subtrochanteric fracture – intramedullary nail (see also **1.47** for acute state).

4.99 A, B Lateral condyle of tibia – two screws inserted to restore the joint surface (see also **1.49** for acute state).

described as consisting of one or two transverse or oblique fragments, it may be suitable for intramedullary nailing (**4.98**), whereas if it consists of multiple fragments, is highly oblique or spiral, a long plate with anchorage in the femoral head may be the preferred choice. With this type of fracture weight bearing is not allowed until at least 12 weeks and after radiographic follow-up, a postfracture routine that is very demanding on the elderly, most of whom cannot quickly master crutches and so need a wheelchair. This lack of mobility leads to further increased bone loss, decreased muscle strength, and thus a high risk of additional fractures.

Proximal tibia fracture

The proximal tibia is rich in trabecular bone and in many respects is similar in structure to the distal radius. Fractures of the lateral condyle occur from relatively mild valgus trauma to the knee. Most fractures require surgical treatment since the articular surface is suppressed and the

fracture needs support in order not to dislocate further. The method of choice is to fasten the lateral fragment with screws in the least severe cases, and with a plate and screws in severe cases (**4.99**). The intra-articular surface is reconstructed by using bone grafts from the iliac crest. Postfracture treatment involves training of the thigh muscles and knee motion without weight bearing for up to 3 months. With this type of fracture, training in a swimming pool is often beneficial, provided the patient does not slip!

Rehabilitation after fracture

The impact of fracture will depend on the fracture site, characteristics and age of the patient, and if comorbidity exists or not. The actual treatment of a fracture in terms of hospital care and surgery is often very short in relation to the time required to regain function; however, adequate fracture

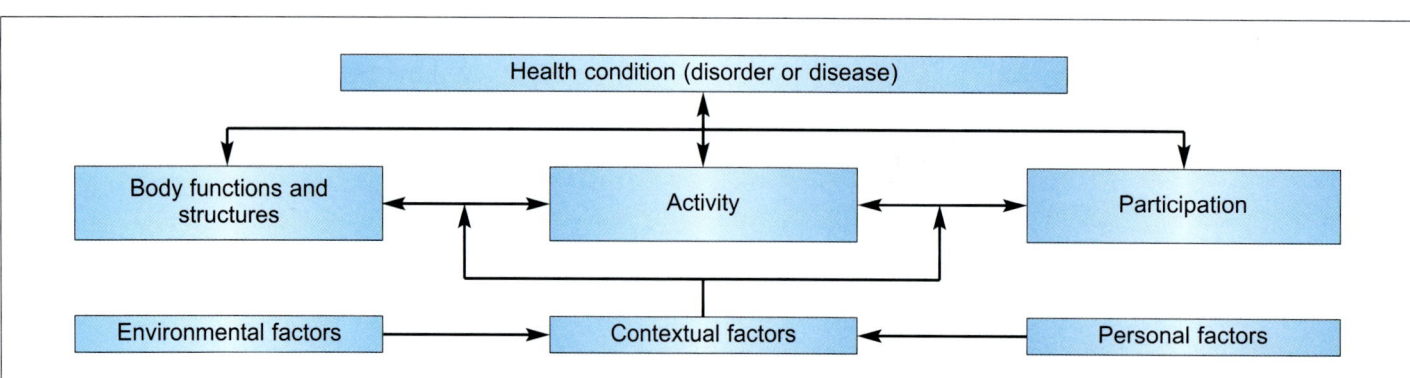

4.100 WHO International Classification of Functioning.

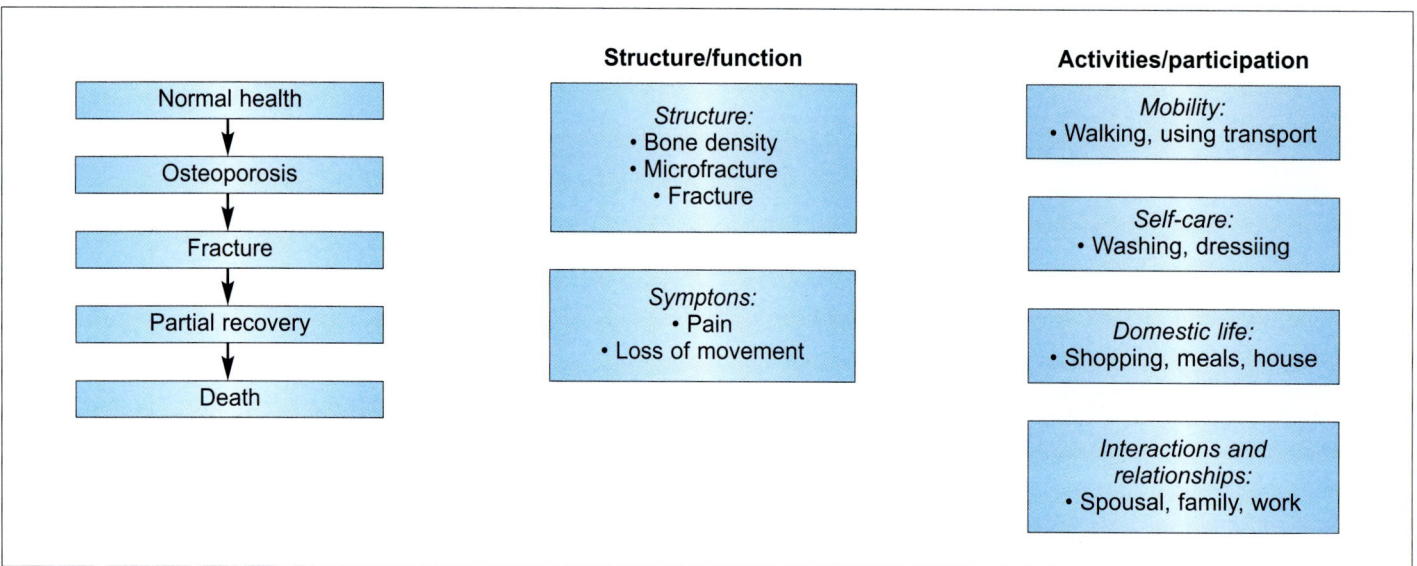

4.101 The impact of osteoporosis and fracture in terms of the WHO International Classification of Functioning.

treatment is a prerequisite for successful rehabilitation.

The nature of the impact of osteoporosis and fracture on the individual can be evaluated within the WHO International Classification of Functioning (ICF) (**4.100**). The concept behind developing the ICF has been the awareness that bodily or structural impairment is only one factor in the perception of what is 'unhealthy' by a person. For example, one person may suffer from what without doubt can be regarded as a minor disorder and still be severely disabled in terms of activity and participation, whereas someone with a severe injury will overcome the restrictions and perceive only marginal limitations to participation in society.

Structural parameters in osteoporosis are reduced bone mass, deterioration in microarchitecture, and loss of strength with subsequent fracture. The structural loss of function is, in the case of osteoporosis and fracture, related to impaired mobility and impaired psychological function due to pain. Loss of function will limit the activities of the individual, such as walking, and restrict their participation in society, such as going to work. The impact on an individual will be influenced by the context in which they live – the complete background of the person's life and living situation, such as their physical, social, and attitudinal environment, and also personal factors, such as sex, age, ethnicity, lifestyle, and social background. The ICF classification can be applied to activity and participation of a person with osteoporosis (**4.101**). Rehabilitation after fracture needs to take all of these factors into account in these commonly elderly patients.

In those with fragility fractures that need in-hospital care, an increasingly successful concept revolves around

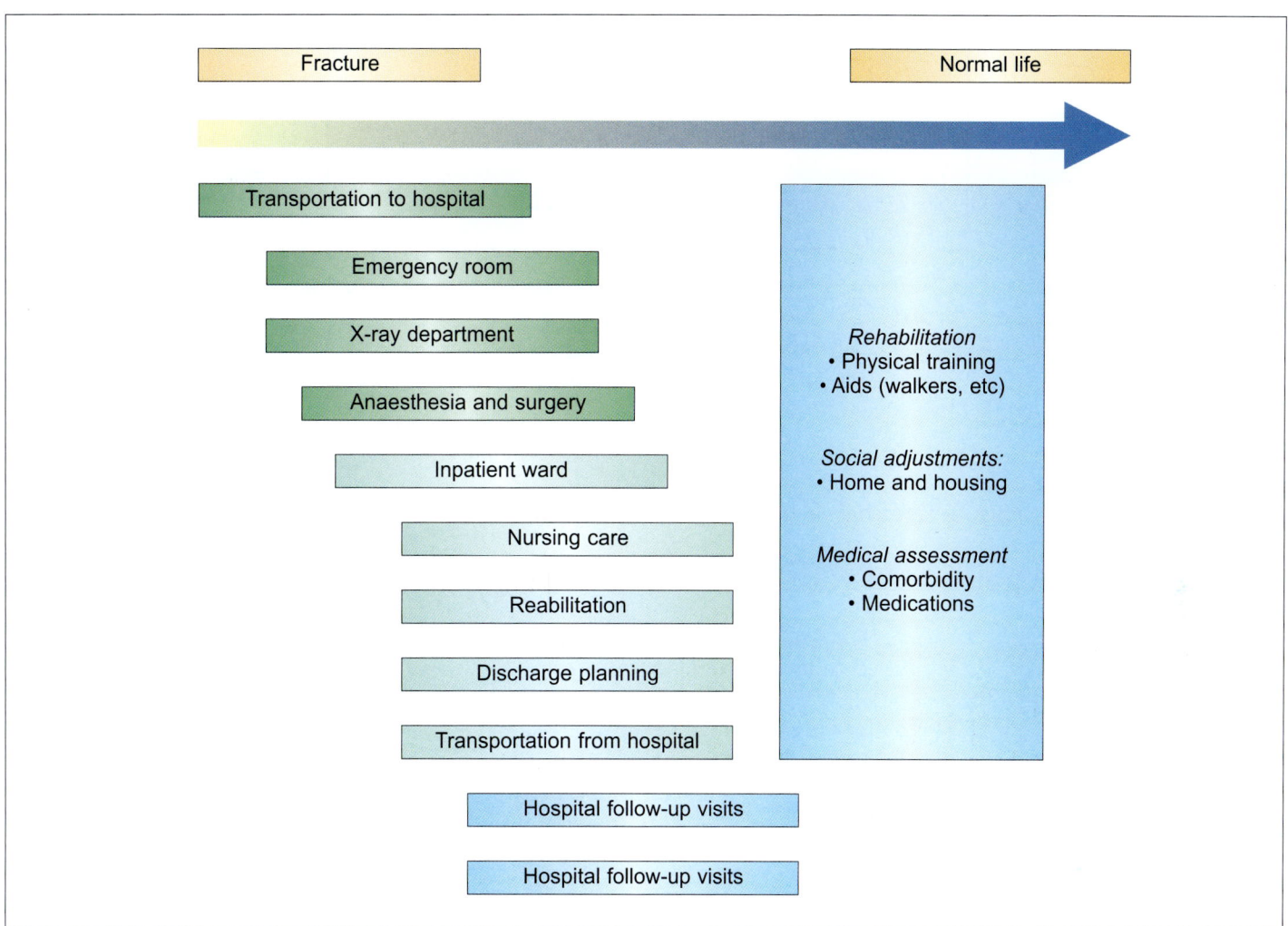

4.102 Fracture treatment path.

multidisciplinary teamwork, each professional contributing with their particular skills and expertise. The health care professionals that are most involved in the care of patients in the hospital are instrumental in initiating rehabilitation after a fracture. Comprehensive management guidelines for hip fracture have been developed in a number of countries, but are virtually nonexisting for other types of fracture. The Scottish Sign guidelines are an example of such guidelines for prevention and management of hip fracture[181].

Most patients suffering a fracture require hospital evaluation, and for patients with severe fractures in-hospital care, with or without surgery, is required. In-hospital care involves a number of steps and collaboration between different departments and professionals before the patient is ready for discharge. Figure **4.102** illustrates the different units and, indirectly, some of the professionals involved in the immediate care process of a person with a fracture.

Many more are involved but rarely mentioned, such as laboratory personnel or the blood bank. Importantly, this process needs to run smoothly and timely so that surgery is not unnecessarily delayed as the latter is associated with poor outcome in the elderly[182, 183].

Establishing 'fracture chains', or having a systematic approach to the treatment and rehabilitation of patients with osteoporotic fractures, will improve the outcome and be cost-effective. The chain needs to be activated at the first point of interaction with the health care system, commonly the ambulance or emergency room personnel, in order to optimize the final outcome and be continued beyond the hospital management of a fracture.

The rehabilitation of a patient begins when the patient enters the hospital doors. All measures taken during the treatment of the patient are steps in the rehabilitative process of restoring function. In-hospital professionals have

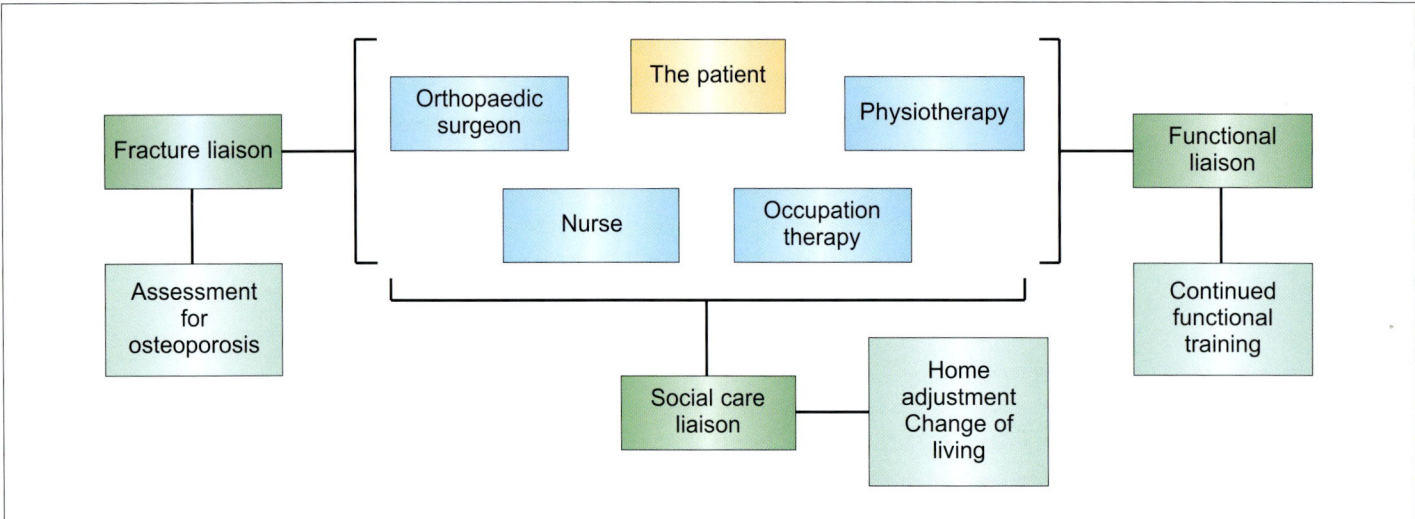

4.103 Team approach – fracture care chain in hospital.

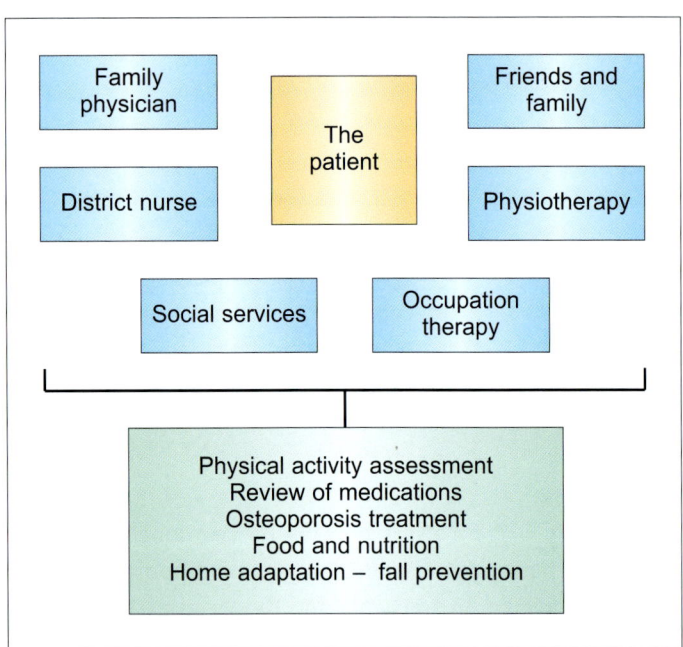

4.104 Team approach – fracture care chain after discharge.

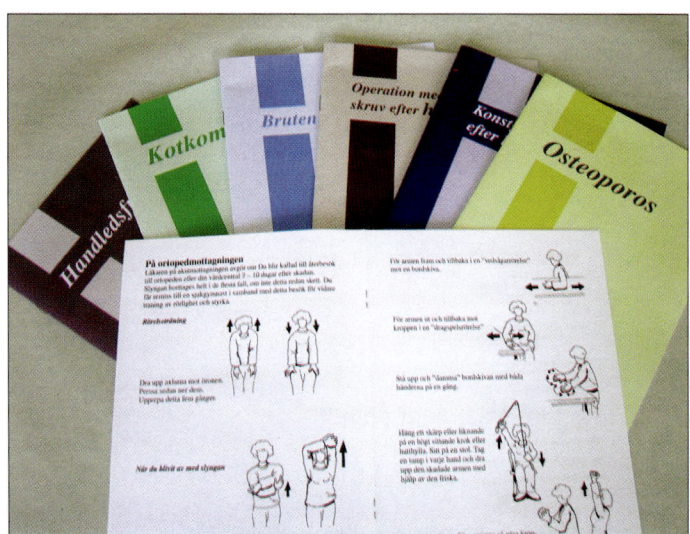

4.105 Examples of brochures giving fracture advice for patients.

counterparts in the out-patient care and in the social service systems, and it is helpful to regard the care process as a chain of initiatives, where each link needs to be established before the patient is admitted (**4.103**). If communication systems are in place, the duration of the hospital stay will be shortened and the patient will be able to return home earlier. One way to improve care chains is to have specifically assigned liaison persons: one for the assessment of osteoporosis, one for functional rehabilitation, and one for living circumstances.

In primary care, a similar structure needs to be established, so that functional gains during in-hospital care are maintained and continue to improve (**4.104**). In addition, most patients need continuous encouragement and reassurance that their training is not harmful, since such anxiety is common. Additional areas (such as medical management of comorbidities and reassessment of pharmacotherapy, initiation of osteoporosis treatment if indicated, the nutrition of the patient, and fall prevention measures especially in the home) need to be addressed by the 'out-patient primary care team' in order to avoid new trauma.

It is important to meet the expectations of the patient, but also to inform the patient correctly of a realistic outcome with each type of fracture. The patient plays the main role in the rehabilitative process – apart from adequate fracture treatment the care givers serve as facilitators and supporters in the process.

Pain is a limiting function in the initial period after sustaining a fracture. Nevertheless, mobility training should in all cases, with the exception of unstable fractures, begin the day after fracture treatment. The extent of training will be determined by the type of fracture. The patient needs to be informed both verbally and in written form. Simple brochures supplying information on each of the major types of osteoporotic fractures, their treatment, and the expected outcome, should provide easy instructions on how to continue training at home (**4.105**). The relevant brochure is given to the patient or their relatives at the time of treatment regardless if a fracture can be fully managed in an out-patient setting or if it needs hospital care.

Few fractures can be managed orthopaedically so that full recovery of prefracture status is regained. The aim of management is to achieve the best possible outcome considering the severity of the fracture and patient-related factors, such as the patient's age, comorbidity, and cognitive function. Hip fractures are often associated with significantly impaired functioning, as is shown in Figure **4.106**[184]. It describes the probability (percent with 95% CI) of events after sustaining hip fracture, given that the patient was not characterized by the event before fracture. Over 55% needed a walking aid or were unable to walk; however, it is a vastly better outcome to be able to walk with a walker compared to needing full-time care. Thus, for some patients, mobility with a walking aid should be the realistic goal of rehabilitation.

Proximal humerus fractures are often associated with a remaining limitation in range of motion. In a study of 376 patients followed over 1 year, 88% achieved an excellent or good outcome *Table 4.13*[185]. Age was the main factor determining outcome, nevertheless, subjectively, the older patients tended to accept functional limitations better and still regard the result as good[186]. This points to the importance of informing the patient of the expected outcome and to define the aim of rehabilitation in terms of what is possible in view of the fracture.

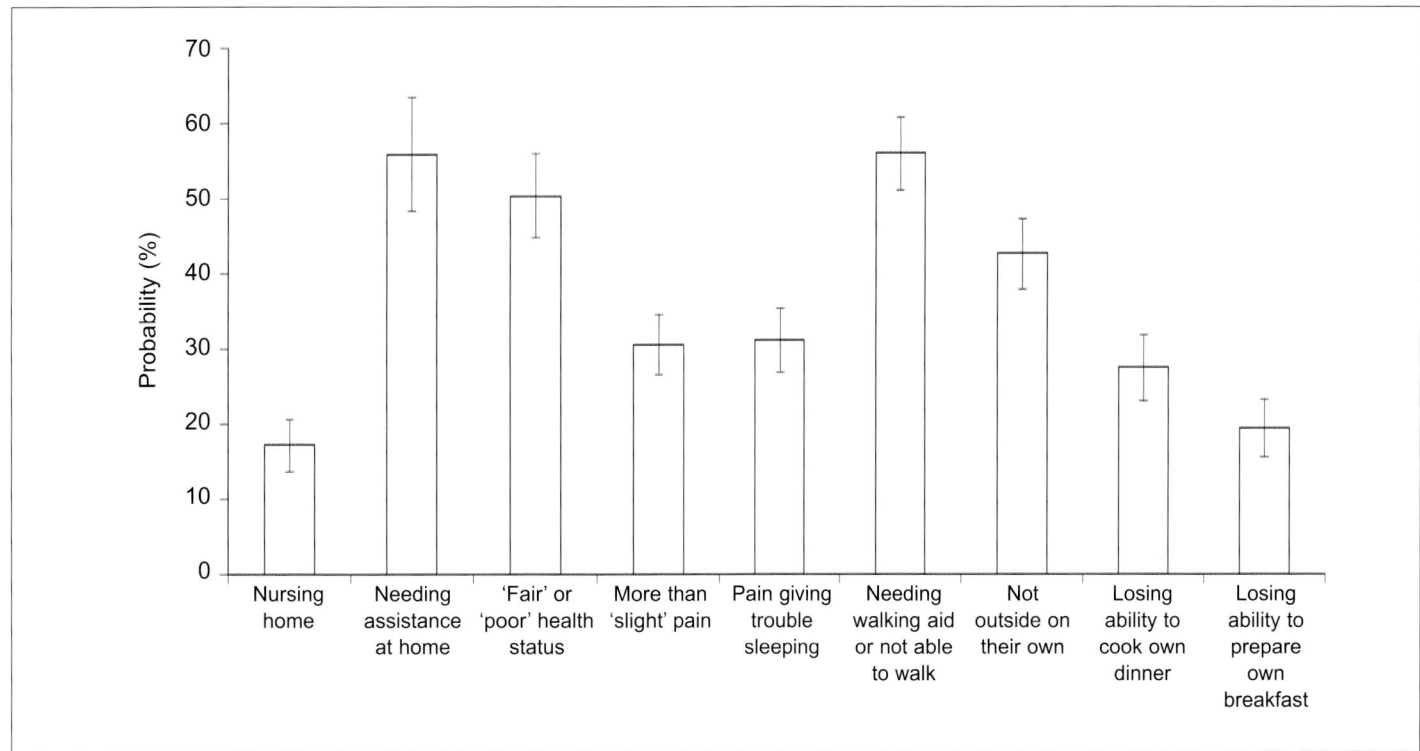

4.106 Probability of events after hip fracture. (Adapted from Osnes EK, *et al.* (2004). Consequences of hip fracture on activities of daily life and residential needs. *Osteoporos Int*, **15**(7):567–574.)

Table 4.13 Relationship of age to functional outcome (expressed in weeks)

Age (years)	<20	20–29	30–39	40–49	50–59	60–69	70–79	80–99	P value
Shopping	4.9	5.9	6.7	6.1	7.5	7.9	7.2	9.1	<0.05
Dressing	1.7	3.7	3.2	2.7	3.3	4.3	4.4	5.7	<0.001
Hygiene	1.7	4.1	3.1	2.9	3.9	4.9	5.2	6.0	<0.001
Housework	2.9	7.1	6.3	5.0	7.9	9.4	7.4	21.0	<0.01
Driving	0	6.9	7.4	8.8	20.0	35.0	17	11.0	<0.001
Employment	3.4	4.0	4.8	8.6	6.8	10.3	–	–	<0.001

(Adapted from Court-Brown CM, *et al.* (2001). The epidemiology of proximal humeral fractures. *Acta Orthop Scand,* **72**(4):365–371.)

References

1 Feskanich D, Willett W, Colditz G (2002). Walking and leisure-time activity and risk of hip fracture in postmenopausal women. *JAMA,* **288**:2300–2306.

2 WHO physical activity fact sheet.

3 Kannus P (1999). Preventing osteoporosis, falls, and fractures among elderly people. Promotion of lifelong physical activity is essential. *BMJ,* **318**:1695–1696.

4 Wolff I, van Croonenborg JJ, Kemper HC, *et al.* (1999). The effect of exercise training programs on bone mass: a meta-analysis of published controlled trials in pre- and postmenopausal women. *Osteopor Int,* **9**:1–12.

5 Kelley GA, Kelley KS, Tran ZV (2001). Resistance training and bone mineral density in women: a meta-analysis of controlled trials. *Am J Phys Med Rehabil,* **80**(1):65–77.

6 Wallace RB (2000). Bone health in nursing home residents. *JAMA,* **284**(8):1018–1019.

7 Specker BL (1996). Evidence for an interaction between calcium intake and physical activity on changes in bone mineral density. *J Bone Mineral Res,* **11**:1539–1544.

8 Valdimarsson O, Alborg HG, Duppe H, *et al.* (2005). Reduced training is associated with increased loss of BMD. *J Bone Mineral Res,* **20**:906–912.

9 Gillespie LD, Gillespie WJ, Robertson MC, *et al.* (2003). Interventions for preventing falls in elderly people. *Cochrane Database Syst Rev,* CD000340.

10 Hillsdon M, Foster C, Thorogood M (2005). Interventions for promoting physical activity. *Cochrane Database Syst Rev,* CD003180.

11 Reid IR (2002). Relationships among body mass, its components, and bone. *Bone,* **31**:547–555.

12 Langlois JA, Mussolino ME, Visser M, *et al.* (2001). Weight loss from maximum body weight among middle-aged and older white women and the risk of hip fracture: the NHANES I epidemiologic follow-up study. *Osteoporos Int,* **12**:763–768.

13 Ensrud KE, Ewing SK, Stone KL, *et al.* (2003). Intentional and unintentional weight loss increase bone loss and hip fracture risk in older women. *J Am Ger Soc,* **51**:1740–1747.

14 WHO (2003). Prevention and management of osteoporosis. *WHO Technical Report Series No. 921.* World Health Organization, Geneva.

15 Bonjour JP, Schurch MA, Rizzoli R (1996). Nutritional aspects of hip fractures. *Bone,* **18**:139S–144S.

16 European Action 2004

17 Wengreen HJ, Munger RG, West NA, *et al.* (2004). Dietary protein intake and risk of osteoporotic hip fracture in elderly residents of Utah. *J Bone Mineral Res,* **19**:537–545.

18 Law MR, Hackshaw AK (1997). A meta-analysis of cigarette smoking, bone mineral density and risk of hip fracture: recognition of a major effect. *BMJ,* **315**:841–846.

19 Vestergaard P, Mosekilde L (2003). Fracture risk associated with smoking: a meta-analysis. *J Int Med,* **254**:572–583.

20 Kanis JA, Johnell O, Oden A, *et al.* (2005). Smoking and fracture risk: a meta-analysis. *Osteopor Int* **16**:155–162.

21 Olofsson H, Byberg L, Mohsen R, *et al.* (2005). Smoking and the risk of fracture in older men. *J Bone Mineral Res,* **20**:1208–1215.

22 Lau EM, Leung PC, Kwok T, *et al.* (2006). The determinants of bone mineral density in Chinese men: results from Mr. Os (Hong Kong), the first cohort study on osteoporosis in Asian men. *Osteoporosis Int,* **17**:297–303.

23 Ward KD, Klesges RC (2001). A meta-analysis of the effects of cigarette smoking on bone mineral density. *Calcif Tissue Int,* **68**:259–270.

24 Cornuz J, Feskanich D, Willett WC, *et al.* (1999). Smoking, smoking cessation, and risk of hip fracture in women. *Am J Med,* **106**:311–314.

25 Kanis JA, Johansson H, Johnell O, *et al.* (2005). Alcohol intake as a risk factor for fracture. *Osteopor Int,* **16**:737–742.

26 Hoidrup S, Gronbaek M, Gottschau A, *et al.* (1999). Alcohol intake, beverage preference, and risk of hip fracture in men and women. Copenhagen Centre for Prospective Population Studies. *Am J Epidemiol,* **149**:993–1001.

27 Felson DT, Kiel DP, Anderson JJ, *et al.* (1988). Alcohol consumption and hip fractures: the Framingham Study. *Am J Epidemiol*, **128**:1102–1110.

28 Espallargues M, Sampietro-Colom L, Estrada MD, *et al.* (2001). Identifying bone-mass-related risk factors for fracture to guide bone densitometry measurements: a systematic review of the literature. *Osteoporos Int*, **12**:811–822.

29 Lau EM, Suriwongpaisal P, Lee JK, *et al.* (2001). Risk factors for hip fracture in Asian men and women: the Asian osteoporosis study. *J Bone Mineral Res*, **16**:572–580.

30 Shea B, Wells G, Cranney A, *et al.* (2002). Meta-analyses of therapies for postmenopausal osteoporosis. VII. Meta-analysis of calcium supplementation for the prevention of postmenopausal osteoporosis. *Endocrinol Rev*, **23**:552–559.

31 Dawson-Hughes B, Dallal GE, Krall EA, *et al.* (1990). A controlled trial of the effect of calcium supplementation on bone density in postmenopausal women. *N Engl J Med*, **323**:878–883.

32 Lips P, Graafmans WC, Ooms ME, *et al.* (1996). Vitamin D supplementation and fracture incidence in elderly persons. A randomized, placebo-controlled clinical trial. *Ann Int Med*, **124**:400–406.

33 Meyer HE, Smedshaug GB, Kvaavik E, *et al.* (2002). Can vitamin D supplementation reduce the risk of fracture in the elderly? A randomized controlled trial. *J Bone Mineral Res*, **17**:709–715.

34 Avenell A, Gillespie WJ, Gillespie LD, *et al.* (2005). Vitamin D and vitamin D analogues for preventing fractures associated with involutional and post-menopausal osteoporosis. *Cochrane Database Syst Rev*, CD000227.

35 Trivedi DP, Doll R, Khaw KT (2003).Effect of four monthly oral vitamin D3 (cholecalciferol) supplementation on fractures and mortality in men and women living in the community: randomized double blind controlled trial. *BMJ*, **326**:469.

36 Ooms ME, Roos JC, Bezemer PD, *et al.* (1995). Prevention of bone loss by vitamin D supplementation in elderly women: a randomized double-blind trial. *J Clin Endocrinol Metab*, **80**:1052–1058.

37 Dawson-Hughes B, Harris SS, Krall EA, *et al.* (1995). Rates of bone loss in postmenopausal women randomly assigned to one of two dosages of vitamin D. *Am J Clin Nutr*, **61**:1140–1145.

38 Bischoff-Ferrari HA, Dawson-Hughes B, Willett WC, *et al.* (2004). Effect of Vitamin D on falls: a meta-analysis. *JAMA*, **291**:1999–2006.

39 Bischoff HA, Stahelin HB, Dick W, *et al.* (2003). Effects of vitamin D and calcium supplementation on falls: a randomized controlled trial. *J Bone Mineral Res*, **18**:343–351.

40 Chapuy MC, Arlot ME, Duboeuf F, *et al.* (1992). Vitamin D3 and calcium to prevent hip fractures in the elderly women. *N Engl J Med*, **327**:1637–1642.

41 Chapuy MC, Arlot ME, Delmas PD, Meunier PJ (1994). Effect of calcium and cholecalciferol treatment for three years on hip fractures in elderly women. *BMJ*, **308**:1081–1082.

42 Grant AM, Avenell A, Campbell MK, *et al.* (2005). Oral vitamin D3 and calcium for secondary prevention of low-trauma fractures in elderly people (Randomized Evaluation of Calcium Or vitamin D, RECORD): a randomized placebo-controlled trial. *Lancet*, **365**(9471):1621–1628.

43 Porthouse J, Cockayne S, King C, *et al.* (2005). Randomised controlled trial of calcium and supplementation with cholecalciferol (vitamin D3) for prevention of fractures in primary care. *BMJ*, **330**:1003.

44 Jackson RD, LaCroix AZ, Gass M, *et al.* (2006). Calcium plus vitamin D supplementation and the risk of fractures. *NEJM*, **354**:669–683.

45 Devine A, Dhaliwal SS, Dick IM, *et al.*(2004). Physical activity and calcium consumption are important determinants of lower limb bone mass in older women. *J Bone Mineral Res*, **19**:1634–1639.

46 Eccles M, Freemantle N, Mason J (1998). North of England evidence based guidelines development project: methods of developing guidelines for efficient drug use in primary care. *BMJ*, **316**(7139):1232–1235.

47 Fleisch H (2000). *Bisphosphonates in Bone Disease. From Laboratory to Patient*. 4th edn. Academic Press, San Diego.

48 Devogelaer JP, Broll H, Correa-Rotter R, *et al.* (1996). Oral alendronate induces progressive increases in bone mass of the spine, hip, and total body over 3 years in postmenopausal women with osteoporosis. *Bone*, **18**(2):141–150.

49 Liberman UA, Weiss SR, Broll J, *et al.* (1995). Effect of oral alendronate on bone mineral density and the incidence of fractures in postmenopausal osteoporosis. The Alendronate Phase III Osteoporosis Treatment Study Group. *N Engl J Med*, **333**(22):1437–1443.

50 Black DM, Cummings SR, Karpf DB, *et al.* (1996). Randomised trial of effect of alendronate on risk of fracture in women with existing vertebral fractures. Fracture Intervention Trial Research Group. *Lancet*, **348**(9041):1535–1541.

51 Cranney A, Wells G, Willan A, *et al.* (2002). Meta-analyses of therapies for postmenopausal osteoporosis. II. Meta-analysis of alendronate for the treatment of postmenopausal women. *Endocr Rev*, **23**(4):508–516.

52 Tonino RP, Meunier PJ, Emkey R, *et al.* (2000). Skeletal benefits of alendronate: 7-year treatment of postmenopausal osteoporotic women. Phase III Osteoporosis Treatment Study Group. *J Clin Endocrinol Metab*, **85**(9):3109–3115.

53 Bone HG, Hosking D, Devogelaer JP, *et al.* (2004). Ten years' experience with alendronate for osteoporosis in postmenopausal women. *N Engl J Med*, **350**(12):1189–1199.

54 Schnitzer T, Bone HG, Crepaldi G, *et al.* (2000). Therapeutic equivalence of alendronate 70 mg once-weekly and alendronate 10 mg daily in the treatment of osteoporosis. Alendronate Once-Weekly Study Group. *Aging (Milano)*, **12**(1):1–12.

55 Rizzoli R, Greenspan SL, Bone G, III, *et al.* (2002). Two-year results of once-weekly administration of alendronate 70 mg for the treatment of postmenopausal osteoporosis. *J Bone Miner Res* **17**(11):1988–1996.

56 A Luckman SP, Coxon FP, Ebetino FH, *et al.* (1998). Heterocycle-containing bisphosphonates cause apoptosis and inhibit bone resorption by preventing protein prenylation: evidence from structure-activity relationships in J774 macrophages. *J Bone Miner Res*, **13**(11):1668–1678.

57 Harris ST, Watts NB, Genant HK, *et al.* (1999). Effects of risedronate treatment on vertebral and nonvertebral fractures in women with postmenopausal osteoporosis: a randomized controlled trial. Vertebral Efficacy With Risedronate Therapy (VERT) Study Group. *JAMA*, **282**(14):1344–1352.

58 Reginster JY, Minne HW, Sorensen OH, *et al.* (2000). Randomised trial of the effects of risedronate on vertical fractures in women with established postmenopausal osteoporosis. *Osteoporos Int*, **11**:83–91.

59 McClung MR, Geusens P, Miller PD, *et al.* (2001). Effect of risedronate on the risk of hip fracture in elderly women. Hip Intervention Program Study Group. *N Engl J Med*, **344**(5):333–340.

60 Eriksen EF, Melsen F, Sod E, *et al.* (2002). Effects of long-term risedronate on bone quality and bone turnover in women with postmenopausal osteoporosis. *Bone*, **31**(5):620–625.

61 Watts NB, Cooper C, Lindsay R, *et al.* (2004). Relationship between changes in bone mineral density and vertebral fracture risk associated with risedronate: greater increases in bone mineral density do not relate to greater decreases in fracture risk. *J Clin Densitom*, 7(3):255–261.

62 Cranney A, Tugwell P, Adachi J, *et al.* (2002). Meta-analyses of therapies for postmenopausal osteoporosis. III. Meta-analysis of risedronate for the treatment of postmenopausal osteoporosis. *Endocr Rev*, **23**(4):517–523.

63 Mellstrom DD, Sorensen OH, Goemaere S, *et al.* (2004). Seven years of treatment with risedronate in women with postmenopausal osteoporosis. *Calcif Tissue Int*, **75**(6):462–468.

64 Brown JP, Kendler DL, McClung MR, *et al.* (2002). The efficacy and tolerability of risedronate once a week for the treatment of postmenopausal osteoporosis. *Calcif Tissue Int*, **71**(2):103–111.

65 Ringe JD, Faber H, Farahmand P, *et al.* (2006). Efficacy of risedronate in men with primary and secondary osteoporosis: results of a 1-year study. *Rheumatol Int*, **26**(5):427–431.

66 Lanza FL, Hunt RH, Thomson AB, *et al.* (2000). Endoscopic comparison of esophageal and gastroduodenal effects of risedronate and alendronate in postmenopausal women. *Gastroenterol*, **119**(3):631–638.

67 Aurich-Barrera B, Wilton L, Harris S, *et al.* (2006). Ophthalmological events in patients receiving risedronate: summary of information gained through follow-up in a prescription-event monitoring study in England. *Drug Saf*, **29**(2):151–160.

68 Muhlbauer RC, Bauss F, Schenk R, *et al.* (1991). BM 21.0955, a potent new bisphosphonate to inhibit bone resorption. *J Bone Miner Res*, **6**(9):1003–1011.

69 Akesson K Beusterien K, Hebborn A, *et al.* (2005). Patient preference for once-monthly over once-weekly bisphosphonate treatment. *Osteoporos Int*, **16**:S83.

70 Emkey R, Koltun W, Beusterien K, *et al.* (2005). Patient preference for once-monthly ibandronate versus once-weekly alendronate in a randomized, open-label, cross-over trial: the Boniva Alendronate Trial in Osteoporosis (BALTO). *Curr Med Res Opin*, **21**(12):1895–1903.

71 Smith SY, Recker RR, Hannan M, *et al.* (2003). Intermittent intravenous administration of the bisphosphonate ibandronate prevents bone loss and maintains bone strength and quality in ovariectomized cynomolgus monkeys. *Bone*, **32**(1):45–55.

72 Chesnut III CH, Skag A, Christiansen C, *et al.* (2004). Effects of oral ibandronate administered daily or intermittently on fracture risk in postmenopausal osteoporosis. *J Bone Miner Res*, **19**(8):1241–1249.

73 Delmas PD, Recker RR, Chesnut CH, III, *et al.* (2004). Daily and intermittent oral ibandronate normalize bone turnover and provide significant reduction in vertebral fracture risk: results from the BONE study. *Osteoporos Int*, **15**(10):792–798.

74 Stakkestad JA, Benevolenskaya LI, Stepan JJ, *et al.* (2003). Ibandronate injections given every three months: a new treatment option to prevent bone loss in postmenopausal women. *Ann Rheum Dis*, **62**(10):969–975.

75 Adami S, Felsenberg D, Christiansen C, *et al.* (2004). Efficacy and safety of ibandronate given by intravenous injection once every 3 months. *Bone*, **34**(5):881–889.

76 Miller PD, McClung MR, Macovei L, *et al.* (2005). Monthly oral ibandronate therapy in postmenopausal osteoporosis: 1-year results from the MOBILE study. *J Bone Miner Res*, **20**(8):1315–1322.

77 Cooper C, Emkey RD, McDonald RH, *et al.* (2003). Efficacy and safety of oral weekly ibandronate in the treatment of postmenopausal osteoporosis. *J Clin Endocrinol Metab*, **88**(10):4609–4615.

78 Ringe JD, Dorst A, Faber H, *et al.* (2003). Intermittent intravenous ibandronate injections reduce vertebral fracture risk in corticosteroid-induced osteoporosis: results from a long-term comparative study. *Osteoporos Int*, **14**(10):801–807.

79 Pavlakis N, Schmidt R, Stockler M (2005). Bisphosphonates for breast cancer. *Cochrane Database Syst Rev*, (3):CD003474.

80 Thompson K, Rogers MJ, Coxon FP, *et al.* (2006). Cytosolic entry of bisphosphonate drugs requires acidification of vesicles after fluid-phase endocytosis. *Mol Pharmacol*, **69**(5):1624–1632.

81 Reid IR, Miller P, Lyles K, *et al.* (2005). Comparison of a single infusion of zoledronic acid with risedronate for Paget's disease. *N Engl J Med*, **353**(9):898–908.

82 Reid IR, Brown JP, Burckhardt P, *et al.* (2002). Intravenous zoledronic acid in postmenopausal women with low bone mineral density. *N Engl J Med*, **346**(9):653–661.

83 Black DM, Delmas PD, Eastell R, *et al.* (2007). Once-yearly zoledronic acid for treatment of postmenopausal osteoporosis. *N Engl J Med*, **356**(18):1809–1822.

84 Lyles KW, Colón-Emeric CS, Magaziner JS, *et al.* (2007). Zoledronic acid and clinical fracture and mortality after hip fracture. *N Engl J Med*, **357**(18):1799–1809.

85 Torgerson DJ, Bell-Syer SE (2001). Hormone replacement therapy and prevention of nonvertebral fractures: a meta-analysis of randomized trials. *JAMA*, **285**(22):2891–2897.

86 Torgerson DJ, Bell-Syer SE (2001). Hormone replacement therapy and prevention of vertebral fractures: a meta-analysis of randomised trials. *BMC Musculoskelet Disord*, **2**(1):7.

87 Black LJ, Sato M, Rowley ER, *et al.* (1994). Raloxifene (LY139481 HCI) prevents bone loss and reduces serum cholesterol without causing uterine hypertrophy in ovariectomized rats. *J Clin Invest*, **93**(1):63–69.

88 Riggs BL, Hartmann LC (2003). Selective estrogen-receptor modulators – mechanisms of action and application to clinical practice. *N Engl J Med*, **348**(7):618–629.

89 Kumar V, Chambon P (1988). The estrogen receptor binds tightly to its responsive element as a ligand-induced homodimer. *Cell 55*(1): 145–156.

90 Gruber CJ, Tschugguel W, *et al.* (2002). Production and actions of estrogens. *N Engl J Med*, **346**(5): 340–52.

91 Riggs BL, Hartmann LC (2003). Selective estrogen-receptor modulators – mechanisms of action and application to clinical practice. *N Engl J Med* **348**(7): 618–629.

92 Draper MW, Flowers DE, Huster WJ, *et al.* (1996). A controlled trial of raloxifene (LY139481) HCl: impact on bone turnover and serum lipid profile in healthy postmenopausal women. *J Bone Miner Res*, **11**(6):835–842.

93 Delmas PD, Bjarnason NH, Mitlak BH, *et al.* (1997). Effects of raloxifene on bone mineral density, serum cholesterol concentrations, and uterine endometrium in postmenopausal women. *N Engl J Med*, **337**(23):1641–1647.

94 Delmas PD, Ensrud KE, Adachi JD, *et al.* (2002). Efficacy of raloxifene on vertebral fracture risk reduction in postmenopausal women with osteoporosis: four-year results from a randomized clinical trial. *J Clin Endocrinol Metab*, **87**(8):3609–3617.

95 Johnell O, Scheele WH, Lu Y, *et al.* (2002). Additive effects of raloxifene and alendronate on bone density and biochemical markers of bone remodeling in postmenopausal women with osteoporosis. *J Clin Endocrinol Metab*, **87**(3):985–992.

96 Michalska D, Stepan JJ, Basson BR, *et al.* (2006). The effect of raloxifene after discontinuation of long-term alendronate treatment of postmenopausal osteoporosis. *J Clin Endocrinol Metab*, **91**(3):870–877.

97 Ettinger B, Black DM, Mitlak BH, *et al.* (1999). Reduction of vertebral fracture risk in postmenopausal women with osteoporosis treated with raloxifene: results from a 3-year randomized clinical trial. Multiple Outcomes of Raloxifene Evaluation (MORE) Investigators. *JAMA*, **282**(7):637–645.

98 Cranney A, Tugwell P, Zytaruk N, *et al.* (2002). Meta-analyses of therapies for postmenopausal osteoporosis. IV. Meta-analysis of raloxifene for the prevention and treatment of postmenopausal osteoporosis. *Endocr Rev*, **23**(4):524–528.

99 Delmas PD, Genant HK, Crans GG, *et al.* (2003). Severity of prevalent vertebral fractures and the risk of subsequent vertebral and nonvertebral fractures: results from the MORE trial. *Bone*, **33**(4):522–532.

100 Kanis JA, Johnell O, Black DM, *et al.* (2003). Effect of raloxifene on the risk of new vertebral fracture in postmenopausal women with osteopenia or osteoporosis: a reanalysis of the Multiple Outcomes of Raloxifene Evaluation trial. *Bone*, **33**(3):293–300.

101 Cummings SR, Eckert S, Krueger KA, *et al.* (1999). The effect of raloxifene on risk of breast cancer in postmenopausal women: results from the MORE randomized trial. Multiple Outcomes of Raloxifene Evaluation. *JAMA*, **281**(23):2189–2197.

102 Cauley JA, Norton L, Lippman ME, *et al.* (2001). Continued breast cancer risk reduction in postmenopausal women treated with raloxifene: 4-year results from the MORE trial. Multiple outcomes of raloxifene evaluation. *Breast Cancer Res Treat*, **65**(2):125–134.

103 Vogel VG, Costantino JP, Wickerham DL, *et al.* (2006). Effects of tamoxifen vs raloxifene on the risk of developing invasive breast cancer and other disease outcomes: the NSABP Study of Tamoxifen and Raloxifene (STAR) P-2 trial. *JAMA*, **295**(23):2727–2741.

104 Land SR, Wickerham DL, Costantino JP, *et al.* (2006). Patient-reported symptoms and quality of life during treatment with tamoxifen or raloxifene for breast cancer prevention: the NSABP Study of Tamoxifen and Raloxifene (STAR) P-2 trial. *JAMA*, **295**(23):2742–2751.

105 Walsh BW, Kuller LH, Wild RA, *et al.* (1998). Effects of raloxifene on serum lipids and coagulation factors in healthy postmenopausal women. *JAMA*, **279**(18):1445–1451.

106 Barrett-Connor E, Grady D, Sashegyi A, *et al.* (2002). Raloxifene and cardiovascular events in osteoporotic postmenopausal women: four-year results from the MORE (Multiple Outcomes of Raloxifene Evaluation) randomized trial. *JAMA*, **287**(7):847–857.

107 Cranney A, Tugwell P, Zytaruk N, *et al.* (2002). Meta-analyses of therapies for postmenopausal osteoporosis. VI. Meta-analysis of calcitonin for the treatment of postmenopausal osteoporosis. *Endocr Rev*, **23**(4):540–551.

108 Reeve J, Meunier PJ, Parsons JA, *et al.* (1980). Anabolic effect of human parathyroid hormone fragment on trabecular bone in involutional osteoporosis: a multicentre trial. *Br Med J*, **280**(6228):1340–1344.

109 Marx SJ (2000). Hyperparathyroid and hypoparathyroid disorders. *N Engl J Med*, **343**(25):1863–1875.

110 Mosekilde L, Sogaard CH, McOsker JE, *et al.* (1994). PTH has a more pronounced effect on vertebral bone mass and biomechanical competence than antiresorptive agents (estrogen and bisphosphonate)—assessed in sexually mature, ovariectomized rats. *Bone*, **15**(4):401–408.

111 Mosekilde L, Danielsen CC, Sogaard CH, *et al.* (1995). The anabolic effects of parathyroid hormone on cortical bone mass, dimensions and strength–assessed in a sexually mature, ovariectomized rat model. *Bone*, **16**(2):223–230.

112 Zanchetta JR, Bogado CE, Ferretti JL, *et al.* (2003). Effects of teriparatide [recombinant human parathyroid hormone (1-34)] on cortical bone in postmenopausal women with osteoporosis. *J Bone Miner Res*, **18**(3):539–543.

113 Dempster DW, Cosman F, Kurland ES, *et al.* (2001). Effects of daily treatment with parathyroid hormone on bone microarchitecture and turnover in patients with osteoporosis: a paired biopsy study. *J Bone Miner Res*, **16**(10):1846–1853.

114 Hodsman AB, Fraher LJ, Ostbye T, *et al.* (1993). An evaluation of several biochemical markers for bone formation and resorption in a protocol utilizing cyclical parathyroid hormone and calcitonin therapy for osteoporosis. *J Clin Invest*, **91**(3):1138–1148.

115 Lindsay R, Nieves J, Henneman E, *et al.* (1993). Subcutaneous administration of the amino-terminal fragment of human parathyroid hormone-(1-34): kinetics and biochemical response in estrogenized osteoporotic patients. *J Clin Endocrinol Metab*, **77**(6):1535–1539.

116 Body JJ, Gaich GA, Scheele WH, *et al.* (2002). A randomized double-blind trial to compare the efficacy of teriparatide [recombinant human parathyroid hormone (1-34)] with alendronate in postmenopausal women with osteoporosis. *J Clin Endocrinol Metab*, **87**(10):4528–4535.

117 Hodsman AB, Hanley DA, Ettinger MP, *et al.* (2003). Efficacy and safety of human parathyroid hormone-(1-84) in increasing bone mineral density in postmenopausal osteoporosis. *J Clin Endocrinol Metab*, **88**(11):5212–5220.

118 Orwoll ES, Scheele WH, Paul S, *et al.* (2003). The effect of teriparatide [human parathyroid hormone (1-34)] therapy on bone density in men with osteoporosis. *J Bone Miner Res*, **18**(1):9–17.

119 Bauer DC, Garnero P, Bilezikian JP, *et al.* (2006). Short-term changes in bone turnover markers and bone mineral density response to parathyroid hormone in postmenopausal women with osteoporosis. *J Clin Endocrinol Metab*, **91**(4):1370–1375.

120 Cosman F, Morgan DC, Nieves JW, *et al.* (1997). Resistance to bone resorbing effects of PTH in black women. *J Bone Miner Res*, **12**(6):958–966.

121 Rittmaster RS, Bolognese M, Ettinger MP, *et al.* (2000). Enhancement of bone mass in osteoporotic women with parathyroid hormone followed by alendronate. *J Clin Endocrinol Metab*, **85**(6):2129–2134.

122 Neer RM, Arnaud CD, Zanchetta JR, *et al.* (2001). Effect of parathyroid hormone (1-34) on fractures and bone mineral density in postmenopausal women with osteoporosis. *N Engl J Med*, **344**(19):1434–1441.

123 Lindsay R, Nieves J, Formica C, *et al.* (1997). Randomised controlled study of effect of parathyroid hormone on vertebral-bone mass and fracture incidence among postmenopausal women on oestrogen with osteoporosis. *Lancet*, **350**(9077):550–555.

124 Finkelstein JS, Klibanski A, Schaefer EH, *et al.* (1994). Parathyroid hormone for the prevention of bone loss induced by estrogen deficiency. *N Engl J Med*, **331**(24):1618–1623.

125 Reeve J, Mitchell A, Tellez M, *et al.* (2001). Treatment with parathyroid peptides and estrogen replacement for severe postmenopausal vertebral osteoporosis: prediction of long-term responses in spine and femur. *J Bone Miner Metab*, **19**(2):102–114.

126 McClung MR, San Martin J, Miller PD, *et al.* (2005). Opposite bone remodeling effects of teriparatide and alendronate in increasing bone mass. *Arch Intern Med*, **165**(15):1762–1768.

127 Black DM, Greenspan SL, Ensrud KE, *et al.* (2003). The effects of parathyroid hormone and alendronate alone or in combination in postmenopausal osteoporosis. *N Engl J Med*, **349**(13):1207–1215.

128 Cosman F, Nieves J, Zion M, *et al.* (2005). Daily and cyclic parathyroid hormone in women receiving alendronate. *N Engl J Med*, **353**(6):566–575.

129 Hodsman AB, Fraher LJ, Watson PH, *et al.* (1997). A randomized controlled trial to compare the efficacy of cyclical parathyroid hormone versus cyclical parathyroid hormone and sequential calcitonin to improve bone mass in postmenopausal women with osteoporosis. *J Clin Endocrinol Metab*, **82**(2):620–628.

130 Black DM, Bilezikian JP, Ensrud KE, *et al.* (2005). One year of alendronate after one year of parathyroid hormone (1-84) for osteoporosis. *N Engl J Med*, **353**(6):555-565.

131 Vahle JL, Sato M, Long GG, *et al.* (2002). Skeletal changes in rats given daily subcutaneous injections of recombinant human parathyroid hormone (1-34) for 2 years and relevance to human safety. *Toxicol Pathol*, **30**(3):312–321.

132 Lane NE, Sanchez S, Modin GW, *et al.* (1998). Parathyroid hormone treatment can reverse corticosteroid-induced osteoporosis. Results of a randomized controlled clinical trial. *J Clin Invest*, **102**(8):1627–1633.

133 Finkelstein JS, Hayes A, Hunzelman JL, *et al.* (2003). The effects of parathyroid hormone, alendronate, or both in men with osteoporosis. *N Engl J Med*, **349**(13):1216–1226.

134 Finkelstein JS, Leder BZ, Burnett SA, *et al.* (2006). Effects of teriparatide, alendronate, or both on bone turnover in osteoporotic men. *J Clin Endocrinol Metab*.

135 Inzerillo AM, Zaidi M, Huang CL (2002). Calcitonin: the other thyroid hormone. *Thyroid*, **12**(9):791–798.

136 Deftos LJ, Powell D, Parthemore JG, *et al.* (1973). Secretion of calcitonin in hypocalcemic states in man. *J Clin Invest*, **52**(12):3109–3114.

137 Chesnut CH, III, Silverman S, Andriano K, *et al.* (2000). A randomized trial of nasal spray salmon calcitonin in postmenopausal women with established osteoporosis: the prevent recurrence of osteoporotic fractures study. PROOF Study Group. *Am J Med*, **109**(4):267–276.

138 Delmas PD, Seeman E (2004). Changes in bone mineral density explain little of the reduction in vertebral or nonvertebral fracture risk with anti-resorptive therapy. *Bone*, **34**(4):599–604.

139 Cranney A, Tugwell P, Zytaruk N, *et al.* (2002). Meta-analyses of therapies for postmenopausal osteoporosis. VI. Meta-analysis of calcitonin for the treatment of postmenopausal osteoporosis. *Endocr Rev*, **23**(4):540–551.

140 Kaskani E, Lyritis GP, Kosmidis C, *et al.* (2005). Effect of intermittent administration of 200 IU intranasal salmon calcitonin and low doses of 1alpha(OH) vitamin D3 on bone mineral density of the lumbar spine and hip region and biochemical bone markers in women with postmenopausal osteoporosis: a pilot study. *Clin Rheumatol*, **24**(3):232–238.

141 Downs RW, Jr., Bell NH, Ettinger MP, *et al.* (2000). Comparison of alendronate and intranasal calcitonin for treatment of osteoporosis in postmenopausal women. *J Clin Endocrinol Metab*, **85**(5):1783–1788.

142 Ljunghall S, Gardsell P, Johnell O, *et al.* (1991). Synthetic human calcitonin in postmenopausal osteoporosis: a placebo-controlled, double-blind study. *Calcif Tissue Int*, **49**(1):17–19.

143 Lyritis GP, Tsakalakos N, Magiasis B, *et al.* (1991). Analgesic effect of salmon calcitonin in osteoporotic vertebral fractures: a double-blind placebo-controlled clinical study. *Calcif Tissue Int*, **49**(6):369–372.

144 Lyritis GP, Paspati I, Karachalios T, *et al.* (1997). Pain relief from nasal salmon calcitonin in osteoporotic vertebral crush fractures. A double blind, placebo-controlled clinical study. *Acta Orthop Scand Suppl*, **275**:112–114.

145 Combe B, Cohen C, Aubin F (1997). Equivalence of nasal spray and subcutaneous formulations of salmon calcitonin. *Calcif Tissue Int*, **61**(1):10–15.

146 Silverman SL, Azria M (2002). The analgesic role of calcitonin following osteoporotic fracture. *Osteoporos Int*, **13**(11):858–867.

147 Lyritis GP, Trovas G (2002). Analgesic effects of calcitonin. *Bone*, 30(5 Suppl):71S–74S.

148 Marie PJ, Ammann P, Boivin G, *et al.* (2001). Mechanisms of action and therapeutic potential of strontium in bone. *Calcif Tissue Int*, **69**(3):121–129.

149 Meunier PJ, Roux C, Seeman E, *et al.* (2004). The effects of strontium ranelate on the risk of vertebral fracture in women with postmenopausal osteoporosis. *N Engl J Med*, **350**(5):459–468.

150 Reginster JY, Seeman E, De Vernejoul MC, *et al.* (2005). Strontium ranelate reduces the risk of nonvertebral fractures in postmenopausal women with osteoporosis: Treatment of Peripheral Osteoporosis (TROPOS) study. *J Clin Endocrinol Metab*, **90**(5):2816–2822.

151 Hofbauer LC, Schoppet M (2004). Clinical implications of the osteoprotegerin/RANKL/RANK system for bone and vascular diseases. *JAMA*, **292**(4):490–495.

152 Bekker PJ, Holloway D, Nakanishi A, *et al.* (2001). The effect of a single dose of osteoprotegerin in postmenopausal women. *J Bone Miner Res*, **16**(2):348–360.

153 Bekker PJ, Holloway DL, Rasmussen AS, *et al.* (2004). A single-dose placebo-controlled study of AMG 162, a fully human monoclonal antibody to RANKL, in postmenopausal women. *J Bone Miner Res*, **19**(7):1059–1066.

154 McClung MR, Lewiecki EM, Cohen SB, *et al.* (2006). Denosumab in postmenopausal women with low bone mineral density. *N Engl J Med*, **354**(8):821–831.

155 Body JJ, Facon T, Coleman RE, *et al.* (2006). A study of the biological receptor activator of nuclear factor-kappaB ligand inhibitor, denosumab, in patients with multiple myeloma or bone metastases from breast cancer. *Clin Cancer Res*, **12**(4):1221–1228.

156 Body JJ, Greipp P, Coleman RE, *et al.* (2003). A phase I study of AMGN-0007, a recombinant osteoprotegerin construct, in patients with multiple myeloma or breast carcinoma related bone metastases. *Cancer*, **97**(3 Suppl):887–892.

157 Hermann J, Mueller T, Fahrleitner A, *et al.* (2003). Early onset and effective inhibition of bone resorption in patients with rheumatoid arthritis treated with the tumour necrosis factor alpha antibody infliximab. *Clin Exp Rheumatol*, **21**(4):473–476.

158 Drake FH, Dodds RA, James IE, *et al.* (1996). Cathepsin K, but not cathepsins B, L, or S, is abundantly expressed in human osteoclasts. *J Biol Chem*, **271**(21):12511–12516.

159 Gelb BD, Shi GP, Chapman HA, *et al.* (1996). Pycnodysostosis, a lysosomal disease caused by cathepsin K deficiency. *Science*, **273**(5279):1236–1238.

160 Lark MW, Stroup GB, James IE, *et al.* (2002). A potent small molecule, nonpeptide inhibitor of cathepsin K (SB 331750) prevents bone matrix resorption in the ovariectomized rat. *Bone*, **30**(5):746–753.

161 Lark MW, Stroup GB, Hwang SM, *et al.* (1999). Design and characterization of orally active Arg-Gly-Asp peptidomimetic vitronectin receptor antagonist SB 265123 for prevention of bone loss in osteoporosis. *J Pharmacol Exp Ther*, **291**(2):612–617.

162 Gerdhem P, Brandstrom H, Stiger F, *et al.* (2004). Association of the collagen type 1 (COL1A 1) Sp1 binding site polymorphism to femoral neck bone mineral density and wrist fracture in 1044 elderly Swedish women. *Calcif Tissue Int*, **74**(3):264–269.

163 Gerdhem P, Ringsberg KA, Magnusson H, *et al.* (2003). Bone mass cannot be predicted by estimations of frailty in elderly ambulatory women. *Gerontology*, **49**(3):168–172.

164 Guideline for the prevention of falls in older persons. American Geriatrics Society, British Geriatrics Society, and American Academy of Orthopaedic Surgeons Panel on Falls Prevention (2001). *J Am Geriatr Soc*, **49**(5):664–672.

165 Falls: the assessment and prevention of falls in older people. NICE Clinical Guideline 21 (2004). NICE.

166 Gillespie LD, Gillespie WJ, Robertson MC, *et al.* (2003). Interventions for preventing falls in elderly people. *Cochrane Database Syst Rev*, (4):CD000340.

167 Bischoff-Ferrari HA, Dawson-Hughes B, Willett WC, *et al.* (2004). Effect of Vitamin D on falls: a meta-analysis. *JAMA*, **291**(16):1999–2006.

168 Lauritzen JB, Petersen MM, Lund B (1993). Effect of external hip protectors on hip fractures. *Lancet*, **341**(8836):11–13.

169 Kannus P, Parkkari J, Niemi S, *et al.* (2000). Prevention of hip fracture in elderly people with use of a hip protector. *N Engl J Med*, **343**(21):1506–1513.

170 Parker MJ, Gillespie WJ, Gillespie LD (2005). Hip protectors for preventing hip fractures in older people. *Cochrane Database Syst Rev*, (3):CD001255.

171 Parker MJ, Gillespie WJ, Gillespie LD (2006). Effectiveness of hip protectors for preventing hip fractures in elderly people: systematic review. *BMJ*, **332**(7541):571–574.

172 van Schoor NM, Deville WL, Bouter LM, *et al.* (2002). Acceptance and compliance with external hip protectors: a systematic review of the literature. *Osteoporos Int*, **13**(12):917–924.

173 Forsen L, Sogaard AJ, Sandvig S, *et al.* (2004). Risk of hip fracture in protected and unprotected falls in nursing homes in Norway. *Inj Prev*, **10**(1):16–20.

174 Hadjipavlou AG, Tzermiadianos MN, Katonis PG, *et al.* (2005). Percutaneous vertebroplasty and balloon kyphoplasty for the treatment of osteoporotic vertebral compression fractures and osteolytic tumours. *J Bone Joint Surg Br*, **87**(12):1595–1604.

175 Bouza C, Lopez T, Magro A, *et al.* (2006). Efficacy and safety of balloon kyphoplasty in the treatment of vertebral compression fractures: a systematic review. *Eur Spine J*, 1-18.

176 Osteoporosis: assessment of fracture risk and the prevention of osteoporotic fractures in individuals at high risk. NICE guideline, 7th wave, final publication date TBC.

177 Rogmark C, Johnell O (2005). Orthopaedic treatment of displaced femoral neck fractures in elderly patients. *Disabil Rehabil*, **27**(18–19):1143–1149.

178 Rogmark C, Carlsson A, Johnell O, *et al.* (2002). Primary hemiarthroplasty in old patients with displaced femoral neck fracture: a 1-year follow-up of 103 patients aged 80 years or more. *Acta Orthop Scand*, **73**(6):605–610.

179 Tidermark J (2003). Quality of life and femoral neck fractures. *Acta Orthop Scand Suppl*, **74**(309):1–42.

180 Blomfeldt R, Tornkvist H, Ponzer S, *et al.* (2005). Comparison of internal fixation with total hip replacement for displaced femoral neck fractures. Randomized, controlled trial performed at four years. *J Bone Joint Surg Am*, **87**(8):1680–1688.

181 SIGN (2002). *Prevention and Management of Hip Fracture in Older People. A national clinical guideline*.

182 Hamlet WP, Lieberman JR, Freedman EL, *et al.* (1997). Influence of health status and the timing of surgery on mortality in hip fracture patients. *Am J Orthop*, **26**(9):621–627.

183 Villar RN, Allen SM, Barnes SJ (1986). Hip fractures in healthy patients: operative delay versus prognosis. *Br Med J (Clin Res Ed)*, **293**(6556):1203–1204.

184 Osnes EK, Lofthus CM, Meyer HE, *et al.* (2004). Consequences of hip fracture on activities of daily life and residential needs. *Osteoporos Int*, **15**(7):567–574.

185 Court-Brown CM, Garg A, McQueen MM (2001). The epidemiology of proximal humeral fractures. *Acta Orthop Scand*, **72**(4):365–371.

186 Gaebler C, McQueen MM, Court-Brown CM (2003). Minimally displaced proximal humeral fractures: epidemiology and outcome in 507 cases. *Acta Orthop Scand*, **74**(5):580–585.

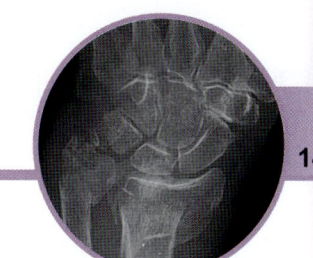

Chapter 5

Osteoporosis in clinical care

Introduction

Osteoporosis is common and the burden of the resultant low-trauma fractures great and increasing. Action must be taken at all stages of life to effectively prevent and treat osteoporosis (**5.1**, *Table 5.1*). Healthy youths may develop osteoporosis in later years – it is not always predictable even in older people. It is therefore the responsibility for all to follow a bone healthy lifestyle at all stages of life, to maximise peak bone mass and prevent loss during older years. There are some who are, however, at higher risk than others of osteoporosis and fracture. These people need to be identified and treated appropriately to reduce that risk (see Chapter 3). There are also those who have osteoporosis and have sustained a fracture. It is important that they regain their independence as much as possible, as well as reduce their risk of further fracture. They need rehabilitation and often pain management. They also need treatment to improve bone strength and to reduce the risk of falls so that the risk of further fracture is reduced. In these ways the impact of osteoporosis can be lessened.

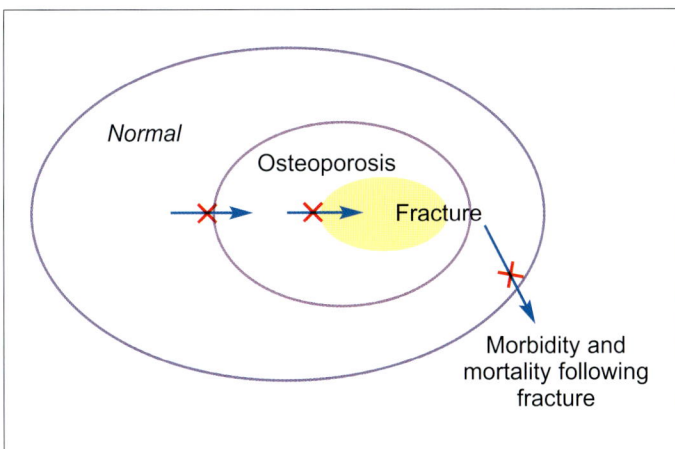

5.1 Schematic to illustrate stages when the burden of osteoporosis on the individual and on society can be reduced.

Table 5.1 When and how to prevent osteoporosis and fracture

When
• At all ages

How
• Bone mass
  – Maximize peak bone mass
  – Delay onset of bone loss
  – Prevent bone loss in older age
• Maintain physical fitness throughout life
• Prevent falls in later life
• Treat those at highest risk close to the time when probability of fracture greatest

Opportunities for prevention and treatment

There are clearly some specific opportunities to recognize those at most risk and to intervene (**5.2**). Some of these will be considered

Childhood and adolescence

Bone mass acquired during childhood and adolescence is a key determinant of bone health in adulthood. Any factor that affects the development of the skeleton during these early years will affect attainment of peak bone mass and will have long-term consequences on bone health in later life, and increase the risk of future osteoporosis and fracture. Osteoporosis in adulthood can, therefore, have its origins already in these early years and detrimental factors to bone health need to be recognized and corrected where possible. Osteoporosis may also (rarely) manifest itself in childhood and adolescence with low-trauma fractures, such as in diseases treated with high doses of corticosteroids.

Bone development requires good nutrition along with physical stimulation in an environment of normal gonadal hormones, without the presence of noxious substances such as from smoking, excess alcohol, or corticosteroid therapy. However, the majority of bone mass and strength is determined by genetic factors which cannot as yet be modified.

In childhood and early adulthood, the commonest specific cause for inadequate bone acquisition relates to gonadal hormone deficiency which can affect both sexes. Females with late menarche and secondary amenorrhoea need to be identified and the underlying cause found and treated. Anorexia nervosa and over-exercise syndrome are common causes of low bone mass leading to premature osteoporosis and fracture. This is a consequence of poor nutrition, low body mass, and gonadal hormone deficiency.

Adequate nutrients during the growth phase are important, and lactose intolerance can result in lifelong low calcium intake. Gluten intolerance also increases the risk of future osteoporosis if not diagnosed early and treated by close adherence to an appropriate diet. Specific nutrients are

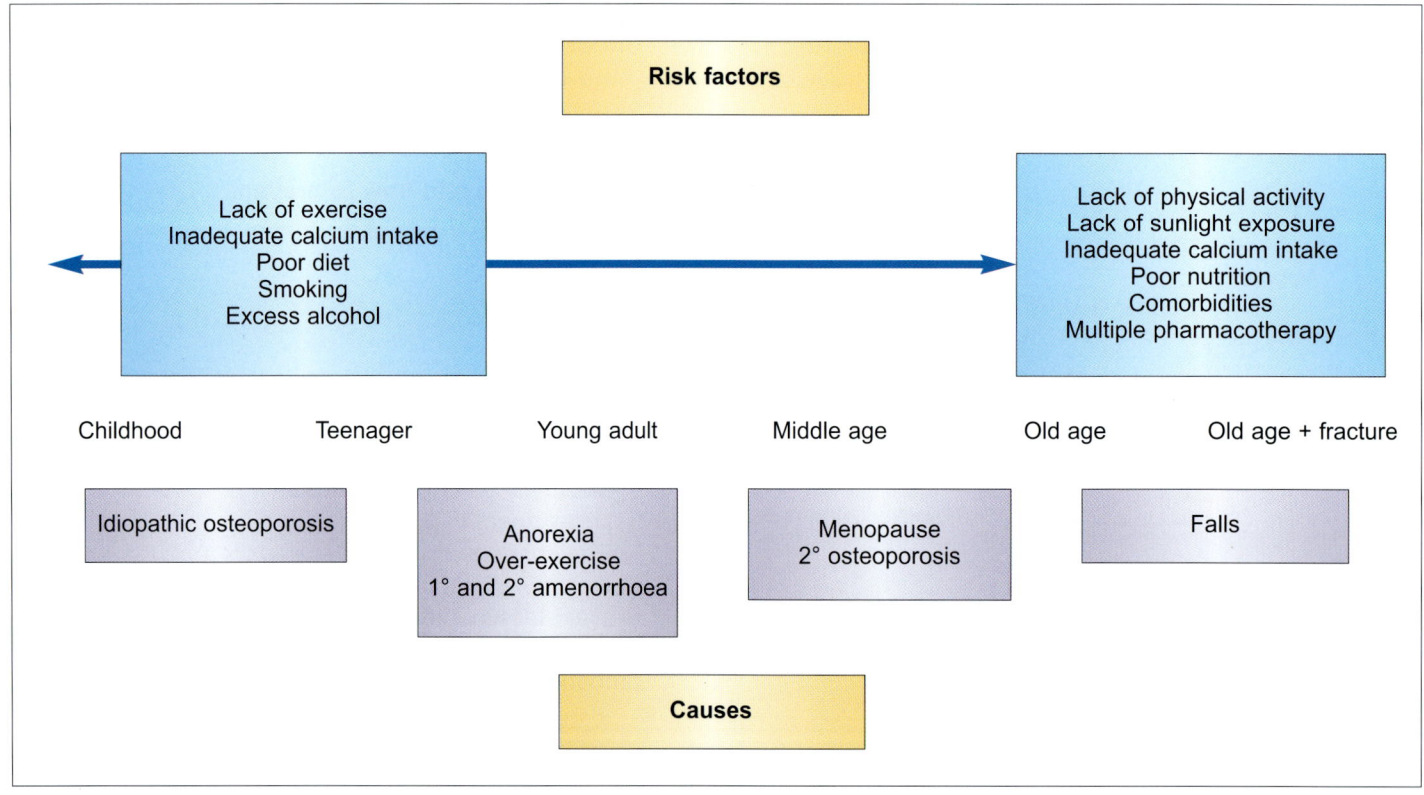

5.2 Risk factors for osteoporosis and fracture.

important, but the body mass index (BMI) is a simple way of estimating the overall adequacy of nutrition; it is recommended that the BMI is 19 or above.

Steroid treatment at these ages, especially if in high doses, for diseases such as asthma, juvenile idiopathic arthritis, systemic lupus erythematosis or rheumatoid arthritis, or related to organ transplantation is a common cause of osteoporosis developing in childhood and presenting with low-trauma fracture. Cystic fibrosis now has a better survival prognosis and the complication of osteoporosis presenting with fracture is now becoming a problem affecting these children's quality of life. Prolonged immobilization can affect skeletal development, such as related to spinal injuries or cerebral palsy.

Diagnosis of osteoporosis is difficult by bone density in the growing skeleton as it is dependent on stage of puberty (Tanner stage), and the relationship of bone density with fracture risk is not established for this age. However, it is an important age to recognize those few young people with these conditions that will put them at future risk of osteoporosis and fracture. Reversing the risk factors is most important, such as minimizing dose and duration of oral steroid use in asthma or maximizing BMI and correcting estrogen deficiency in anorexia nervosa. The evidence for specific treatments such as bisphosphonates is small and the outcome used is bone density. This is used as a surrogate for future fracture risk, but the value of bone density at this age in predicting events that may not happen for many years is not established.

Children and adolescents should be made aware of the importance of bone health and encouraged to follow a bone healthy lifestyle with regular weight-bearing exercise, adequate dietary calcium, sufficient sunlight exposure and oily fish in the diet for vitamin D, and avoiding smoking and excess alcohol. Those at specific risk need to be recognized and managed appropriately.

Case study 1

At 22 years of age, a young female was referred for assessment of bone mineral density (BMD) because of an eating disorder throughout her adolescence. She had a late menarche at 16 years and then irregular periods for 3 years and had since been receiving deoprovera injections for contraception. She had always been thin and her BMI was 16.4 when she was 18 years old. When she was assessed at 22 years her BMI was 18.5. She admitted to anorexia and also periods of bulimia. Her bone density was low with a Z-score of -2.19 in the lumbar spine and -2.05 in the proximal femur. She was counselled about her poor bone health and future risk of fracture and she was strongly recommended to improve her nutrition, to gain weight, and to use the oral combined contraceptive pill. As her grandmother had recently fractured her hip and lost her independence as a result, she followed the advice; when reassessed 2 years later she had gained 6 kg in weight, achieving a BMI of 21.5, was taking oestrogen in the form of the oral contraceptive pill, and had increased her bone density in the lumbar spine by 5.74% per annum and in the proximal femur.

Comment: Anorexia nervosa is a very important cause of low bone mass in adolescence that can lead to osteoporosis in later life. Sometimes it is severe enough to cause osteoporosis and fracture at an early age. Management is to improve diet and body weight and ensuring adequate oestrogen levels. It is often very challenging to treat as the person often has a resistance to gaining weight and they frequently do not wish to take oestrogens. Concern about osteoporosis and fracture can sometimes help encourage the person to accept a higher weight.

The gain in bone mass demonstrated in this case is exceptional with an initial rapid increase in bone density but sustained improvement, but this shows what can be achieved if there is good concordance with recommendations.

Case study 2

This 17-year-old boy has cystic fibrosis and was seen in the Osteoporosis Clinic for assessment of risk of future osteoporosis. His bone density in the lumbar spine was Z score -2.29. He had a calcium-poor diet and was not able to do a lot of physical activity, being limited by breathlessness. He was encouraged to do more weight-bearing activities and advised how he could achieve this despite impaired respiratory capacity by a physiotherapist. He was given calcium and vitamin D supplements. His bone density will be repeated in 2 years and if it worsens further compared to what would be expected for his age, then pharmacological treatment may be considered.

Comment: The outcome of cystic fibrosis has improved but with improved survival the complication of osteoporosis due to the condition, its effects on mobility and its treatment has become more of a problem. Low BMD can occur as a consequence of decreased exercise, glucocorticoid therapy, malabsorption, low body weight, and chronic infection. Adequate calcium and vitamin D is important in the diet or through supplementation, along with maximising weight-bearing activities. This will need physiotherapy advice. If bone density is very low during adolescence or early adulthood, then pharmacological treatment is used to improve it, with the aim of preventing fractures at an early age.

Case study 3

A 12-year-old boy had developed systemic juvenile inflammatory arthritis (Still's Disease) at the age of 4 years. He required corticosteroids to control his disease adequately from a year from its onset, often at high doses. At the age of 11 years he suddenly developed severe back pain, initially localized to the low back, but after a day he had pain radiating around the whole torso. His mobility was further reduced. X-ray showed a wedge fracture of T11 and loss of anterior height of several lower thoracic and lumbar vertebrae. He was commenced on alendronic acid.

Comment: The need for high-dose corticosteroid treatment in childhood is not common but can lead to major skeletal complications with osteoporosis, fracture, and avascular necrosis. Antiresorptive therapy is used to prevent and treat steroid-induced osteoporosis, and this should be considered at the initiation of high-dose corticosteroid therapy. Parenteral bisphosphonate in the form of pamidronate has often been used. It is also important to minimize the dose and duration of corticosteroid in disease suppressing therapy. The consequent fractures will add to the problems of the child and need to be managed in terms of pain control and minimizing disability.

Adulthood

Peak bone mass is achieved in early adulthood. This is dependent on genetic factors and other personal and lifestyle factors during the first 2–3 decades. Bone mass declines from mid-life onwards, due to an imbalance between formation and resorption. Any factors which cause an imbalance between formation and resorption or increased bone turnover will lead to bone loss and future osteoporosis with increased fracture risk.

Premature loss of sex hormones will result in the early onset of bone loss, such as associated with secondary amenorrhoea or premature menopause (i.e. before 45 years of age). Infertility is often associated with low oestrogen levels that need to be treated beyond the management of infertility. Pregnancy can be rarely associated with osteoporosis with rapid loss of spinal bone mass and fracture, but may also relate to surgical removal or chemical ablation of the ovaries or testes.

Conditions may develop which increase the risk of osteoporosis due to factors such as their inflammatory nature, resultant reduced mobility, impaired nutrition, or treatment with corticosteroids (*Table 2.8*). Lifestyle factors continue to be very important at this age. Smoking and excess alcohol will continue to have a harmful effect on the skeleton throughout life and need to be avoided. This is currently a major problem as the current trend is an increase in these risk factors in young adults. Maintaining physical activity is very important at this stage of life for bone and general health, and there is a similar current trend to increasing physical inactivity and loss of fitness. Regular exercise is recommended, but it should not be promoted in a way that discourages those who are not wishing to go to a gym or go jogging. Weight-bearing exercise such as brisk walking is also of value and may be more sustainable into later life.

This is an important age to promote a bone healthy lifestyle to establish patterns of behaviour that will continue throughout the rest of life. It is also important to recognize those situations which arise during this age that will increase the risk of osteoporosis and fracture in later life. Risks need to be reduced by the best management of the condition that increases the risk, such as good control of rheumatoid disease with suppression of inflammatory disease activity, avoiding long-term corticosteroids, and maintaining physical function. Bone active drugs such as bisphosphonates are sometimes used at this age if the risk of future fracture is considered high enough, although there are little data about the long-term benefits of such an approach.

Case study 4

A 33-year-old woman has primary amenorrhoea due to a rare condition, Kallman's syndrome. Her bone density in the lumbar spine was T -3.23 and in the proximal femur was T -3.37. She had sustained low-trauma fractures of her wrist and metatarsals. This was despite taking hormone supplements in the form of the combined oral contraceptive pill for over 12 years from 18 years, and then combined hormone replacement therapy. In Kallman's syndrome, there is a specific lack of gonadotrophin-releasing hormone (GnRH) which normally stimulates excretion of both luteinizing hormone (LH) and follicle-stimulating hormone (FSH). These gonadotrophins are necessary to stimulate ovarian follicular development and ovulation and absence results in amenorrhoea, infertility, and the consequences of oestrogen deficiency. GnRH therapy is now possible.

Comment: Sex hormones are important for the normal development of bone mass and any deficiency during the years of skeletal growth and consolidation will increase the risk of future osteoporosis. This needs to be recognized and treatment given to ensure normal oestrogen levels throughout adolescence and adulthood until the expected age of menopause. Sometimes amenorrhoea or oligomenorrhoea is associated with a low BMI and/or over-exercise syndrome. Inadequate oestrogen levels may present as infertility and, after treatment for this, the use of ongoing oestrogen needs to be considered to benefit bone health.

Case study 5

A 51-year-old woman had a bilateral salpingo-oophorectomy and partial hysterectomy for tuberculosis at the age of 23 years. She received oestrogen replacement therapy for 2 weeks following surgery. Her aunt had breast cancer and she was advised against taking prolonged oestrogen replacement therapy. At the age of 51 she was markedly osteoporotic, with a bone density in the lumbar spine of T -3.28 and in the proximal femur of T -3.19.

Comment: She is now at high risk of future fracture. It would have been advisable for her to have taken oestrogen replacement therapy up to the expected age of menopause to ensure she developed and maintained her peak bone mass. Treatment with an antiresorptive drug to improve and maintain bone mass is now indicated but the duration of therapy for someone at this age to prevent fracture effectively in later life is unclear. A 10-year period of treatment with reassessment of fracture risk at that stage to decide on ongoing therapy would be a reasonable approach.

Case study 6

A 41-year-old man developed asthma at the age of 18 years which was treated with inhaled steroids and occasional courses of high-dose oral steroids. He then required regular oral steroids with doses of 10–20 mg prednisolone daily. At 30 years, he twisted his right ankle and fractured the distal tip of the left maleolus, and he also fell that year and fractured the right clavicle. At 33 years, he had avascular necrosis of the right hip leading to a total hip replacement. He also fractured several ribs during karate. He works as a scaffolder but has not had any major accidents.
 At 35 years his bone density was assessed with T score lumbar spine of -4.61 and T score of the proximal femur of -1.04. He has taken bisphosphonates for the last 6 years and his bone density has increased in the lumbar spine by 2.96% per annum and in the proximal femur by 0.46% per annum. He has been advised about avoiding trauma such as karate and also at his work. He has not sustained any further fractures.

Comment: Secondary causes of osteoporosis commonly present in men. Corticosteroid therapy is a common cause and this needs to be recognized more in clinical practice so that prevention can be considered. As is common in younger men, various work and leisure activities can put these patients at risk of fracture and advice needs to be given about this along with treatment to improve bone strength.

Midlife: peri- and postmenopausal years

Specific causes of increased bone loss may develop in later life. However, most people identified as having osteopenia and osteoporosis at this age do not have a specific cause. They may have a variety of risk factors that have increased their likelihood of having a low bone mass and of sustaining a fracture in the future; these risk factors can be used to identify who should be formally assessed for bone density and whether or not to treat. Identification of those at risk and assessment by bone densitometry is, however, only appropriate if the person is prepared to, and capable of, taking any recommended treatment for long enough to achieve its goal of fracture prevention.

Age is the most important risk factor for fracture and it is most cost-effective to assess people for their risk when over 65 years, although those with specific causes of osteoporosis should be recognized at all ages. Some of these causes are more common at this stage of life (see *Table 2.8*). Aromatase inhibitors used for treating postmenopausal breast cancer will increase the risk of future osteoporosis.

Women and men at high risk can either be found by a systematic approach at a health check or opportunistically when being seen for an intercurrent problem. Risk factors may be documented on health records. A low-trauma fracture at this age, such as a Colles's fracture, is a strong risk factor for future fracture. Many people are not in routine contact with their family physicians and public awareness campaigns are needed to encourage them to enquire about their individual needs for preventive therapy for osteoporosis. Simple checklists such as the International Osteoporosis Foundation One-Minute Test (**3.13**) can be used.

A bone healthy lifestyle is recommended at all ages, although the level of physical activity that is possible may be reduced. In those with a high probability of future fracture, specific treatments such as bisphosphonates, strontium, and parathyroid hormone (PTH) have been shown to be effective in reducing the risk of fracture.

Case study 7

A 57-year-old woman fell onto her outstretched hand and sustained a Colles' fracture. Her primary care physician was concerned about her risk of sustaining a subsequent fracture. As her mother fractured her hip at 82 years, she was also concerned and wanting to reduce her risk. She kept fit, taking regular walks, and had a good diet including dairy products. She smoked occasionally and drank 14 units of alcohol weekly. She was referred for bone densitometry which was lumbar spine T -2.32 and proximal femur T -2.75.

Comment: She has a high probability of future fracture because of experiencing a low-trauma fracture, a maternal history of hip fracture, and a low bone density. However, any further fracture may not occur for several years. She needs to improve her lifestyle by stopping smoking but she is already taking regular exercise and has a good dietary calcium intake. Pharmacological treatment with an antiresorptive drug should be recommended to reduce fracture probability. The ideal duration is unclear at this age from present evidence, but 10 years of treatment followed by reassessment of fracture probability to decide on ongoing therapy would be an approach.

Case study 8

A 72-year-old woman had presented with pain and morning stiffness across her shoulders, in the upper arms and in the thighs. Her erythrocyte sedimentation rate (ESR) was 53 mm/h. A diagnosis of polymyalgia rheumatica was made and she was commenced on prednisolone. She took 15 mg daily for a month and then 12.5 mg daily, but after 3 weeks she suddenly developed severe low back pain and wedging of T11 was noted on X-ray. She had a bone density assessment which was lumbar spine T -2.45 and proximal femur T -2.37.

Comment: Corticosteroid therapy is associated with increased bone turnover, bone loss, and increased risk of fracture. The increase in bone turnover following the initiation of corticosteroids can occasionally result in the early manifestation of a low-trauma fracture, in particular if bone density was previously low. The increased fracture risk is, however, in part, independent of bone density. The decision to use prophylactic treatment to reduce fracture risk is therefore based on dose of corticosteroids, age, and a lower threshold of bone density. Some guidelines suggest preventative treatment if T score is lower than -1.5; or if corticosteroid dose is ≥15 mg/day: or previous low-trauma fracture; or age over 65 years.

Case study 9

A 67-year-old woman developed coeliac disease at the age of 5 years and was treated by diet but was never very consistent about complying with it and has not been strictly gluten free until recent years. She was found to have endomysial antibodies and 5 years ago was still found to have subtotal villous atrophy despite apparently being on an appropriate diet. She has always had a low body weight. Her menarche was 13 and she had an early menopause at 41 years. She has not sustained any fractures. Her bone density was assessed at the age of 67 years and in the lumbar spine the T score was -5.41 and in the proximal femur, -3.29. She was encouraged to comply with her gluten-free diet and was being treated with alendronate 70 mg weekly.

Comment: She has severe osteoporosis and is at high risk of fracture. Treatment is indicated with an antiresorptive agent but an alternative treatment to consider with such a low bone density is PTH, in particular if an X-ray of the spine shows any vertebral deformity. Evidence shows benefit from PTH therapy in this situation, but access to this treatment may vary in countries dependent on reimbursement criteria. This case also demonstrates the importance of adhering to a strict gluten-free diet in coeliac disease.

In old age

In the more elderly, the potential gain from any intervention is greater because of the high probability of fractures in the later decades of life. The opportunities for case finding are greater at this age as many will be in contact with health professionals for routine procedures such as flu vaccination or as a result of various intercurrent problems.

It may become apparent that they have had events such as a previous Colles' fracture, an early menopause, or had a fall in the last year that will increase their risk of sustaining a fracture. The person may present with a low-energy fracture of the limb bones or pelvis, a sudden onset of back pain, or a gradual loss of height and stoop. Once a fracture has occurred in the presence of low bone density, it is considered established osteoporosis.

Risk of future fracture needs to be considered, including the potential contribution of bone fragility and propensity to fall. In addition, if they have recently sustained a fracture, following a diagnostic workup (see page 68), any pain needs to be controlled and function and independence restored as far as possible through rehabilitation (see page 135). If they are at high risk of further fracture, then prevention through increasing bone strength and reducing risk of falls is necessary.

Maintaining physical activity is important at this age, not so much to increase bone strength but to reduce risk of falling and to preserve general fitness. Balance and coordination exercises should be considered, especially if these are poor. Ensuring adequate calcium intake and that vitamin D levels are adequate is important, but the evidence for suggesting supplementing these further is not established. The frail institutionalized elderly appear to benefit most from calcium and vitamin D supplementation.

There are now several options for increasing bone strength at this age with strong evidence-bases demonstrating fracture prevention within 1 year in older people, including the very elderly. Since life expectancy in an 80-year-old woman in Western Europe is over 5 years, treatment of those at high risk is appropriate. There is little comparative data between the different treatment options to help decide which is most appropriate in each circumstance. An important factor is the likelihood of the person taking the treatment for the necessary duration to gain benefit; factors such as mode and frequency of administration will influence this.

Case study 10

At 81 years, a previously fit woman tripped over a toy of her visiting grandchild, fell and sustained an undisplaced cervical fracture of her right hip. It was pinned, she was mobilized and discharged to her home. She was in good general health but had impaired vision. She had not fallen previously in the last year and had good balance and coordination. She did not like dairy products, did not smoke or drink excess alcohol. She took very little outdoor exercise, never having been a keen walker. Her menopause was at 45 years and she had never taken hormone replacement therapy. Her mother had also fractured her hip when she was 79 years.

Comment: She has sustained a low-trauma fracture which may relate to underlying osteoporosis. She has made a good recovery but is at risk of further fracture. Mortality is increased following hip fracture but mainly in frailer individuals who have comorbidities and are biologically aged. Risk factors for osteoporosis and fracture include early menopause, poor lifestyle for bone health, maternal history of hip fracture, and having sustained a low-trauma fracture. Her lifestyle needs to improve with adequate dietary calcium and regular physical activity such as a daily brisk walk for 30 minutes. If she is willing to take long-term treatment then her probability of further fracture can be better estimated by also performing bone density assessment. If this confirms osteoporosis (T ≥ -2.5), then the probability of further fracture is very high and treatment will be cost-effective. Even without a bone density measurement, the probability of a further fracture at this age is high; however, some people will not be osteoporotic and may not benefit so much from pharmacological treatment. It would have been appropriate to assess her for fracture probability by bone densitometry before she sustained the hip facture in view of the maternal history of hip fracture.

Case study 11

At 73 years, a frail woman with a long-standing history of obstructive airways disease spontaneously developed severe back pain at the level of her waist. She had become stooped over the previous 4 years with height loss of about 5 cm. She had not fallen. She was feeling bloated after eating. She had been treated with inhaled steroids for many years for obstructive airways disease and usually needed 2–3 courses of high-dose oral steroids each year for the last 15 years when she had exacerbations associated with chest infections. She had smoked heavily until the age of 57 years. Her mobility has been limited by her breathlessness for many years. She was thin, with a BMI of 18.5. She had loss of anterior vertebral body height at T11, L2, and L4 and had a wedge fracture at L1.

Comment: She almost certainly has osteoporosis causing her to sustain spontaneous vertebral fractures. Long-standing obstructive airways disease and corticosteroid therapy are contributory factors. It is important to exclude other causes such as myeloma and secondary malignancy. A bone density measurement will add little to the clinical decision making and the result in the spine difficult to interpret because of the vertebral deformities. She has a high probability of further vertebral of appendicular fracture. Pharmacological treatment is indicated if she is willing and able to take it long-term. She should also take adequate calcium and vitamin D, and supplements may be the best way of ensuring this in the present situation. Physical activity should be increased if possible. Balance and coordination need to be reviewed and improved if necessary and feasible. Use of systemic corticosteroids should be avoided if possible.

Conclusion

Osteoporosis can be effectively prevented and treated. As it is so common, all people at all ages should be encouraged to follow a bone healthy lifestyle. This will not only reduce the future burden due to osteoporosis but will also reduce the burden of other musculoskeletal conditions[3] and chronic diseases[4].

Situations may arise at any age that will increase the probability of future osteoporosis and fracture and these need to be recognized and action taken to minimize the risk. As people get older and the 10-year probability of fracture becomes high, then those at most risk should be identified and treated if indicated. Once a fracture has occurred related to osteoporosis, following appropriate fracture management including pain control and rehabilitation, steps need to be taken to prevent further fracture. This includes improving bone strength and reducing the risk of falling. We are now fortunate to have a range of effective interventions to achieve this.

References

1 Eccles M, Mason J (2001). How to develop cost conscious guidelines. *Health Technology Assessment,* **5**:16(5).
2 NICE (2004). Clinical Guidelines on the Assessment and Prevention of Falls in Older People. 3.
3 European Action Towards Better Musculoskeletal Health: A Public Health Strategy to Reduce the Burden of Musculoskeletal Conditions. The European Bone & Joint Health Strategies Project. ISBN 91-975284-0-4. A Bone and Joint Decade Report. The Bone and Joint Decade, Lund, Sweden, 2004. Available at URL: http://ec.europa.eu/health/ph_projects/2000/promotion/fp_promotion_2000_frep_15_en.pdf
4 World Health Organization (2006). *Gaining Health. The European Strategy for the Prevention and Control of Noncommunicable Diseases.* WHO, Copenahgen. ISBN 92-890-2179-9. Available at URL: http://www.euro.who.int/document/E89306

Index